LAPAROSCOPIC
ABDOMINAL SURGERY

NOTICE

Medicine is an ever-changing science. As new research and clinical experience broaden our knowledge, changes in treatment and drug therapy are required. The editors and the publisher of this work have checked with sources believed to be reliable in their efforts to provide information that is complete and generally in accord with the standards accepted at the time of publication. However, in view of the possibility of human error or changes in medical sciences, neither the editors nor the publisher nor any other party who has been involved in the preparation or publication of this work warrants that the information contained herein is in every respect accurate or complete, and they are not responsible for any errors or omissions or for the results obtained from use of such information. Readers are encouraged to confirm the information contained herein with other sources. For example and in particular, readers are advised to check the product information sheet included in the package of each drug they plan to administer to be certain that the information contained in this book is accurate and that changes have not been made in the recommended dose or in the contraindications for administration. This recommendation is of particular importance in connection with new or infrequently used drugs.

LAPAROSCOPIC
ABDOMINAL SURGERY

Editors

John N. Graber, M.D., F.A.C.S.

Director, Institute for Minimally Invasive Surgery, and
Chairman, Department of Surgery
Abbott Northwestern Hospital
Minneapolis, Minnesota

Clinical Instructor in Surgery
University of Minnesota
Minneapolis, Minnesota

Leonard S. Schultz, M.D., F.A.C.S.

Clinical Assistant Professor of Surgery
Department of Surgery
University of Minnesota
Minneapolis, Minnesota

Past Chairman of Department of Surgery
Abbott Northwestern Hospital
Minneapolis, Minnesota

Joseph J. Pietrafitta, M.D.

Director of Research
Institute for Minimally Invasive Surgery
Minneapolis, Minnesota

Director of the Surgical Endoscopy Fellowship Program
Abbott Northwestern Hospital
Minneapolis, Minnesota

David F. Hickok, M.D., F.A.C.S.

Clinical Associate Professor of Surgery
University of Minnesota
Minneapolis, Minnesota

McGraw-Hill, Inc.
HEALTH PROFESSIONS DIVISION

New York St. Louis San Francisco Auckland Bogotá Caracas Lisbon London Madrid Mexico
Milan Montreal New Delhi Paris San Juan Singapore Sydney Tokyo Toronto

LAPAROSCOPIC ABDOMINAL SURGERY

Copyright © 1993 by McGraw-Hill, Inc. All rights reserved. Printed in the United States of America. Except as permitted under the United States Copyright Act of 1976, no part of this publication may be reproduced or distributed in any form or by any means, or stored in a data base or retrieval system, without the prior written permission of the publisher.

1234567890 KGP KGP 98765432

ISBN 0-07-023989-4

This book was set in Caslon by Arcata Graphics/Kingsport.
The editors were Michael J. Houston and Lester A. Sheinis;
the production supervisor was Richard C. Ruzycka;
the cover designer was Marsha Cohen/Parallelogram;
the indexer was Alexandra Nickerson.
Arcata Graphics/Kingsport was printer and binder.

Library of Congress Cataloging-in-Publication Data

Laparoscopic abdominal surgery/editors, John N. Graber . . . [et al.].
    p. cm.
  Includes bibliographical references and index.
  ISBN 0-07-023989-4
  1. Abdomen—Endoscopic surgery. 2. Laparoscopic surgery.
3. Laparoscopy. I. Graber, John N.
  [DNLM: 1. Abdomen—surgery. 2. Peritoneoscopy. WI 900 L299]
RD540.L277 1993
617.5'5059—dc20
DNLM/DLC
for Library of Congress   92–48730
                                                          CIP

Contents

Contributors vii
Preface ix

INTRODUCTION	The Future of Surgery Is "Less Invasiveness" *John N. Graber*	1

PART ONE	Basic Considerations	5
1	THE BASICS OF LAPAROSCOPY *David L. Hill*	7
2	VIDEO SYSTEMS IN LAPAROSCOPY *John Cartmill/Dean Aamodt*	31
3	LASERS AND CAUTERY IN LAPAROSCOPY *Gregory T. Absten*	41
4	OPERATING ROOM, STAFF, AND ADMINISTRATIVE CONCERNS IN LAPAROSCOPIC ABDOMINAL SURGERY *Patricia Hartwig*	57
5	PREOPERATIVE PATIENT EDUCATION *W. Jean Reavis*	65
6	ANESTHETIC CONSIDERATIONS IN LAPAROSCOPIC ABDOMINAL SURGERY *Jonathan T. Gudman/David A. Plut*	69
7	COMPLICATIONS OF LAPAROSCOPY *Edward M. Beadle*	75
8	ERGONOMICS AND LAPAROSCOPIC GENERAL SURGERY *Michael Patkin/Luis Isabel*	83

PART TWO	Laparoscopic Abdominal Surgery	89
9	INITIAL SURVEY OF THE PERITONEAL CAVITY, DIAGNOSTIC LAPAROSCOPY, LYSIS OF ADHESIONS, AND TUMOR BIOPSIES *John N. Graber*	91
10	LAPAROSCOPIC APPENDECTOMY *Joseph J. Pietrafitta*	103

Contents

11	**LAPAROSCOPIC CHOLECYSTECTOMY** *Leonard S. Schultz*	119
12	**LAPAROSCOPIC CHOLANGIOGRAPHY** *Joseph J. Pietrafitta*	137
13	**BLEEDING, ACUTE CHOLECYSTITIS, AND OTHER PROBLEMS ENCOUNTERED DURING LAPAROSCOPIC CHOLECYSTECTOMY** *John N. Graber*	149
14	**LAPAROSCOPIC COMMON BILE DUCT EXPLORATION** *Stephen J. Shapiro/Leo Gordon/Leon Daykhovsky*	169
15	**SHEATH ACCESS VIA THE CYSTIC DUCT FOR COMMON BILE DUCT CHOLEDOCHOSCOPY** *John N. Graber*	189
16	**CHOLELITHIASIS: THE ALTERNATIVES TO SURGERY** *Robert Mackie*	203
17	**COMPLICATIONS OF LAPAROSCOPIC CHOLECYSTECTOMY** *John N. Graber*	217
18	**LAPAROSCOPIC PEPTIC ULCER SURGERY** *Joseph J. Pietrafitta*	233
19	**LAPAROSCOPIC TREATMENT OF GASTROESOPHAGEAL REFLUX** *Joseph J. Pietrafitta/Ronald A. Hinder*	245
20	**LAPAROSCOPIC INGUINAL HERNIORRHAPHY** *Leonard S. Schultz*	255
21	**LAPAROSCOPIC PELVIC LYMPHADENECTOMY** *John C. Hulbert*	271
22	**LAPAROSCOPIC VARICOCELECTOMY** *Keith W. Kaye/Deborah J. Lightner/Leonard S. Schultz*	279
23	**LAPAROSCOPIC SURGERY OF THE UPPER URINARY TRACT AND RETROPERITONEUM** *John C. Hulbert*	295
24	**LAPAROSCOPIC BOWEL RESECTION** *Joseph J. Pietrafitta*	307
25	**LAPAROSCOPIC SURGERY IN CHILDREN AND INFANTS** *Hock L. Tan*	327
26	**REIMBURSEMENT FOR LAPAROSCOPIC PROCEDURES** *Shelley R. Coupanger*	339
Index		341

Contributors

Dean W. Aamodt [2]
Surgical Video Coordinator
Abbott Northwestern Hospital
Roseville, Minnesota

Gregory T. Absten, M.D. [3]
President, Advanced Laser Services
 Corporation
Clinical Instructor, The Ohio State University
 College of Medicine
Columbus, Ohio
Scientific Fellow, American Society for Laser
 Medicine and Surgery

Edward M. Beadle, Jr., M.D., F.A.C.O.G. [7]
Clinical Assistant Professor
Department of Obstetrics and Gynecology
University of Minnesota
Minneapolis, Minnesota

**John A. Cartmill, B.Sc. (med.) M.B., B.S.,
 M.M., F.R.A.C.S. [2]**
Fellow in Laparoendoscopic Surgery
Abbott Northwestern Hospital
Minneapolis, Minnesota

Shelley R. Coupanger [26]
Business Manager
Hickock, Schultz, and Graber, P.A.
Minneapolis, Minnesota

Leon Daykhovsky, M.D. [14]
Medical Director, Laser Research and
 Technology Development
Cedars-Sinai Medical Center
Los Angeles, California

The numbers in brackets following the contributors' names refer to the chapters written or co-written by the contributors.

Clinical Instructor in Surgery, University of
 California at Los Angeles
Clinical Instructor in Surgery, Veterans'
 Administration Hospital
Los Angeles, California

Leo A. Gordon, M.D., F.A.C.S. [14]
Attending Surgeon, Cedars-Sinai Medical
 Center
Los Angeles, California

**John N. Graber, M.D., F.A.C.S.
 [Introduction, 9, 13, 15, 17]**
Director, Institute for Minimally Invasive
 Surgery, and Chairman, Department of
 Surgery
Abbott Northwestern Hospital
Minneapolis, Minnesota
Clinical Instructor in Surgery
University of Minnesota
Minneapolis, Minnesota

Jonathan T. Gudman, M.D. [6]
Staff Anesthesiologist
Abbott Northwestern Hospital
Minneapolis, Minnesota

Patricia A. Hartwig [4]
Director, Laser Center
Institute for Minimally Invasive Surgery
Abbott Northwestern Hospital
Minneapolis, Minnesota

David F. Hickok, M.D., F.A.C.S.
Clinical Associate Professor of Surgery
University of Minnesota
Minneapolis, Minnesota

David Llewellyn Hill, M.D. [1]
Hill, Hzislet, Wzvrin & Wright, P.A.
Minneapolis, Minnesota

Ronald A. Hinder, M.D. [19]
Professor
Creighton University School of Medicine
Omaha, Nebraska

John C. Hulbert, M.D., F.R.C.S. [21, 23]
Professor of Urology
University of Minnesota
Edina, Minnesota

Luis Isabel, M.B., B.S., F.R.A.C.S. [8]
Department of Surgery
The Whyalla Hospital
Whyalla, South Australia

Keith W. Kaye, M.D., F.R.C.S. [22]
Clinical Professor of Urology
University of Minnesota
Minneapolis, Minnesota
Abbott Northwestern Hospital
Minneapolis, Minnesota

Deborah J. Lightner, M.D. [22]
Staff Urologist
Abbott Northwestern Hospital
Minneapolis, Minnesota

Robert D. Mackie, M.D. [16]
Director, Biliary Center at Abbott
  Northwestern Hospital
Minneapolis, Minnesota
Practicing Gastroenterologist with Digestive
  Healthcare
Minneapolis, Minnesota
Clinical Professor, Department of
  Gastroenterology
University of Minnesota Hospitals
Minneapolis, Minnesota

Michael Patkin, M.B., B.S., F.R.A.C.S. [8]
Department of Surgery
The Whyalla Hospital
Whyalla, South Australia

Joseph J. Pietrafitta, M.D. [10, 12, 18, 19, 24]
Director of Research
Institute for Minimally Invasive Surgery
Minneapolis, Minnesota
Director of the Surgical Endoscopy
  Fellowship Program
Abbott Northwestern Hospital
Minneapolis, Minnesota

David A. Plut, M.D. [6]
Department of Anesthesiology
Abbott Northwestern Hospital
Minneapolis, Minnesota

Weyma Jean Reavis, M.A. [5]
Surgical Coordinator
Hickock, Schultz, and Graber, P.A.
Minneapolis, Minnesota

Leonard S. Schultz, M.D., F.A.C.S. [11, 20, 22]
Clinical Assistant Professor of Surgery
Department of Surgery
University of Minnesota
Minneapolis, Minnesota
Past Chairman of Department of Surgery
Abbott Northwestern Hospital
Minneapolis, Minnesota

Stephen J. Shapiro, M.D., F.A.C.S. [14]
Attending Surgeon, Cedars-Sinai Medical
  Center
Los Angeles, California
Assistant Clinical Professor
University of California at Los Angeles School
  of Medicine
Los Angeles, California

Hock L. Tan, M.B., B.S., F.R.A.C.S. [25]
Consultant Pediatric Surgeon and Urologist
Royal Children's Hospital, Parkville
Victoria, Australia

Preface

Laparoscopic abdominal surgery is developing at an extraordinary pace. Surgeons are challenged with the need to keep up with the changes and to learn the new procedures. Although the premiere laparoscopic procedure is cholecystectomy, the technology has been pushed into the management of other abdominal pathologies: colon and rectal surgeries, herniorrhaphy, management of peptic ulcer and gastroesophageal reflux, diagnostic oncology, urologic procedures, and common bile duct exploration.

This text is designed for the surgery resident and the practicing surgeon wishing to gain an understanding of the theory and technique of laparoscopic surgery. Written by experts in each area who were instrumental in the development of laparoscopic approaches, the book is designed to give a clear and encompassing review of the field. The detailed line drawings, color photographs, and extensive index will make it a valuable reference.

Acknowledgments

We should like to thank our wives, Susan, Michele, Nancy, and Hope, for their patience and support of our ambitions. Also we thank Priscilla Kilibarda, Sheila Lawrow, and Mary Kamel for their assistance in the preparation of this text and Mercil Communications, Inc., and Medical Art Services for the photographs and artwork. And, finally, we thank Peter Scott, who introduced us to McGraw-Hill, making this publication possible.

Introduction: The Future of Surgery Is "Less Invasiveness"

John N. Graber

The public knows what it wants from medicine—and in many ways the last people to know it have been surgeons. When balloon angioplasty was first introduced, surgeons uniformly balked, noting that "the only way to fix arterial lesions is to operate on them." There are still some surgeons who argue against gastroenterologists placing percutaneous endoscopic gastrostomy tubes. Angioplasty and endoscopy have become more refined, and despite some remaining questions, when compared with incisional surgery, these procedures are the clear choice of the public.

What is the appeal? In the case of angioplasty it is not improved long-term patency; to the contrary, bypass surgery has repeatedly been shown to be better. It is not that the gastroenterologist's percutaneous gastrostomy (PEG) tube functions as a better gastrostomy tube over the incisionally placed counterpart. The real appeal is in the "less invasive" character of the procedures. Surgeons are just becoming aware of the importance of this trend.

If a procedure can be done with less pain, less incision, less scar, less hospitalization, less time off work, and above all less cost, and still deliver a relatively similar outcome, it will be viewed as better. This vision of an "improved surgical product" will force a change in the way surgeons operate in two basic ways.

First, since information moves much more quickly now than it used to, many patients soon ask for the new and "better" procedure. If one surgeon doesn't offer the procedure, then the patient will go to another one who does.

Secondly, the procedures that surgeons will be doing in 10 years are ones that offer a demonstrable overall cost savings—procedures that the public can pay for through their insurance plans or their employers' plans. These two factors, less invasive benefit and overall cost to society, combine to direct surgery with the most weight given to cost. The changes in surgical practice that they will effect are already being realized.

There will be a continued trend toward less

hospitalization and more outpatient surgeries. This will be dictated by third-party payers. Home health care will become more prominent. Home nursing, intravenous (IV) therapy, and medication will be available routinely not only for procedures such as cholecystectomy and appendectomy, but also for bowel resections, vagotomies, and antireflux operations.

More "high-tech" procedures will be developed, but they will not be used routinely unless their initial up-front costs can be balanced by an overall cost savings by reducing hospital days, shortening time off work, or preventing progressive disability.

Surgeons will have to travel more to attain new information and learn new techniques as these techniques become available. No longer will surgical residency alone be the only training needed to keep pace with the surgical practice of the future. These factors will combine further to centralize the availability of futuristic surgical procedures.

A procedure that exemplifies these points well seems to be laparoscopic cholecystectomy. Surely, the possible use of laser and laparoscopic instrumentation adds to the operative cost of cholecystectomy; however, the routine reduction of hospital length of stay by 2-to-4 days makes up for any added cost. Also, by allowing patients to return to work within 7

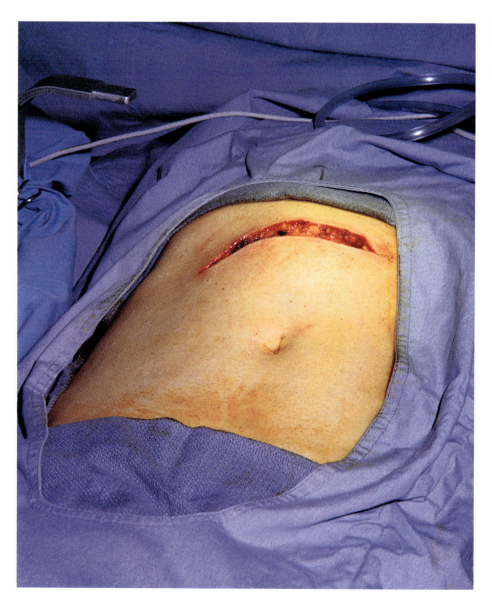

Figure I-1
A large right subcostal incision, traditionally commonplace, will become a rarity as the times and surgical procedures change.

days, the new procedures allow employers to realize a dramatic savings in prolonged disability payments and increased employee productivity. Training programs have been developed and thousands of surgeons have traveled to learn the technique. It has been estimated that 70 percent of all cholecystectomies done in the United States in 1992 were done via laparoscopic technique—the figure was less than 1 percent in 1989! The subcostal incision that surgeons knew well in the past will become a rarity as the times change (Fig. I-1).

This book is in response to the overwhelming interest in the new and expanding field of laparoscopic abdominal surgery. The field is driven by the engine of "less invasiveness," and dramatic changes in surgery have arrived. The first section of the book is dedicated to the basics of the newer technologies applied to abdominal pathology. Laparoscopy, lasers, cautery, and operating room requirements are reviewed. The second section deals with specific laparoscopic abdominal procedures. The authors have extensive experience in the field. Their techniques are reviewed in a step-by-step fashion, and each author injects specific observations derived from his and her clinical experience and research endeavors.

Although we have done all that we can to provide as much detail and nuance to these operations, no amount of study will replace hands-on laboratory training and well-supervised initial procedures. The reader is encouraged to gain as much information as possible from this text and other referenced readings, but clearly he or she must develop the skills and abilities required in a setting that has the best interest of the patient as the primary goal.

One thing that the feverish interest in laparoscopic abdominal surgery points out is that surgeons are much more keenly aware of ground that they gave up in the past when new procedures were being developed. Surgeons have begun to understand that less may be better—and that it will be better for a long time.

PART ONE

Basic Considerations

1

The Basics of Laparoscopy

David L. Hill

Modern laparoscopy began in the early 1960s with the replacement of the incandescent bulb with fiberoptic light sources. Urologists and otolaryngologists were already using endoscopy. Gynecologists had been struggling with a procedure called *culdoscopy*. To enable the physician to look inside the pelvis, the patient was given an intravenous sedation and then placed in the knee chest position. A culdoscope was placed through a puncture in the posterior cul-de-sac of the vagina. Then, with the aid of a hot incandescent light, attempts were made to see the uterus, tubes, and ovaries. Controlled pneumoperitoneum was not available until the development of automatic insufflators. It is no wonder that laparoscopy was welcomed so enthusiastically.

Initially, the gynecologist was primarily interested in using laparoscopy as a diagnostic procedure. Tubal sterilization and ovarian biopsy were about the most aggressive procedures performed. Literally years were spent at this level obtaining expertise at insufflating the abdomen and exposing pelvic organs. When diagnostic laparoscopy became routine, more surgical procedures were then attempted.

Laparoscopy was recognized as a minimally traumatic method of performing many surgical procedures. Its evolution follows the development of optics, fiberoptics, insufflation devices, instruments, lasers, electrocoagulation devices, and video equipment. As each of these technologies has developed, the range of application of laparoscopy has increased.

This chapter is intended to introduce the different technologies required to perform laparoscopy. In order to become an expert in operative laparoscopy, you must understand the mechanics and function of each of the components of the system.

Pneumoperitoneum

The first step in obtaining a pneumoperitoneum is the insertion of the Verres needle (a special needle that is spring-loaded with a blunt central core) (Fig. 1-1). The blunt core is intended to protect the bowel from injury from a sharp needle tip at the time of the blind insertion of the needle. The Verres needle has a stopcock that can open and close the lumen of the needle. There are also disposable needles that have the advantage of guaranteed sharpness. An extra

Part One Basic Considerations

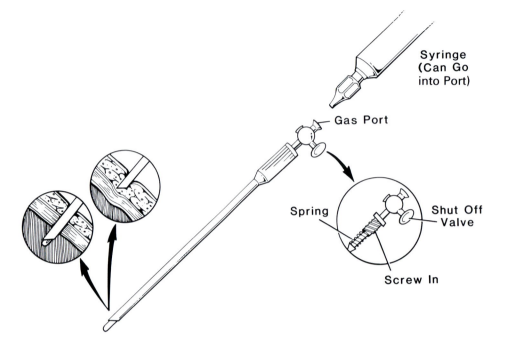

Figure 1-1
The Verres needle provides safety during insufflation of the peritoneal cavity. The inner spring mechanism allows the protective blunt inner trocar to retract and expose the sharp needle when fascial resistance is encountered.

long needle can be helpful in the obese patient. Insertion of the Verres needle is made at the umbilicus. This area is where the abdominal wall is the most thin and is away from any significant anatomical hazard. The puncture can be made above or below the umbilicus in the midline. There are anatomical advantages to supraumbilical insertion (Fig. 1-2A). If the patient has a surgical scar, it is wise to stay away from that immediate area.

A no. 11 blade is used to make a puncture in the skin. This puncture should be no larger

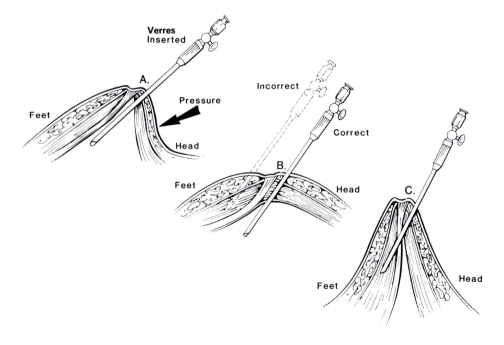

Figure 1-2
A. Supraumbilical insertion has the advantage of perpendicular penetration of tissue planes. B. Infraumbilical puncture penetrates at an angle, requires more distance, and more frequently ends up in the preperitoneal space. C. Too much initial elevation can lead to improper placement.

than needed because large incisions can lead to unnecessary bleeding and slippage of the trocar sheaths. Also, beware of going too deep with the no. 11 blade because the aorta and vena cava can be quite close to the navel in a slender patient. Check the pressure resistance of the Verres needle before it is inserted into the abdominal cavity to see if it has an unusually high resistance to flow. If so, then it should be replaced.

When inserting the needle, you must grasp the abdominal wall near the puncture site and lift as the needle is inserted (Fig. 1-2A, B, and C). This gives effective countertraction and helps direct the needle safely toward the pelvis. There will be two layers to penetrate, the fascia and the peritoneum. Resistance will be encountered at each of these levels and a definite snap of the needle can be heard or felt. There are several ways of checking the placement of the needle to confirm that the tip is in the peritoneal cavity.

A small syringe of saline can be injected and if the tip is in the peritoneal cavity, no fluid would return with aspiration (Fig. 1-3A). If it is in a confined space, fluid will return (Fig. 1-3B). Another method is to place a drop of saline on the needle inlet and lift the abdominal wall (Fig. 1-3C). The negative pressure produced in the peritoneal cavity will aspirate the drop. A third method is by feel. Grasp the needle as close to the skin as possible. With the abdominal wall acting as a fulcrum of a lever, the tip of the needle is allowed to fan freely back and forth if properly placed (Fig. 1-3D). If there is no free movement of the needle tip, remove the needle and reinsert it.

The most common misplacement of the Verres needle is into the preperitoneal space. In this situation, you will not obtain a normal expansion of the abdomen above the navel. Once again, you can feel by placing a hand above and below the navel and alternating pressure to get a real sense of intraperitoneal gas.

Figure 1-3
A. Injected saline cannot be aspirated from the peritoneal space, but **(B.)** will be aspirated if injected into a confined space (preperitoneal). **C.** A droplet of saline is aspirated into the peritoneal cavity, but not the preperitoneal space. **D.** The tip should "fan" freely if in the peritoneal cavity.

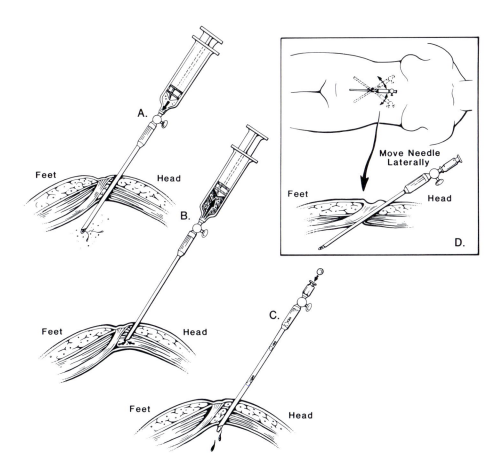

The patient should be completely paralyzed and the abdominal wall should distend uniformly and feel soft to compression in all quadrants. If the gas is installed in the preperitoneal space, the abdomen may feel as though it is not paralyzed. Also notice that liver dullness to percussion should disappear after 0.5 to 1 liter of CO_2 administered. This is an absolute indicator that the gas is intraperitoneal. With preperitoneal inflation, the pressures will be higher than expected—in the range of 15 to 25 mmHg. If you are uncertain about the needle placement, remove and reinsert it.

The CO_2 insufflator required for operative laparoscopy is a high flow device. This allows for rapid vapor and smoke removal by suction. The insufflator automatically regulates the speed of flow related to the intraperitoneal pressure (Fig. 1-4). The maximum rate of flow can be adjusted. It is safest to use a slow insufflation rate until you have confidence in Verres needle placement. At first, the 1 liter rate should be used. When you have more experience, the higher flow rates will save time and also will be necessary when suction devices are used. Even with these high flow rates, excessive suctioning will rapidly deplete the pneumoperitoneum. Experience is necessary to use suction and maintain a pneumoperitoneum.

The maximum intraperitoneal pressure needs to be set on the insufflator. When this set maximum is reached, the flow into the patient is stopped. The recommended setting is 15 mmHg. A continuous readout of the actual intraperitoneal pressure is displayed. This reading is checked when connecting the Verres needle to the insufflator at the start of the insufflation. Readings should be less than 10 mmHg. If the needle is attached to the insufflator before insertion, the resistant pressure should be 0. Another measured component is the flow rate. This can be observed as constantly changing in relationship to the intraperitoneal pressure. As the intraabdominal pressure goes up and the flow rate goes down, the flow rate will not exceed the rate that has been set.

An equipment check should be made on the insufflator and Verres needle before insertion. Turn on the insufflator and confirm that the tank pressure is adequate. Set the flow rate to 1 liter per min (low) on the dial and completely obstruct the tubing. The intraperitoneal pressure reading should rise above 20 mmHg and the flow rate should be 0. Now discontinue the obstruction and the intraperitoneal pressure should drop to 0 and the flow rate should be 1 liter per min. Then attach the Verres needle to the tubing and the pressure reading should relate to the resistance to flow of the needle's lumen. This should be almost 0. If it is higher, it suggests that the lumen is obstructed and another needle should be used. Consider how confusing this would be if the needle had already been placed and the pressure was high. When

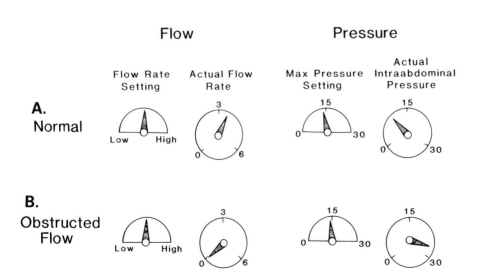

Figure 1-4
The laparoscopic insufflator: **A.** The maximum pressure is set at 15 mmHg and the flow rate is medium for general use. Intraabdominal pressure is average at 7 mmHg and the flow rate is 3 liters/min. **B.** Inflow obstruction is demonstrated by an intraabdominal pressure of 25 mmHg and a flow rate of 0.

using high flow rates, a less than desired flow will usually result from an obstructed inflow. Sometimes it is necessary to change inflow ports or even remove an instrument from the sheath in order to decrease inflow resistance.

A final readout on the insufflator is the running total of how many liters of CO_2 have been insufflated. This is useful only when initially insufflating before inserting the laparoscope. An adequate insufflation before insertion of the laparoscope can vary from 1 to 5 liters of gas depending on the size of the patient. The feel of fullness or attaining of an intraabdominal pressure of 10 to 15 mmHg is a better indicator of adequate insufflation than a set number of liters.

Trocars and Cannulas

Cannulas are the devices that are placed into the peritoneal cavity through which laparoscopes and various instruments can be passed during the procedure (Fig. 1-5A and B). Trocars are the sharp removable inserts that are used for the placement of the cannulas. Cannulas come in sizes ranging from 5 to 18 mm. Basic features include a connection for gas insufflation and a valve to prevent the escape of gas when exchanging instruments. Reusable models usually have trumpet valves to prevent gas escape. Large models are not easily adaptable to smaller-sized instruments. Their major advantage is cost.

The disposable models have several additional features (Fig. 1-6A and B). Caps are available so that the larger models can be adapted for smaller instruments. The disposable trocars guarantee sharpness. A spring-loaded shield gives additional protection against inadvertent bowel injury. Recently developed cannulas have external threads that screw into the abdominal wall and fix them in a permanent position. This very important feature prevents the cannula from slipping out of the abdominal wall with removal of an instrument. Too much cannula inside the peritoneal cavity can also be a hindrance to opening instruments. Disposable cannulas have automatic spring-loaded flap valves to prevent loss of pneumoperitoneum.

Placement of the cannulas is one of the most important steps in laparoscopy. The site of placement varies with each type of procedure. The initial puncture is usually for the laparoscope and is almost universally placed above or below the umbilicus. The skin incision for the Verres needle is simply enlarged. The abdominal wall is lifted, similarly to the technique used for insertion of the Verres needle. The cannula and trocar are then inserted with a controlled thrust toward the pelvis (Fig. 1-7A). Another method is to compress the upper abdomen while at the same time inserting the trocar in the direction of the pelvis (Fig. 1-7B). This elevates the lower abdominal wall and provides an ideal angle for the trocar puncture. The laparoscope is then inserted and the video camera is attached. With your view of the peritoneal cavity, placement of the remaining cannulas is more safely accomplished. Significant blood vessels and adhesed bowel are avoided. Transillumination of light can also help in avoiding major blood vessels (Fig. 1-8). The size of the cannula depends on the largest instrument to be used at that site. The site is selected based on the procedure to be performed, with consideration given to instrument crossover, internal operative site, and location of the laparoscope. Wide separation of sites is an advantage in knot tying; however, the instruments must reach the field. Placement of cannulas is very individualized as is the number of sights. An additional site can be very useful to gain better access, better suction, or a better insufflation rate.

Open laparoscopy refers to a technique of direct insertion of the cannula without the use of a Verres needle or pneumoperitoneum (Fig. 1-9A and B). A small incision is made through the skin, fascia, and peritoneum. A special cone-shaped cannula is then tied in place to seal the fascial incision tightly and prevent loss of intraperitoneal gas. This method was developed to avoid inadvertent injury of bowel with blind insertion techniques. Because bowel injury has been such an infrequent problem with closed techniques, this open method has never gained widespread popularity. Special situa-

Part One Basic Considerations

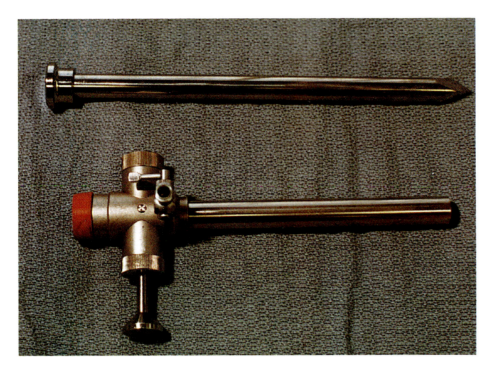

Figure 1-5
A. Reusable cannulas will cost less over time.

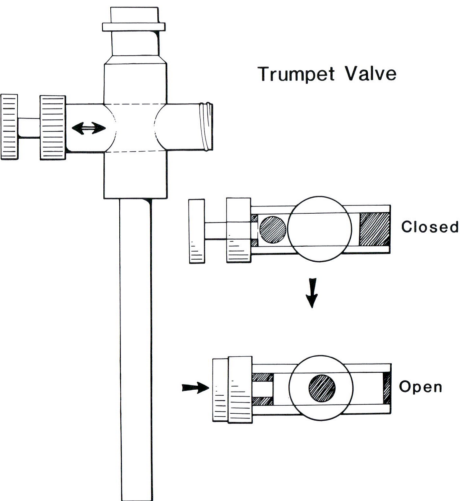

Figure 1-5
B. They generally use a trumpet valve to prevent gas loss when the instrument is removed.

Chapter 1 The Basics of Laparoscopy

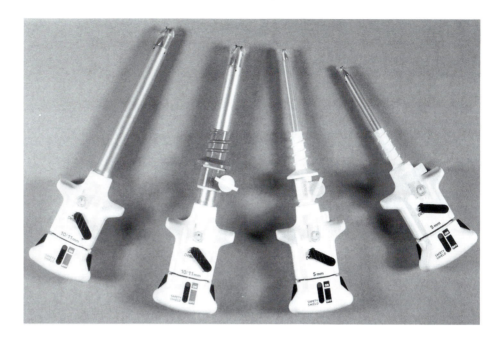

Figure 1-6
A. Disposable cannulas come in various sizes and have multiple features.

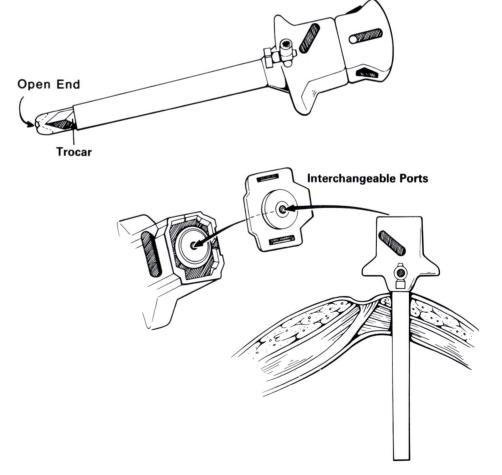

Figure 1-6
B. A spring-loaded sheath protects the sharp trocar. A threaded cannula holder is available for all cannula sizes. Adjustable caps make large cannulas functional with small instruments.

Part One Basic Considerations

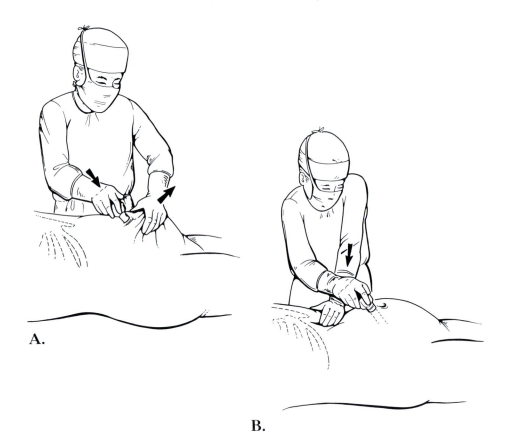

Figure 1-7
Two techniques of inserting the initial trocar. **A.** After obtaining a pneumoperitoneum, lifting the hypogastric abdominal wall gives countertraction against the considerable force necessary to insert the trocar. **B.** An alternative method is to apply epigastric compression. This elevates the lower abdomen, gives counterpressure, and creates a much safer angle of penetration.

tions, such as multiple previous surgeries with adhesions, will benefit by this technique.

Laparoscopes

Laparoscopes consist of lenses and fiberoptic viewing and illumination channels. The bigger the laparoscope, the more fibers, the more light, and the better the view (Fig. 1-10A and B). The small "pediatric" model is 6 mm in diameter. This model is used when there is need for a small puncture sight but the field of vision is smaller and the amount of light is considerably less. It is not adequate for video. It can be used through a small puncture site to inspect the umbilical puncture from within for bleeding or bowel adhesions. The 10-mm laparoscope is used with the video camera. Almost always it is inserted through an umbilical puncture whether the operative field is in the upper or lower abdomen. The placement needs to be close enough to the field to see well but far enough away so as not to get in the way of the operative instruments.

Laparoscopes also come with different angles of view. The standard is a 0° laparoscope in which the view is not angled but straight out of the end of the scope. Other scopes will have an angled view up to 45° (Fig. 1-11A, B, and C). This enables you to look around corners and into holes, depending on the procedure being done. It also helps you to keep the laparoscope above and away from the operative field and, thus, out of the way of operative instruments. When using an angled laparoscope, attention must be paid to orientation of the field of vision. Almost all laparoscopes have the angled view directed opposite to the insertion of the light source. When initially using an angled laparoscope, turn the light source through 360° and observe the changing field. Although the video camera is attached to the laparoscope, it has to be held still while the scope is rotated in order to maintain orientation. A video camera must be kept in proper position or all ori-

Chapter 1 The Basics of Laparoscopy

15

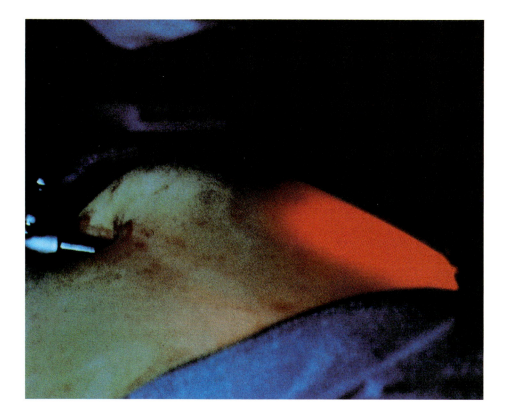

Figure 1-8
Transillumination of the abdominal wall reveals a blood vessel to be avoided during cannula insertion.

entation will be lost. On some chip cameras, the connecting cord will be angled out of the rear of the camera. In these models, the cord angle must remain at the 6-o'clock position in order to retain proper orientation. If the cord is in the 12-o'clock position, the video image will show up as down and show right as left. If the cord comes straight out of the chip camera, there will be a mark at 12 o'clock on the camera. Maintaining proper orientation is a major concern of the camera operator. Familiarity with this instrument is best obtained in the laboratory setting before being used in patients. When using an angled scope in the laboratory, be sure to try different positions of the camera and the laparoscope. The importance of orientation is readily apparent. The experienced camera operator is a very important part of the team.

Losing a sharp clear image is a common problem and can be due to many different reasons. Simple fogging can occur on any lens, including the video camera, the eyepiece, or the tip of the scope. This problem can be reduced by using various antifogging agents. If the laparoscope is at a lower temperature than the intraabdominal environment, the lens will fog. Laparoscopes are always colder than the abdominal cavity. Heaters are very helpful to minimize this problem. If the laparoscope is at body temperature when inserted, its environment usually maintains its temperature.

A fogged lens can sometimes be cleared by just touching the tip of the scope to bowel. If this fails, however, the scope must be removed, cleaned, and more antifog solution applied. If the image is still blurred, remember that it may be the eyepiece or the camera lens. As the operation proceeds, another reason for loss of clarity is related to vapor and smoke accumulation in the abdominal cavity after cauterization. In these situations, gas exchange is important. Inflow must be unrestricted. Check the flow gauge to see if the flow corresponds to the set rate. When the setting is high and the flow is low, there is either inflow obstruction or high in-

Part One Basic Considerations

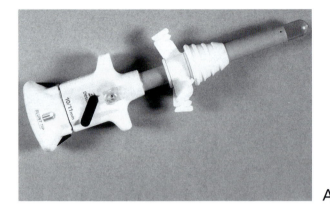

Figure 1-9
A. The Hasson cannula has a blunt-tipped trocar, and the cannula travels through a beveled outer ring.

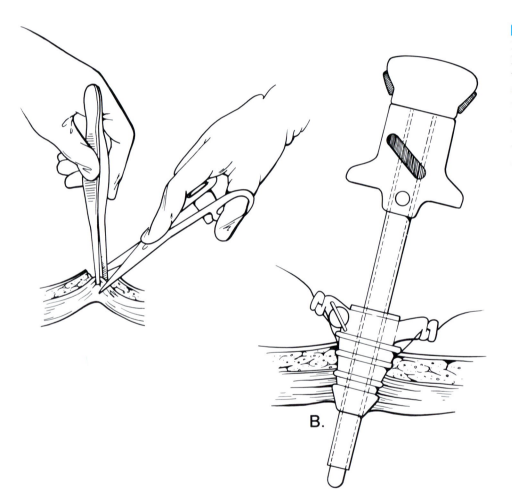

Figure 1-9
B. It is held to the fascia with sutures to prevent air loss. It is placed through a minifascial and peritoneal incision under direct visualization rather than a blind puncture.

traabdominal pressure. Inflow may be restricted by cannula size. The highest inflow is through a cannula that has no instrument in it. Changing the inflow site may be necessary. With increased intraabdominal pressure, the solution is simply to suction the gas and smoke. Time will be saved if the procedure is stopped and all the fog and smoky gas is removed. The pneumoperitoneum can be readily reestablished by high flow insufflation.

Chapter 1 The Basics of Laparoscopy

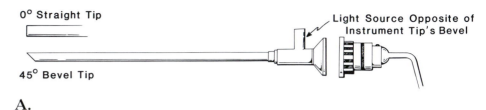

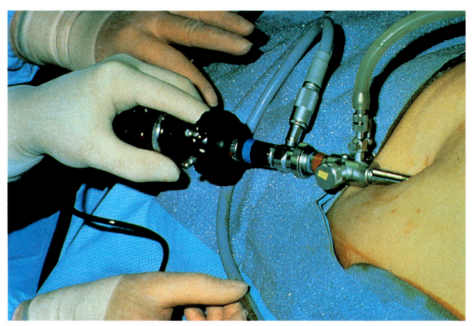

Figure 1-10A and B
The laparoscope consists of an eyepiece and a light source connection. The video camera typically has a connection mechanism and a focus adjustment.

Mechanical Laparoscope Holders

Mechanical devices to hold laparoscopes (and other instruments) are now available. These devices attach to the operating table frame and can be adjusted to hold the camera in any conformation (see Fig. 20-7B). Visualization is dramatically improved, and the stable image is very beneficial during dissection.

Light Sources

Fiberoptic light sources provide an intensity of light that allows split beams to be used and photographs to be taken. But the high intensity of light is most beneficial in allowing the use of the video camera. Light sources are fairly straightforward. They are, however, "high tech" and once again you need to understand them to benefit from their potential completely. The delivered light is only as good as the cord transmitting it. Fiberoptic cords are very vulnerable to fiber breakage. Close attention to connections and the condition of the cord is necessary. Every connection will lose light. To minimize this, ends of the cord should fit well and be clean. If there is poor light, always check the integrity of the cord fibers (Fig. 1-12). Enough of the fibers may have been damaged to effect light transmission significantly. Newer light sources have devices that regulate the amount of light to optimize visibility. These include automatic irises and automatic light intensity regulators that are helpful in keeping glare from being a problem. Bulbs also have a definite life span. Bulb changes should be dated. New bulbs must be immediately available. Someone in the operating room has to know how to change the bulb.

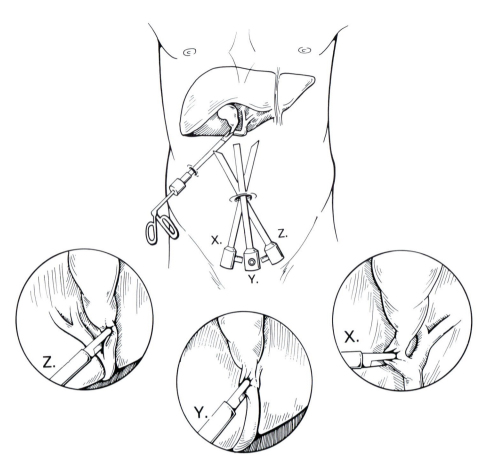

Figure 1-11
The view from the laparoscope can vary from 0° to 45°. **A.** The angle gives the advantage of enabling you to look into holes and around corners, as well as to stay out of the way of instruments being used.

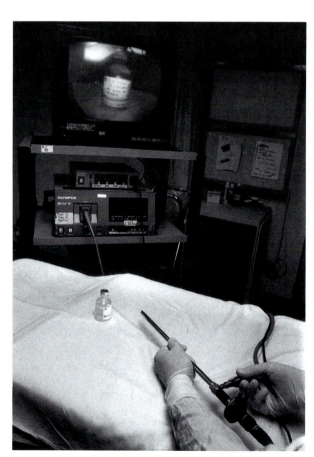

Figure 1-11 B. The angle of vision is opposite the light source connection.

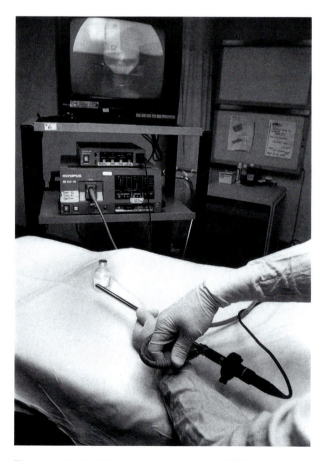

Figure 1-11 C. When the scope is rotated 180° to change the viewing angle, the camera must be held still to prevent turning the video image upside down.

Chapter 1 The Basics of Laparoscopy

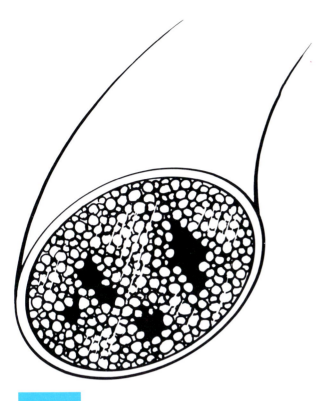

Figure 1-12
Sources for fiberoptic delivery of light are vulnerable to wear and tear over time. Broken fibers are seen as black "holes" in the light spot that the cable projects on a white surface.

Coagulation Methods

Although laser has become a very useful modality in operative laparoscopy, electric cautery remains the basic method of coagulation and hemostasis. A practical as well as theoretical understanding is necessary in order to maximize benefits and safety. The two basic types of electric cautery, monopolar and bipolar, will be considered separately.

Monopolar cautery involves an electric current passing through the patient's body. The intensity of effect of this current is related to the amount of current and the cross-sectional area of the conducting material through which the current flows. The cutting or coagulating needle has a small area of contact compared with the large area of the ground plate. Monopolar cautery is the method used in virtually all major surgery. Its use is also standard in operative laparoscopy, but there are additional considerations for patient safety. There is a close relationship of cautery wires and cautery instruments to metal laparoscopes and instruments. This close relationship can lead to short circuits and arcing that can cause significant tissue injury. The early laparoscopic experience in the gynecologic literature reports many bowel burns, both recognized and unrecognized. A case has been made by some to use only laser because of this risk. This, however, seems extreme because cautery can be safely used for both cutting and coagulating. Special care must be taken to keep instruments and power sources in perfect working condition to maximize safety. Consideration must always be given to the area where coagulation is being used. Deep tissue injury is a recognized effect of monopolar cautery. Monopolar cautery is simply not used near tissue that would be harmed by coagulation.

Bipolar cautery is a less hazardous method than monopolar cautery. This is because the current in bipolar cautery does not pass through the patient's body but from only one paddle to the other. This eliminates the risk of arcing and short-circuiting to adjacent tissue. There is not the deep coagulation effect as well, making bipolar a much more controlled method. It allows bipolar to be used in areas where it would not be safe to use monopolar. The desiccation effect of bipolar cautery can safely seal blood vessels as large as the ovarian or cystic artery. When vessels of this size are cauterized, it is helpful to have an ammeter connected to your power source. After adequately skeletonizing the vessel, current is passed through the tissue between the paddles. When the ammeter shows no current flow, the desiccation is complete.

Bipolar and monopolar instruments come in a wide variety of configurations. Bipolar instruments are most often grasping devices with two paddles, but now there is a bipolar "hook" cautery tool as well (Fig. 1-13A and B). The most basic monopolar device is a ball tip that gives coagulation at the point of contact (Fig. 1-14A, B, and C). Most useful for dissecting are heavy wire hooks of various shapes. The smallest wire needles can serve as microcoagulators or as electronic scalpels, depending on the type of

Part One Basic Considerations

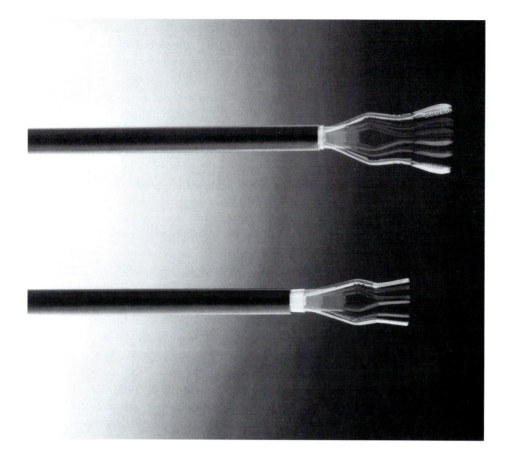

Figure 1-13
A. The paddle grasping bipolar cautery device.

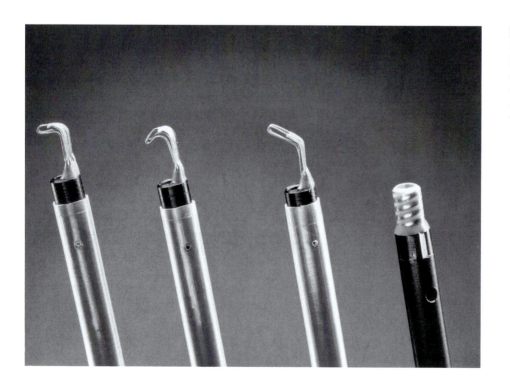

Figure 1-13
B. Other bipolar devices can be used like the unipolar hook but do not affect surrounding tissue. (Everest Medical.)

Figure 1-14
A. There are multiple heads available for the unipolar cautery devices: hook, needle, spatula, and blunt.

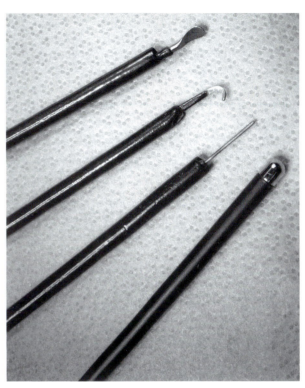

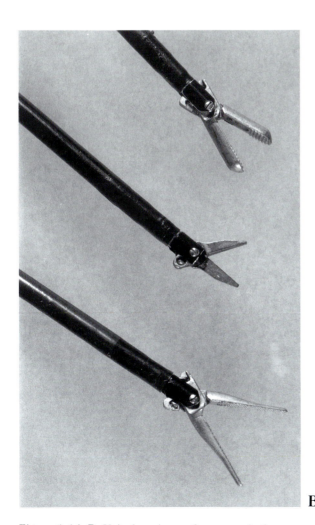

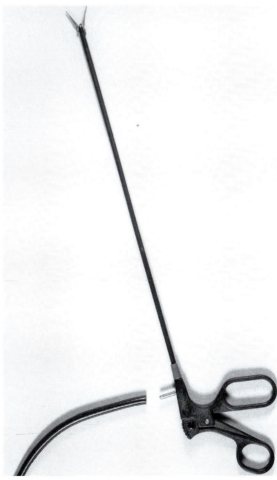

Figure 1-14 B. Unipolar scissors, forceps, and other instruments are also available.

Figure 1-14 C. They are connected to the generator by a detachable cable.

current used. Also available are unipolar cautery scissors, dissectors, and clamps.

A very helpful exercise is to test all of the different monopolar and bipolar coagulation equipment in the laboratory. A state of the art power source should be used but only by someone who understands how to use it. A whole frying chicken is a good model. Learn all the functions of the power source and then try all of the instruments. Test all the different power settings and blends. The needle electrode is a very impressive scalpel. The bipolar coagula-

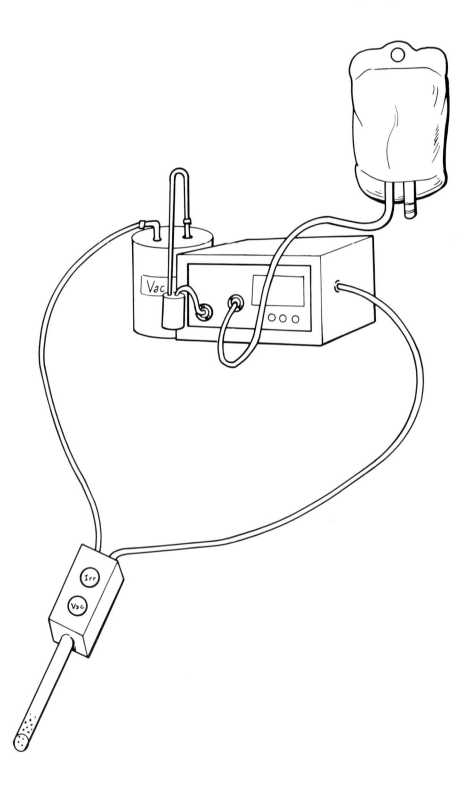

Figure 1-15
Suction and irrigation devices work through a common channel.

tion will completely desiccate with little deep or lateral injury. Invaluable experience is obtained if proper power settings are learned. Virtually all cutting and coagulating can be safely done with electrocautery.

Mention should be made of another method of coagulation called *endocoagulation*. This is a strictly thermal method that heats tissue to temperatures high enough to coagulate proteins but not higher than necessary. The rationale behind this method is the attempt to injure no more tissue than necessary to obtain the desired hemostasis. The benefits of this method have not overshadowed its limitations. Use of this method has been limited.

Irrigation and Suction

In order to do any procedure, exposure of the operative field is essential. Irrigation and suction make this possible. There are many different models available for laparoscopy, all having their positive and negative features (Fig. 1-15). Many procedures require large volumes of irrigation fluid; therefore, the source needs to deliver large volumes. Irrigation is necessary to free the field of blood or other material that interferes with a clear view. It also helps identify bleeding sources. Fluid under pressure is also a helpful method of dissection when separating tissue planes.

Suction must be variable in strength. It is desirable to have gentle aspiration in order not to obstruct the tip immediately with omentum or bowel. Small multiple openings minimize this problem, but these instruments do not have large enough openings to remove blood clots. It is also advantageous to have a fairly strong suction to remove blood clots. However, the stronger the aspiration, the faster the pneumoperitoneum is lost. The balance of suction and maintenance of pneumoperitoneum comes with experience.

Any relatively isotonic intravenous (IV) fluid solution can be used for the irrigation solution. Some surgeons advocate adding 5000 units of heparin to each 1000 mL of irrigating solution in order to inhibit clotting and fibrin formation. They feel that this allows for easier aspiration of blood and lessens the formation of adhesions. This is most popular in fertility surgery. Some investigators feel that copious irrigation is more effective than antibiotics in the solution.

Instruments

The instruments for operative laparoscopy are very basic. Other than the above-mentioned instruments for cauterization, irrigation, and suction, the only requirements are graspers, scissors, and dissectors. The variations of instruments are endless. Grasping instruments with teeth are very effective in holding tissue; however, they can be used only on tissue that is to be removed because of the trauma they inflict (Fig. 1-16). Toothless graspers are available in all shapes in an effort to hold tissue firmly in an atraumatic manner. Some handles have ratchets; some are spring-loaded. A round handle that has recently been developed allows for easier maneuverability.

Scissors are a special consideration. They come in different shapes and sizes, but the most important thing about scissors is their sharpness. It is very hard to maintain sharpness, even with meticulous care, thus the recent availability of disposable instruments. Cost effectiveness of throwaway items has always been subject to fluctuations in the cost of labor for maintaining reusable instruments. Now an additional unmistaken advantage are the scissors with guaranteed sharpness. All other instruments can be easily reused, but their care is critical. Again, it should be emphasized that operative laparoscopy is extremely high-tech. Any procedure is limited by the availability of functional equipment.

Suturing and Knot Tying

Suturing and knot tying are the most difficult parts of operative laparoscopy. Technology is behind in these techniques because coagulation and clips have almost eliminated the need for suturing. There are, however, several methods of suturing and ligating that need to be learned for the occasional indication.

Suture material, needle selection, and needle

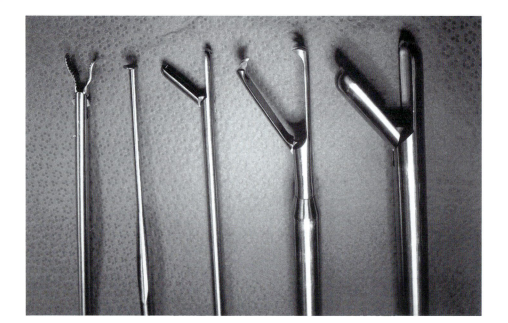

Figure 1-16
There is a variety of reusable instrumentation.

holders have all progressed with the development of operative laparoscopy. Original suture material consisted of very heavy gut that is useful in ligating heavy pedicles but worthless for any more delicate suturing. Early attempts with lighter material were with monofilament synthetics that proved tedious to tie. The best suture material seems to be a multistranded synthetic of an appropriate size. Original needles were all straight because the narrow diameter of the cannula would not accept any available curved needles. The early needle holders could hold only straight needles. A recently designed needle is in a ski shape that takes advantage of the benefits of both the straight and the curved needle. There are new curved needle holders that, when combined with certain tying techniques, make suturing a much more practical consideration.

The simplest method of ligation is the original loop ligature. This is a prepackaged plain-gut single-application slipknot with its own plastic pusher. It is introduced through a small cannula by means of a special introducer that allows the suture material to be protected from getting caught in the gas trap of the cannula. The method of introduction is shown in Fig. 1-17. All suture material needs the protection of an introducer. Anything the pretied loop can get around can be secured, such as an ovary or an appendix. The loop has a slipknot that can be tightened with the pusher. The suture material absorbs moisture and becomes even more secure. Disadvantages of these loops have been their expense and their availability only in heavy gut. Recently they have been introduced with other absorbable materials.

Loops can also be made by tying a slipknot externally with any type of suture material. This requires a special pusher. The loop is first introduced intraabdominally, then placed around the tissue to be ligated. The knot is then tightened with the pusher. An alternative technique is to place a suture, withdraw the needle, and have both ends of the suture externalized. A slipknot is then tied externally and slipped into place with the special pusher. The major problem with this technique is the necessity to drag a great length of suture material through the sutured site when tightening the slipknot. The suture will frequently tear out unless great care is taken to minimize the shear affect. A similar and yet more practical technique involves tying sutures that have been placed internally with each end of the suture available externally. This technique uses a pusher that acts as a finger

Chapter 1 The Basics of Laparoscopy

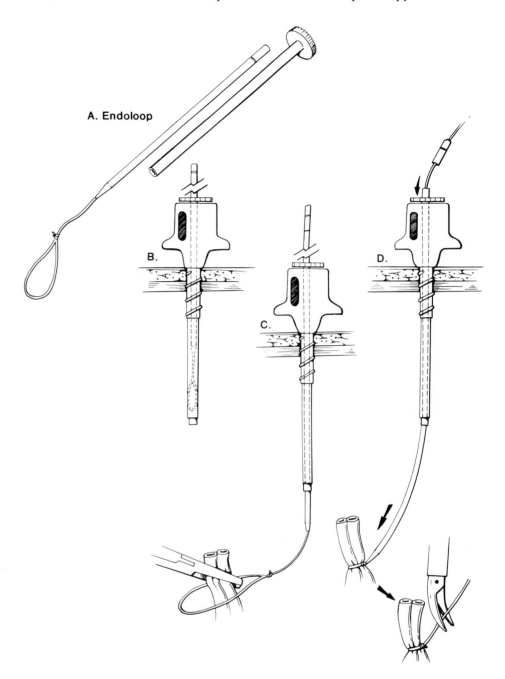

Figure 1-17
The Endoloop is the easiest internal tie, made for a medium-sized pedicle. **A.** It is prepackaged with a throwaway pusher. **B.** An inserter is needed to protect it from the trap valve of the cannula. **C.** The tissue pedicle must be passed through the loop internally. **D.** The knot is then pushed to secure the loop around the pedicle as the end of the suture is pulled from above.

extension to place each throw of the knot. This method is called *extracorporeal knot tying* (Fig. 1-18). Sutures are not dragged through tissue with this technique, resulting in less tissue disruption at the site of the knot.

The most complex technique is internal knot tying, referred to as *intracorporeal knot tying* (Fig. 1-19). These knots are simple square knots. Two needle holders are used in tying these knots. Initially this should be done with no restriction to familiarize the routine. The most important step is always to reach to the opposite side for the short end through the looped end. When this technique is familiar, proceed to the clear laparoscopic trainer. This allows direct visualization while movement of the needle holders is restricted. When this level is mastered, the ultimate practice simulation is the black-box trainer with video allowing only two-dimensional vision.

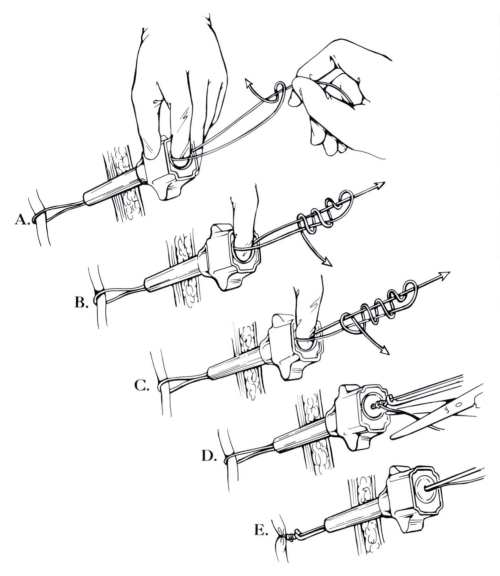

Figure 1-18
The extracorporeal knot-tying technique consists of passing a suture around or through tissue and bringing it back out through the cannula before tying it. The assistant holds a finger over the cannula to prevent air loss. When the knot is completed, a special "knot pusher" is needed to push the slip knot down and snug around the tissue. Some sutures come with an attached pusher similar to the one used with the Endoloop.

Removal of Tissue

As operative laparoscopy has been extended to more and more procedures, the inevitable problem of tissue removal had to be considered. The gallbladder, the stone, the cyst, or the ovary are often larger than the cannula lumen. If the tissue to be removed is benign, there is no reason to remove the specimen intact. The specimen is cut into pieces that will fit through the biggest puncture site. Immediately after tissue has been detached, attention must be paid either to remove the tissue or store it in a place for future retrieval. Specimens are easily lost in the multiple folds of bowel. A lost specimen does not harm the patient simply by being there, but tissue diagnosis is always desirable. Many surgeons feel that any benign material can be left in the abdominal cavity with no significant consequence.

If the specimen needs to be removed intact, as in the case of a questionable malignancy, there are several options. An Endobag, which is a small plastic bag that can be inserted through a cannula, can be used by placing the specimen into it (Fig. 1-20A and B). It can then be pulled out of the abdomen, keeping the tissue intact and preventing contamination of abdominal wall. If it is too large to pull through the

Chapter 1 The Basics of Laparoscopy

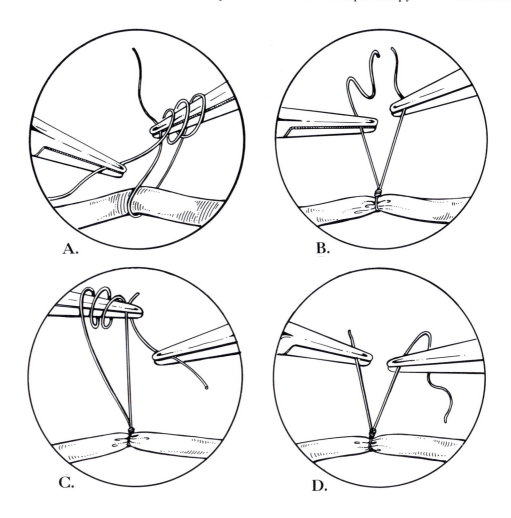

Figure 1-19
The internal instrument tie begins with a long and short end after the suture has been placed. Always cross the instruments when grasping the suture so that when the knot is pulled down the instruments are uncrossed.

largest cannula site, one of the puncture sites can be enlarged. For this, the umbilical site is best because of the single layer of fascia as opposed to several layers of muscle.

There are a number of ways to do this, all of which are equally successful. The fascia and skin incisions need to be extended to the size of the specimen. The most popular incision to extend is the umbilical incision because there is only one layer of fascia that is easy to access. Since this incision has been used for the laparoscope, it can be reinserted through one of the other cannulas. A closure of the fascia in these instances is definitely required.

A third way to remove larger objects is available in the female. An incision can be made in the posterior cul-de-sac of the vagina. Fairly large specimens can be removed in this manner. Care must be taken to consider measures to maintain the pneumoperitoneum. The cul-de-sac also must be closed.

Lastly, a new device is presently in design to assist in removal of large specimens (Fig. 13-14). It is called the *Tissue and Organ Extractor,* and it uses a sheath or a shroud into which the specimen can be withdrawn. Then the entire device, cannula, and specimen are pulled out through the abdominal wall in unison. This device appears to be ideal for removal of fragile tissues that tear when pulled through small holes. Also it is helpful for removal of infected tissues (for example, the appendix) that may contaminate the cannula tract if pulled through uncovered.

Each specific procedure will have its own special techniques for tissue removal. Individual experience will lead the surgeon to his or her preference.

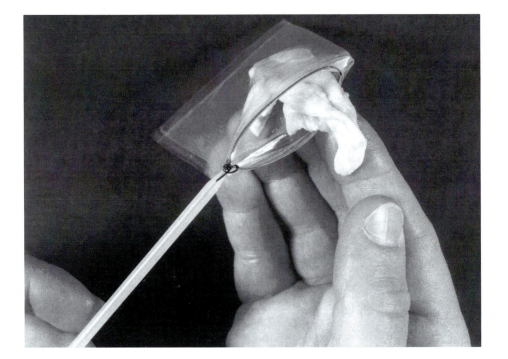

Figure 1-20
A. The Endobag is a small plastic bag inserted through a cannula with a special inserter.

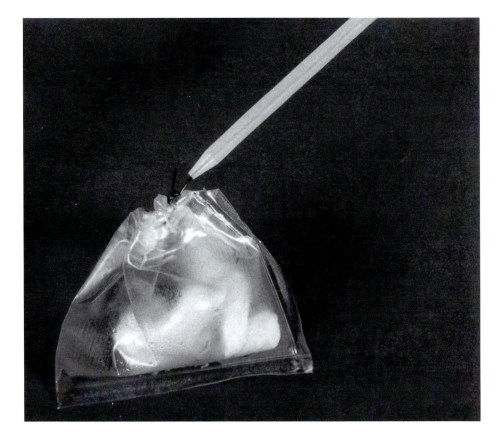

Figure 1-20
B. Tissue can be placed into it and the purse string drawn up before pulling the bag and its contents out of the abdomen.

Bibliography

Gaskin TA et al: Laparoscopy and the general surgeon. *Surg Clin North Am* 71(5):1085–1097, 1991.

Dorsey JH: Operating room organization: Laser and advanced operative laparoscopy. *Obstet Gynecol Clin North Am* September:569–574, 1991.

Semm K: *Operative Manual for Endoscopic Abdominal Surgery.* Chicago, Year Book Medical Publishers, 1987, pp 1–254.

Hulka JF: *Textbook of Laparoscopy.* Orlando, FL, Grune and Stratton, 1985, pp 1–88.

Bruhat MA et al: *Operative Laparoscopy.* New York, McGraw-Hill, 1992.

2

Video Systems in Laparoscopy

John Cartmill
Dean Aamodt

Introduction

The video system converts the optical image provided by the laparoscope into an electronic signal that can be duplicated, transmitted, recorded, and displayed on a screen. Duplication of the image allows coordination of more pairs of hands in increasingly complex cases. Screens can be placed for comfortable viewing, allowing other personnel to be involved in the procedure. The video image may be recorded on tape or a still image generator for subsequent analysis, teaching, or medicolegal purposes.

The video systems used for laparoscopy use the same technology that runs a domestic television set and video recorder; in many cases, the components are identical. The parameters that govern the current system reflect the technology (and expectations) that were available when television was introduced. These parameters limit the absolute resolution that current video systems can hope to approach.

The convenience of a video image comes at a price (Fig. 2-1). Image degradation occurs at each step of the data coding and transmission chain, from operative field to laparoscope, through the camera to camera control unit and its connections to recorders, monitors, and still-image generators. The extent to which data is lost (and the image degraded) depends on the design, quality, and maintenance of the equipment but also on optimizing the performance of each component and the system as a whole. A high resolution monitor will not compensate for a fogged lens, an out of focus camera, or the unnoticed reflection of ambient room light on a monitor. "If you can't see it, you can't fix it!" The surgeon should not forget that the final optical step is through his or her prescription lens and eyes.

Video system performance failures are frustrating. Most of these failures are due to errors in setting up and running the system. They are human errors not electronic ones. A working knowledge of the components of the video system will allow the surgeon to optimize its performance and solve common problems systematically and quickly. A basic understanding of the principles of video technology will make tuning and troubleshooting the system a satisfying process and enable the surgeon to discuss current and future needs with industry representatives in an informed way. Increasing

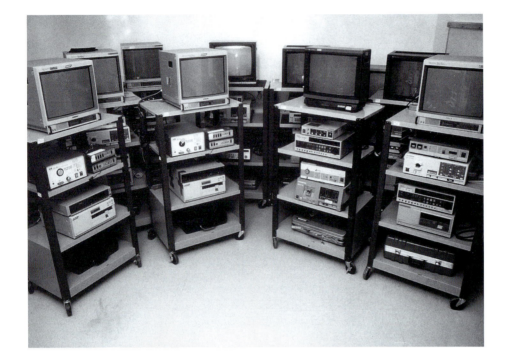

Figure 2-1
A section of the video cart "garage" at Abbott Northwestern Hospital.

knowledge will also bring an awareness of the limitations of current video technology and how this might affect operative strategy.

Video Basic Principles

Video technology grew from the television broadcasting industry and its terminology and standards, and in some cases, its limitations still apply to medical video systems.

Television was developed in the era of pickup tubes and analogue signals. The image was read by a scanning beam from right to left, top to bottom, and this information transmitted to a monitor that reproduced the image in the same number of scanning lines. In the United States, the image was and still is read by 525 scanning lines scanning 30 frames per second, transmitted in two sets of "field," one of the odd lines and one of the even lines, so that the information on the receiving screen changed 60 times per second. This "common language" was called *National Television Systems Committee* (*NTSC*). For the image, 485 of the 525 lines are used, and for framing, 40. To transmit this much information required a bandwidth of 4.3 MHz. Each station was allocated 6 MHz, using the remainder for transmission of an audio signal and boundaries between adjacent stations.

The NTSC standard was used in the United States, Japan, Canada, and Mexico. Other coding systems are available, for example, Phase Alternation Line (PAL) in Germany, England, Australia, Italy, Western Europe, and much of South America and *Séquentiel Couleur à Mémoire* (SECAM) in France, the Commonwealth of Independent States (CIS) (the former Soviet Union), and Eastern Europe. Both PAL and SECAM are based on 625-line, 25-frame per/s systems. These systems are called compound because they combine color and brightness information into one signal.

Stand-alone video systems do not have bandwidth restrictions and can carry multiple channels of information. S-video, also called Y/C, consists of two channels, one for color (chrominance [C]) and one for brightness (luminance [Y]). It is a component signal rather than a compound one. The RGB system consists of separate channels for each of the primary colors (red, green, and blue).

Resolution

Lines of resolution, scanning lines, pixels, and dot pitch govern the detail of the video image. Pixels are "picture elements." Each point of information on a picture is a pixel, and no picture can have more detail than it has pixels. A pixel is represented by an individual photodiode on the camera chip. A row of pixels is the digital equivalent of a scanning line. The number of scanning lines refers to the total number of lines of information on the screen, and dot pitch refers to the size of the phosphor elements on the monitor. Dot pitch limits the amount of information that can fit along a scanning line.

Within the limits imposed by pixels, scanning lines, and dot pitch, clarity or sharpness of image is a function of contrast, brightness, color balance, frequency response, and edge enhancement; it is measured as resolution, subjectively, using a test pattern. Edge enhancement is an electronic device introduced to emphasize edges, compensating for some of the limitations of the system. Some three-chip cameras are able to increase the resolving power of the black and white component of their pickup by effectively overlapping pixels.

Lines of resolution (television lines of resolution) refer to the number of alternate black and white lines that a system discriminates between. Vertical lines of resolution measure the ability to distinguish between a "stack" of alternating white and black lines, and horizontal resolution, between a row of alternating black and white lines. The vertical resolving power is limited by the number of scanning lines. The vertical resolving power of a monitor is theoretically 485 lines but is usually only 350 lines, while poor quality systems and often home television may deliver only 200 lines of vertical resolution. More detail can fit along a line (if the frequency response of the system and its bandwidth can support it), but nothing more can be added between the lines. Stand-alone systems with high frequency response and a broad bandwidth may be able to distinguish between up to 600 or even 750 alternating black and white vertical lines along the scanning line. Convention reduces this absolute number of resolvable lines by a factor of one-quarter because the screen is 1.33 times wider than it is high. A system able to resolve 600 vertical lines across the screen would have a horizontal resolution of 600 × 0.75 or 450 horizontal television lines of resolution.

Product specification tables can be confusing if one is quoting absolute lines of resolution, and another, television lines of resolution.

High Definition Television

High definition television is a separate technology. It has yet to be standardized, and several companies are working on systems with more than 1000 scanning lines.[1] When the standard is decided, it will represent a quantum leap in image quality and probably not have downward compatibility to current systems. To put this in the context of the eye and other imaging systems, fine 35-mm film is said to have a resolution equivalent to that of about 2300 scanning lines, while the eye can perceive improvements in resolution up to the equivalent of 1600 scan lines.[2] Advertising that promises high resolution on standard systems may be a little misleading if it is alluding to high definition systems.

High definition television uses a broader bandwidth (30 MHz), higher frequency response, and computer-aided image enhancement to provide a wider picture with about five times the information provided by current systems. Laparoscopic frames are round and will be able to take advantage of about 80 percent of this expanded capacity, which is designed for the wide rectangular screen consumer.

Color

The human eye relies on contrast rather than color for appreciation of fine detail. It is the black and white information (brightness or luminance) rather than color (chrominance) that imparts detail to an image, any image, not only video images. Color in video is made up of various brightnesses of red, green, and blue. Three-chip cameras split light into each color before converting its luminance into a video signal (or signals) carrying a summary of the luminance and chrominance information of each of the picture elements it is able to resolve. The red, green, and blue are produced on the monitor by activation of individually colored phosphors that give off the color when hit by the scanning electron beam.

In its simplest form, the information derived from each of the color pickup chips can be sent to the monitor in three separate channels (red, green, and blue chrominance [RGB]). A fourth channel carries luminance information derived from an appropriately weighted sampling of the colored channels. This method of carrying the signal is wasteful of bandwidth when one considers the relative unimportance of color to the fine detail or resolution of the final image, but it remains the most accurate way of getting information from the camera control unit (CCU) to the monitor. Bandwidth is not a problem in a self-contained video system, but four separate channels worth of information are too much for standard video recorders to record. A compromise is made by combining the color signals together and using two channels, luminance and chrominance (called Y/C, S-video or component). Historically (and today), the color signal information of a television broadcast had to fit within the channel bandwidth allocated to that broadcasting station as well as being able to be read as a simple black and white signal by a black and white receiver. The NTSC system achieved this by mixing the color information with the black and white signal into a single channel. Detail is lost during this compacting process, and parts of the color (chrominance) signal may be interpreted as black and white (luminance) signal with subsequent blurring of edges (chroma creep) causing a loss of fine detail. The differences are not theoretical and can be confirmed when you try each of the available options on your video cart.

Single-chip cameras use a color mosaic or vertical-striped filter of the so-called complementary video colors (yellow, cyan, and magenta) to present different combinations of the video primary colors to small groups of adjacent pixels on the chip. The camera control unit compares the signal from adjacent pixels and derives a luminance measure for each of the colors at each position. This information is coded as Y/C or NTSC (or PAL or SECAM) and sent to the monitor. Some single-chip cameras provide an RGB output, but it lacks the detail of a three-chip camera's RGB output because of the averaging used to derive the signal.

In practice, it is useful to have each of the systems connected permanently on the video cart and to select between them. Some applications such as arthroscopy suit themselves to the RGB image, while laparoscopy in the vicinity of the very red liver can produce an overly red image (this can be compensated for by washing out some of the red of the image by white balancing against a pink object and in effect tricking the camera into downplaying the red).

Laparoscopes

Laparoscopes have a depth of field and distortion that varies greatly between manufacturers. There is no focus adjustment on a laparoscope. The focus adjustment on the camera places the camera's chip at the laparoscope's image. A good way to explore the limitations and confounding characteristics of straight and angled scopes is to examine a sheet of graph paper at different angles and from different distances, looking directly down the laparoscope. The image at this point is the cleanest and least degraded. It is the best time to take a still photographic image. The resolving power of emulsion photography is much higher than that of video, and a still image captured further along the system will show up the limited resolving power of the system. The camera may be clamped directly to the scope or coupled with a beam-splitting prism.

It is worth remembering that the 300 lines of resolution image seen with a video system attached can be sharpened considerably by simply removing the camera and looking through the laparoscope with the naked eye.

Flexible Scopes

Some flexible scopes like choledocoscopes carry their image along fiberoptic bundles. The image they carry is broken into as many picture elements as there are fibers. In the case of a scope small enough to pass down a cystic duct, the image will be delivered down about 6000 fibers. This image is then magnified with an optical system similar to a microscope to allow each of the fibers to present to more of the camera's pixels and appear larger on the monitor. The image appears larger but not more detailed; the detail has already been limited by the number of fibers. It is clear that the quality-limiting step of this image chain is the fiberoptic bundle and that it would not be cost effective to add high resolution elements further down the image path. Flexible laparoscopes are available that do away with the fiber bundle by mounting the chip at the flexible end of the scope.

Camera and Camera Control Unit (CCU)

The basis of the modern medical video camera is the $\frac{1}{2}$- or $\frac{2}{3}$-in. solid state (rather than bulky tube) charge coupled device (CCD) or chip. The CCD functions as an electronic retina and can be seen by unscrewing the body of the camera. Medical equipment companies use proprietary circuitry and optics to manufacture cameras using CCDs made by a very limited number of companies. The resolution of the CCD is determined by the density of the picture elements (pixels); each pixel is an individual photodiode. The pixels are converted to a conventional horizontal scanning line by the CCU. Commonly, cameras are running at about 300,000 pixels.

The latitude of a video camera refers to the range of contrast it can support. The ratio of the brightest value to the darkest value is the contrast range of a scene. Video cameras have a latitude of about 5 conventional camera stops and a contrast range of 32:1. Color negative film has a contrast range of 128:1, or 100 discernible shades of gray. The human eye at any set iris aperture can probably accept a contrast ratio of 100:1, but in practice it is much higher than this because the iris can adjust rapidly. Camera performance can be optimized if it is allowed to use all of its latitude. The eye will be able to appreciate this range wherever it lies as long as it is being produced. In other words, not enough light will handicap the camera by limiting the maximum range of detail revealing steps of brightness, while too much light will have the same effect at the top of the brightness scale. A gain control or so-called automatic shutter in the CCU regulates the chip to keep it at an optimal level. Not enough light causes the lower brightness steps to be lost in the noise of the system, and the image becomes grainy, while too much light pushes the information into highlights or glare where it is lost. Highlights also cause loss of some surrounding information in a phenomenon known as *blooming,* which is due to overflow of charge from overstimulated photodiodes of the chip to adjacent photodiodes.

The white balance function allows the CCU to adjust the luminance of each of the color components to produce white, compensating for the color spectrum (temperature) produced by the light source. Color is somewhat arbitrary and can be altered to suit individual tastes or situations by white balancing against colors other than white. For example, an overly red image can be toned down by balancing against a low chrominance red (pink) card. Do not white balance on a glaring white "highlight." Some CCUs also offer black balance.

CAUTION: The CCD can be destroyed by a power surge if it is unplugged without turning off the CCU.

Monitor

Phosphors on the monitor screen emit color when excited by a scanning electron beam. Detail is limited by the size and number of red, green, and blue phosphor clusters.

Half an hour devoted to setting up and familiarizing oneself with the video monitor is a worthwhile effort. Not all CCUs produce a color bar but if possible, have the CCU display one, turn down the chroma, and note the gray scale that lies "under" it. This gray scale is a reflection of the different sensitivities of the human eye to red, green, and blue light—most sensitive to green, less sensitive to red, and least sensitive to blue. A color bar can be videoed if the CCU does not produce its own.

Brightness control sets the black bar. Adjust it from gray until the black bar is as black as it gets without going further. Going further will submerge in black some of the dark end detail present in the signal.

Contrast control sets the white bar. Dial contrast down until the white is gray, and then turn it up until the white ceases to become whiter.

Hue, phase, or tint refers to that part of the signal that is interpreted as representing a particular color (in a composite signal like NTSC or PAL). The color bar was designed in such a way that the blue signal would appear in alternate strips. The blue-only setting on the monitor will display those strips as black, and the phase control can be adjusted to produce balanced alternate bars. The hue or phase can also be determined subjectively by selecting the color bar or using the camera-generated image and adjusting hue/phase until it looks "right."

Video Recorder

Video cassette recorders (VCR) are useful for analyzing the procedure and critically evaluating technique. Video presentations are popular at meetings and a good way of getting information across.

VCR format should be one that is commonly available. It can be useful to have it the same as one has at home. An S-VHS deck will allow both standard NTSC and the higher resolution S-video recording. They both use ½-in. tape. A professional deck will be easier to repair, stand up to the extended use it will receive, and have simple controls (domestic VCRs can be confusing to operate with their time delay and simultaneous recording functions and may not allow "loop through" of a Y/C or S-video signal).

No readily available videotape format can record the high resolution detail of an RGB signal, but component systems such as High 8 and S-video can provide higher resolution than standard VHS.

Consider the logistics of a library. Tapes are more bulky than medical records, but the information they hold can be useful.

Still-Image Generator

Still-image generators overcome the problems of photographing a video image. Photographing an image on the monitor shows the scanning fronts and a poor rendition of brightness. The image generator builds the image up a line at a time on sensitive paper. It records less information than a tape, but the image is of higher resolution and is easily stored in the patient record. Still-image generators can record the high resolution RGB signal.

Setting Up the Cart or Trolley

The cart should be a way of keeping everything together. If it has drawers, have these come out the back of the cart so that accessories are available during the case. It should have a wide wheel base because it will be tall and unstable. Large wheels will allow it to negotiate cracks and cables smoothly. Computer workstation ergonomic studies show that the top of the monitor should be at eye level or slightly below.[3] Most video carts have the monitor much higher than this, placing unnecessary strain on the surgeon's neck and back. The light source should be at table level because it has the shortest cable. The VCR and still-image generator can be more out of the way on the bottom of the cart (Fig. 2-2A).

Connect the components in series so that the monitor is last. This is a fail-safe for the other components; if the message is getting to the monitor, then it must have got through the VCR and still-image generator. Some components will not allow true "loop through" of the video signal and will degrade the final image if connected in series. This can be checked with a resolution test card.

For flexibility, use every option possible (NTSC, S-video, RGB) when connecting the cart (Fig. 2-2B). Radio frequency generators such as electrocautery devices should be as far from the video electronics as possible to avoid interference.

Preoperative Check

The cart should be in ideal position with room to move if necessary. The main power board

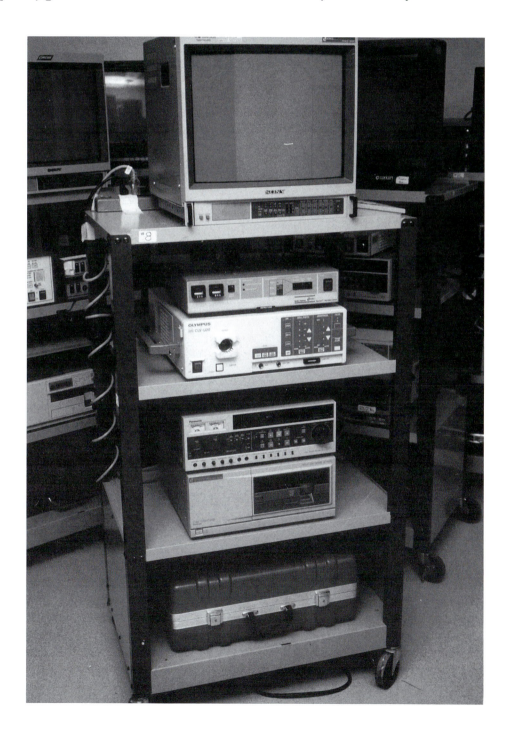

Figure 2-2
A. A typical multilevel video cart. Note the monitor below eye level, the easily accessible camera control unit, the light source at operating table level, and the wide wheel base.

Part One Basic Considerations

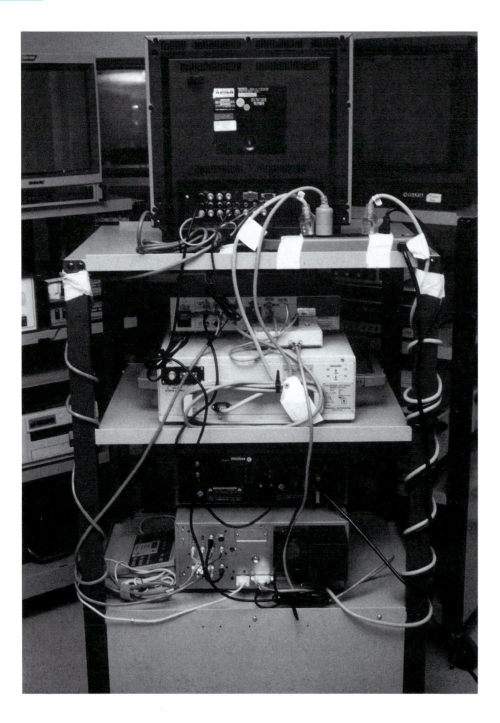

Figure 2-2 **B.** Rear view of the same video cart. Note the common power board and multiple format connections between components.

should be plugged in and switched on. Components should be turned on and off independently of the main switch. The CCU should be on standby or off until the camera is connected.

Check the light cable for broken fibers by looking at a light through it.

The scope must be warm and dry, obsessively so because even a small drop of water or condensation will cause refraction errors and degrade the image. Look down the scope because scopes can be damaged, and it is better to discover that a scope is unusable before a case begins.

Dry the camera. Attach it to the scope and light source and white balance.

The monitor should have been set up as described earlier. It will not usually require setting up prior to every case.

All lights that reflect off the monitor or appear in peripheral vision should be turned off. Light reflecting off the video monitor will alter the detail of the perceived image. X-ray screens are brighter than monitors.

Troubleshooting Common Problems

Problems will almost always be due to a failure in one of the preoperative steps. They are human errors rather than electronic or mechanical ones. Problems are more likely to occur when one is rushed or agitated. Preflight checklists work for 747 pilots and would for the video cart as well.

It is important to start where the image starts at the intraabdominal part of the scope and follow it systematically through the system. It is not always obvious where the cause of the degraded image lies, and a systematic approach will save time.

The most common mechanical problem is a short circuit in the flexible camera cable between camera and CCU that is recognized by intermittent interference or loss of picture.

Fogging can occur wherever there is a glass/air interface, the laparoscope or camera is cold, and the local humidity high; fogging occurs at the laparoscope's objective lens, at the eyepiece, and on the camera. Look down the eyepiece, having disconnected the camera to check the objective lens and eyepiece. If both ends of the laparoscope are clean, the fogging is occurring within the laparoscope. Condensation within the camera coupler or laparoscope can occur and requires formal service.

Focus is adjusted after fogging has been excluded.

Grainy image is caused by a low signal to noise ratio and is usually the result of low light. Check the connections of the light cable, the light cable itself, and the gain control or shutter settings of the CCU.

Highlighting or glare is due to too much light in relation to the proximity and angle of reflecting surfaces. Highlighting is an insidious cause of lost detail because it usually extends over a wider area than the reflecting surface alone would cover.

Color balance. Follow the steps of the color image. Start by white balancing again carefully. If the color is still unsatisfactory, vary the hue/phase control of the monitor (this is probably best done formally with a test pattern produced by the CCU).

In every case, persevere until the system is performing perfectly. Conditions are unlikely to improve during a case.

At another level, do not be afraid to use the industry representative. The companies are becoming increasingly aware of the value "service" adds to their product and realize that selling a complex electronic system carries a different obligation than selling a set of steel retractors. Postsales support is part of the deal or should be—use it!

Virtual Reality

Currently available laparoscopic video systems are moderately useful afferent imaging devices that carry a representation of the operative field to the surgeon's senses. They are limited by the lack of a third dimension and poor resolution.

Dramatic advances are being made in each part of the afferent imaging chain. High resolution pickups, high definition television, dual optic channel laparoscopes (to allow stereo vision), computer image enhancement, and the ability to display volumetric and spatial information convincingly are examples of the multifaceted approach to contemporary imaging. At the same time, understanding of human perception is growing and providing insights into the relative roles of resolution, depth, and color perception to the usefulness of a computer- or video-generated image. Imagine seeing a three-dimensional representation of a lesion within a solid organ during an operation and you will have some idea of the scope of the developing field.[4]

Tactile, force, and auditory feedback are being used to enhance and optimize sensory input. A fighter pilot uses headup displays, auditory alarms, and color cues to optimize his limited human potential. This technology will become available to the surgeon.

On the efferent side, in-built limitations of human performance are being taken into account in the development of performance enhancing robotic devices—machines that can change the order of movement, eliminate tremor,[5] and allow operation at a distance through a computerized electronic coupler.[6,7]

Virtual reality is one of the final common paths of this technology and serves as a focus to bring proponents of its various parts together. Laparoscopic surgery will benefit from advances in virtual reality. The surgeon of the future may be able to operate from a distance, even another city. The technique, teleoperating,[6,7] would rely on robotic instruments equipped with force feedback sensors and a video image in two or three dimensions being sent to a work station. At the work station, a computer would present the operation to surgeons in such a convincing manner in terms of visual, auditory, and tactile feedback that they would be able to interact with the system, directing robotic controls, unaware that they were anywhere but at an operation.

References

1. Toffler A: *Powershift*. New York, Bantam, 1990, pp 131–133.

2. Mathias H, Patterson R: *Electronic Cinematography*. Belmont, CA, Wadsworth, 1985.

3. American National Standard for Human Factors Engineering of Visual Display Terminal Workstations. ANSI/HFS 100–1988. Santa Monica, Human Factors Society, 1988.

4. Kelly PJ: Computer interactive neurosurgery (abstract). *Medicine Meets Virtual Reality,* San Diego, Aligned Management Associates, 1992.

5. Charles ST: Dexterity enhancement in microsurgery using telemicrorobotics (abstract). *Medicine Meets Virtual Reality,* San Diego, Aligned Management Associates, 1992.

6. Green PS: Telepresence: Advanced teleoperator technology for enhanced minimally invasive surgery (abstract). *Medicine Meets Virtual Reality,* San Diego, Aligned Management Associates, 1992.

7. Satava R: Surgery 2001: A technologic framework for the future (abstract). *Medicine Meets Virtual Reality,* San Diego, Aligned Management Associates, 1992.

3

Lasers and Cautery in Laparoscopy

Gregory T. Absten

High Energy Surgery

Lasers and electrosurgical units both utilize high energy waves to produce surgical effects of cutting and coagulation. Both of these modalities are waves of energy within the electromagnetic spectrum and ultimately effect their work by producing heat.[1] In order to exploit these high energy effects most safely and effectively, the laparoscopic surgeon should be knowledgeable of the physical principles that govern the safe and expeditious use of these modalities. Even though any operative laparoscopic procedure may be effectively performed with no high energy assistance, the reward for those who learn to harness these energy sources surgically is extended "reach" through smaller endoscopic access, convenience, and timesaving in fewer required mechanical instruments and greater confidence in maintaining hemostasis and precision.

---

[1] Some laser modalities use effects other than generating heat, but these are specialized applications that are not included in general surgical techniques of cutting, ablation, or photocoagulation.

Heat and Heat Transfer

Whether created by electrosurgical electrodes or laser devices, cutting, ablation, and photocoagulation are caused by heat. The advantages of these high energy modalities lie in their ability to create and localize this heat effectively to produce desired surgical effects with associated hemostasis.

Heat was once thought to be a substance. It was believed that when a hot object was placed in contact with a cooler object, an invisible entity called *phlogiston* entered the cooler object to make it hotter. Actually, heat is the result of continuous motion and vibration of the atoms and molecules that constitute all matter. The transfer of heat between objects of different temperatures involves a reduction in the average motion of the particles of the hotter object and an increase in the average motion of the particles of the cooler object.

Heat energy may be measured quantitatively as either calories or British thermal units (Btu). *TEMPERATURE IS NOT HEAT.* Temperature is a measurement of the intensity of heat, although an object at high temperature does not necessarily contain more heat than an object at lower temperature. Larger or heavier objects can contain more heat, at the same temperature, than smaller objects. This is why larger diameter contact laser fibers or probes can contain more heat, and accomplish more work, than smaller diameter contact devices at the same temperatures.

The transfer of heat from one object to another occurs through one or more of three basic mechanisms: conduction, convection, and radiation.

Conduction heat transfer is the flow of heat energy in matter as a result of molecular collisions. In other words if you touch a hot object to tissue, the object can burn the tissue through direct conduction of heat. This is the mechanism of the classic "cautery" of tissue by hot objects. The word *cautery* however does not describe current electrosurgical monopolar and bipolar units. Instead, *cautery* applies to simple hot objects that touch tissue.

During the Civil War era, iron skillets were heated to "cauterize" the stumps of amputated limbs to provide hemostasis. Present day cautery units include the Semm endocoagulator, where the electricity is used simply to heat up the end of the probe. It is true electrocautery because the electricity heats only the device and does not conduct into tissue. This is used laparoscopically to provide contact hemostasis to tissue but requires a large 10 mm portal for access. The large sizes and relative inefficiencies have been the major drawbacks of electrocautery units.

"Contact" laser fibers and sapphire probes typically used on Nd:YAG lasers are another type of "cautery" that works by direct conduction of heat from an object into tissue by direct contact. These might be truly termed *photocautery* units because the laser supplies the energy required to heat the tip of the fiber or sapphire. This is much more effective than electrical methods and results in significantly smaller devices—less than 1.0 mm. Laser light does transmit through these fiber and sapphire devices, but the major mechanism of action is conduction heating from the crystal material to tissue directly through contact.

An area where conduction heating can become a problem is where laser or electrodes are left in contact with tissue for excessive periods of time because of low power applications. Unwanted heat conducts from the target tissue into adjacent tissues and may cause excessive thermal injury.

Neither noncontact type of laser devices nor electrosurgical devices are cautery units because the devices themselves are not hot.

Convection is the second method of heat transfer and involves larger scale quantities of matter than conduction, such as is seen in the heating of gases and liquids in boiling a pan of water. Convection heating is not really very relevant to high energy surgery.

Radiation heat transfer is very important to electrosurgical and laser modalities. This involves the transfer of thermal energy by electromagnetic waves. Things do not have to touch to transfer heat this way. Heat may even be transmitted across a vacuum by radiation because it does not depend on the presence of matter. This is the essential mechanism of laser and electrosurgical devices. Lasers (all light) are of higher frequency than electrosurgical units (radio frequency electricity), but both are electromagnetic radiation.

Radiation transfer means that laser beams contain no inherent heat—and the electrodes of "bovie" units are not hot! They both transmit only radiation energy. Heat is created only when the tissue absorbs the transmitted radiation and converts it to motion in its atoms and molecules. This is exactly the way a microwave oven works—only at different frequencies.

The last pertinent concept of heat and heat transfer is that of the heat capacity of an object. Heat capacity and specific heats of objects are closely related and have to do with how much heat is required to produce a certain temperature change. In other words, biological objects of high heat capacity require much more heat to cause any given surgical effect. Highly vascular tissues have a higher heat capacity than other tissues and consequently require higher laser or electrical powers to effect the same surgical outcome.

Vascular tissues have the ability to absorb large amounts of heat without destructive tissue effects because of the "heat sink" effect of the blood flow in dispersing the localized heating.

A graphic example of this occurs in the ceremonial practice of a religious group of "washing" their hands in fire. If one is faithful and believing they say, then you won't be burned by placing your hands in the flames. In a sense it is true! There are those who are able to "wash their hands" in the fire and not be burned. The blood flow significantly increases to the hands and the act of "rubbing" distributes the heat more evenly. This results in the high blood flow absorbing and dispersing the heat of the flames throughout the circulation and preventing a localized burn!

A practical surgical example is that liver will require significantly more heat (read higher laser or electrosurgical powers) to achieve hemostasis than cutting through filmy vascular adhesions because of the relative blood flows and heat capacity.

Laser

Laser is an acronym that stands for **l**ight **a**mplification by **s**timulated **e**mission of **r**adiation.[2]

Light (photons of energy) is contained within the forces that hold together atoms and molecules. By tapping into these atomic and molecular bonds, we can release the light that is stored there. Such regular light sources as light bulbs release this light energy in a random, chaotic type process of spontaneously emitting the light. Photons of all energies (wavelengths or colors) are released in all directions with no coordination between them. This results in incoherent white light (all colors combined radiating in all directions).

Laser light consists of the same photons of light as from ordinary light sources but releases them in an organized fashion called *stimulated emission*. The laser tube, with a mirror at each end, serves to propagate this process and build a very intense beam of light. The light is emitted of one energy (wavelength and color) and travels in one direction through space as a tight beam. The result is a coherent beam of bright light of one color or at least pure colors.

Various materials emit characteristic colors of light, and the laser is named after the material used. The five primary laparoscopic lasers are the carbon dioxide (CO_2), which emits far infrared light at 10,600 nm; neodymium: yttrium-aluminum-garnet (Nd:YAG), which emits near infrared light at 1064 nm; argon, which emits blue-green light of 488 and 515 nm; the similar KTP[3] laser, producing green light at 532 nm; and the mid-infrared holmium: yttrium-aluminum-garnet (Ho:YAG) laser at 2100 nm. The table above lists these common laparoscopic lasers and associated wavelengths.

Three unique characteristics differentiate laser light from regular light, not all of which are important for surgical use.

Laser light is monochromatic, or of pure color. Lasers may produce more than one color of light from the same laser, but they are individually pure lines of color. This is very different from such white light sources as sunlight. The color of an incident laser beam can effect tissue absorption, but the "color purity" of the laser is really irrelevant to most surgery. If you get the light beam intense enough, it will create the heat to cut, vaporize, and coagulate. Developing areas of medicine such as photodynamic therapy, which use photosensitizing drugs and lasers to activate them, will be very important in the future. This is a photopharmacological effect used to treat cancers and a

TABLE 1 Common Laparoscopic Lasers

Laser	Color	Wavelength
Argon	Blue	488 nm
	Green	515 nm
KTP	Green	532 nm
Nd:YAG	Near infrared	1064 nm
Ho:YAG	Mid-infrared	2100 nm
CO_2	Far infrared	10,600 nm

---

[2] Radiation here does not refer to such ionizing type radiation as x-ray. It refers to a "radiant" body or one that "shines" light. Ionizing radiation is not a hazard with conventional medical laser units.

[3] KTP is potassium titanyl phosphate. This laser takes the near infrared output of the Nd:YAG and passes it through this KTP crystal. The effect is of frequency doubling, which changes the Nd:YAG wavelength to green 532 nm.

variety of cellular disorders. The pure color of the laser becomes more important here because of the photochemistry.

Lasers are also classified as coherent light waves. That is, the peaks and troughs of the light waves are all in phase. This is almost totally irrelevant to surgery; though for future non-invasive scanning and diagnostic applications, it is critical. This coherence gives the light a mathematical orderliness that may be used to sense the motion and structure of objects it irradiates.

Collimation is what really makes lasers useful for surgery. The beam is transmitted as a tightly aligned beam of parallel rays of light. Because this beam does not appreciably diverge with distance from its source, as do ordinary light sources, it retains the same amount of power anywhere along its path. Regular light sources lose power rapidly as distance increases from the source. Even more importantly, the collimated laser beam, when passed through a focusing lens, will converge the beam to a highly intensified point (like a magnifying glass with sunlight). This is not possible with regular light sources. Consequently, a laser is able to deliver the power efficiently that is generated and intensify this light in fine points. This intensity creates the ability to generate high temperatures within the spot and cut, vaporize, and coagulate.

Several parameters control the delivery of laser energy to tissue. These include the power (watts), total energy delivered (watts and time), power density (how small is the focused spot used to intensify the light), the color of the light, and the color and vascularity of the tissue.

In some ways these energy concepts are intuitive. An analogy is the use of a magnifying glass to focus sunlight and create a burn. The brighter the sun (power), the more it burns. The smaller the spot created with the lens (power density), the "hotter" it burns. The longer the sun is focused in one place (total energy), the more extensively it burns. The wetter the target you are trying to burn (vacularity and heat capacity), the more energy it takes to create the same effect.

Surgical lasers have evolved into two broad basic mechanisms: free beam or hot tip applications. Hot tip mechanisms have been described above as "photocautery" and encompass the popular sapphire tip and sculptured fiber devices. Free beam applications rely on radiation transfer and absorption by tissue to create their heating effects. This may be deliv-

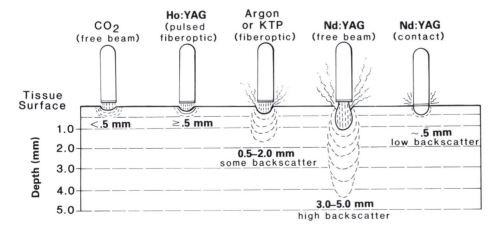

Figure 3-1
The absorption depths of the various lasers determine how well localized the vaporization or thermal injury will be, depending upon how the laser is used (i.e., power, spot size, exposure time, delivery system, etc.). Actual surgical effects can be varied from this simplified diagram and are explained in the text.

ered by a straight beam, such as a CO_2 laser, or by any of the fiberoptic lasers, such as Nd:YAG, argon, KTP, or Ho:YAG.

The color (wavelength) of the various lasers determines how effectively the light is absorbed by soft tissue. Figure 3-1 illustrates the relative absorption depths of the common laparoscopic lasers. If the light is absorbed over a broader volume of tissue (i.e., noncontact Nd:YAG), then diffuse tissue destruction can occur over this area—but it creates tremendous hemostasis. The CO_2 laser is highly absorbed, producing intense cutting and vaporizing effects but highly limiting any adjacent thermal damage.

In practice, these effects can be changed from the simplified diagram in Fig. 3-1. Argon and KTP lasers, when used to cut at high power densities at the fiber tip, can confine any lateral damage to under 1.0 mm or so. By using contact type of heated tips, the highly diffuse effects of the Nd:YAG can be made to mimic the highly confined effects of the CO_2 laser.

Energy Concepts (Watts, Power Density, Joules, Fluence)

Power is simply a measure of the *rate* of energy delivery in joules/second (J/s) and is expressed in watts (W). This applies equally to lasers or electrosurgery.

Of greater importance is the amount of power that can be focused into a spot. This *power density*, or irradiance (sometimes called *spot brightness*), of a laser is the number of W/cm^2 of a spot and is the single most important factor in the effective application of a laser. The surface area of the spot (spot size controlled by the surgeon in the field) and the total power in watts (set at the laser by the operator) determine the power density as follows:

$$\frac{(W \times 100) \times 0.86}{Pi \times r^2} = W/cm^2$$

Power density over a spot determines the rate of tissue removal within that spot. Therefore, it is not the power that determines the "controllability" of the beam but rather the power density. One can effectively change the size of the "paintbrush" (spot size) with which you are working without changing the overall rate of tissue removal (power density) within that spot by varying the spot sizes and power. The larger the spot, the greater the power required to maintain the same power density, shown as follows:

$1900 \ W/cm^2 = 10 \ W/0.6 \ mm \ spot = 60 \ W/2.0 \ mm \ spot$

Power density is also a critical concept in electrosurgery but is expressed as current density and will be discussed shortly.

Laparoscopic delivery devices are divided into two groups. The CO_2 laser is in a group of its own because it uses a dedicated laparoscopic coupler tube to deliver the beam. The rest of the lasers—argon, KTP, Nd:YAG, and Ho:YAG—all use fibers in one way or another. These fibers may be passed through conventional laparoscopic probes, unlike the CO_2 laser. Contact fibers and probes may also be added to the fiber systems to alter effects if desired.

Figure 3-2 illustrates how spot size changes with distance from the end of the laser device. The primary difference between the two systems is that fibers emit a beam that immediately begins to diverge, while a CO_2 laser laparoscope first comes to a focal point, then diverges after this. This means that the fiber systems "range of effect" is only an inch or two off the end of the fiber. Not much happens past this distance. CO_2 laser systems maintain a relatively long depth of field[4] and can burn or vaporize tissue some distance behind the target if a suitable backstop is not selected.

The advantage of fibers is that different effects can be accomplished quickly with only a slight motion of the fingers that are holding the

---

[4] Depth of field is a concept that might be familiar to amateur photographers. This is the horizontal distance, or "depth," where the focal point of the lens system stays in focus. With a laser, this means that the focal point may extend virtually unchanged for 1 or 2 in. on either side of the focal point. This means that the "range of effect" of this device is much longer than with a fiber system.

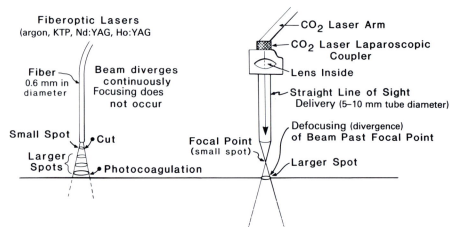

Figure 3-2
Control of spot size fundamentally differs between the focusing mechanism of a CO_2 laser and the divergent one of a fiber laser. If the power is kept constant, the spot size will change the power density and hence surgical effect and control. Fiber systems diverge rapidly so that all of the surgical effects are confined to within 1 in. or so of the fiber tip. The CO_2 laser focuses to a smaller spot (highest power density) within about $\frac{1}{2}$ in. from the end of the tube. However, it does not diverge as rapidly as a fiber system and still "packs a punch" several in. distal to the instrument. The text describes waveguides that somewhat alter this effect.

fiber handpiece. A small pinch back with the fingers allows a small blood vessel to be photocoagulated, then a small pinch forward to bring the fiber end just over tissue results in a cut—both at the same power settings on the machine. The short "range of effect" also reduces the need for intraabdominal backstops. Many times these fibers are actually touched into tissue when cutting, but this should still not be confused with the contact type of fibers and probes that must be touched to create an effect. These fiber systems may also be delivered through any conventional portal including 3-mm sites or even needle puncture sites. The argon and KTP are the primary fiber lasers, besides contact type modalities.

The CO_2 laser provides a great deal of versatility in the "reach" it provides from the end of the laparoscope, the number of angles where it can work, and the speed at which it can vaporize if desired. In this sense it is probably more versatile than a fiber system but has a significantly longer learning curve and does not provide the hemostasis that fiber systems provide. It also requires a specialized laparoscope set and coupler to mate the laser with the scope.

CO_2 laser waveguides are available for laparoscopic use and somewhat resemble a fiber. Unlike regular fibers that are of one filament of quartz around 0.6 mm in diameter, a CO_2 laser waveguide is actually a slender hollow tube around 3 mm in diameter with an internal hollow ceramic insert or coating. The laser is focused into the proximal end of this tube and, through hundreds of internal glancing reflections, bounces down the tube until it is emitted from the end. This does destroy the focusing property of the beam and instead diverges somewhat like a fiber. It does not diverge as rapidly as a fiber, however, and has a longer "range of effect."

Fibers that terminate in some device such as a metal tip, sapphire probe, or even an altered shape of the fiber tip (Fig. 3-3) generate a significant amount of heat at this tip, and are referred to as hot tip devices. They act as a very intense, but precise, thermal knife. Energy concepts such as power density do not really apply to contact devices, since they rely on simple heat conduction. The Nd:YAG laser is the primary one used for hot tip devices, and this is a popular way to use the laser laparoscopically.

Some of the hot tip devices, such as rounded or chisel sapphire tips, do actually focus some of the laser light so that combination effects may occur. A combination rounded tip fiber is also available that may be backed off tissue to vaporize or coagulate as free beam or touched to tissue to cut as a hot tip.

Sculptured fibers have increased in popular-

Figure 3-3
Sapphire tips (synthetic ceramics) are an attachment that screw onto the laparoscopic fiber handpiece. Sculpted fibers simply have the shapes of their distal ends modified by heat or in manufacturing. The mechanism of either device is the same—high temperatures of the material cause direct vaporization of soft tissue upon contact. They provide the touch control of electrosurgery but can more precisely localize their tissue effect.

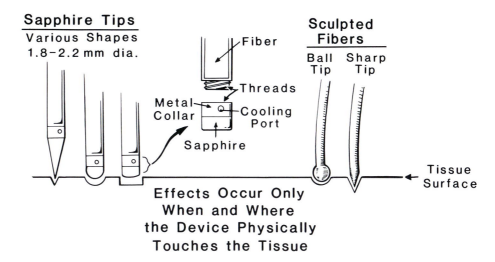

ity as a laparoscopic tool. These are not as expensive as the sapphire tips but are single-use items compared with multiple use of the sapphires. With either of these tips, one must be careful not to fire the laser for extended periods (several seconds) when not in contact with tissue. This will burn up the tip.

Because larger objects have higher heat capacities than smaller objects, larger fibers or sapphires seem to cut better and are less fragile than smaller ones. This does not refer to the size of the very tip of the device, but to the bulk behind it. For instance a 1.0+ mm sapphire, which is tapered to 0.2 mm at the tip, creates an exceptionally clean, controlled cut.

A laser may be used with either free beam or hot tip technique, depending on the fiber or device connected to the laser. The argon or KTP lasers can be used either way, for instance. Laparoscopically, the effects of argon and KTP are indistinguishable. The KTP laser though, because it uses Nd:YAG laser light shot through a KTP crystal to make green light, has the capability of the green KTP and near infrared Nd:YAG, both from the same machine. Even though the Nd:YAG laser could be used free beam intraabdominally, sapphires or sculptured fibers are preferred for a contact technique to limit the lateral and deep damage to fractions of a millimeter. Otherwise much deeper damage could occur with the free beam Nd:YAG laser.

The total energy dosage within any laser beam is expressed in joules (J). Power multiplied by delivery time equals the number of joules—10 W delivered for 3 s is 30 J of energy. A joule describes the total energy delivered but does not by itself indicate how concentrated this dose of light is. This also applies to electrosurgery in exactly the same way.

Fluence combines the concepts of power density (spot brightness) and dosage (joules), and is expressed in J/cm^2. A high fluence is like a bolus of light. It gets the job done without allowing enough time for excessive heat conduction to occur—thereby limiting lateral damage.

Pulsing a laser is a way to achieve high fluence. This delivers high peak power bursts of light but for very short periods—usually in microseconds per burst—and may be repeated as

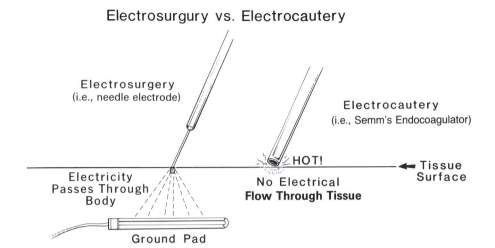

Figure 3-4
Electrosurgery, both monopolar (unipolar) and bipolar, involves electrical current actually passing through tissue. The phrase "bovie"—though technically incorrect—is customarily used to describe electrosurgery (usually monopolar). Electrocautery utilizes the electricity only to heat an element. The electricity does not pass through tissue and is a true "hot cautery."

fast as 1000 times per s. CO_2 lasers provide this feature in superpulse modes. Average powers are not high. The mode is very controllable and produces an exceptionally clean tissue effect.

A new type of Nd:YAG laser, which is a pulsed system, has recently been introduced for laparoscopic use. This provides a much cleaner cut than would be provided by ordinary continuous wave Nd:YAG lasers and significantly reduces concern about deep coagulation damage. Additionally, the laser incorporates an internal sensor to sense fiber tip temperatures and prevent overheating. When the tip is not in tissue, excessive powers will cause it to overheat. The laser immediately reacts by automatically throttling back the power. This is a major advantage in using contact type fibers and an additional safety feature to prevent high laser powers from "free beaming" in the abdomen.

Once proper use is learned, lasers add a significantly useful tool for the laparoscopic surgeon by providing better tissue precision and control than electrosurgery, good hemostasis, and the convenience of a tool that accomplishes several tasks. However, they are not a better choice than electrosurgery in all circumstances, and sometimes the ease and simplicity of electrosurgery make it the tool of choice when the advantages of laser are not required.

Electrosurgery

As we discussed previously, "cautery" is not the correct description of current day electrosurgical units, even though these terms are often used to mean the same thing. Bovie is the name of the gentleman who first devised the electrosurgical unit for neurosurgery earlier in this century. Older "bovie" units (the big green machines) work in a different manner than today's electrosurgical units (ESUs).

Figure 3-4 illustrates the difference between electrosurgery and cautery. Semm's endocoagulator is a true cautery unit for laparoscopy, which fits through a 10-mm trocar sleeve. Because the unit simply gets hot, it is used to press against bleeding sites to induce hemostasis or alternately provide prophylactic hemostasis before dissection is performed.

Electrosurgery involves electric current passing through the tissue. Since electricity is a form of electromagnetic radiation (like light but of a different frequency), radiation heat transfer becomes the mechanism of action,[5] not simply

---

[5] The effect might also be partially mediated through the temperatures involved in the short sparks that are thrown from the electrode when an electrical incision is done correctly.

Chapter 3 Lasers and Cautery in Laparoscopy

49

conduction heating like cautery. This also means that heat damage can occur anywhere in the body where the electricity travels if conditions are right (high current density).

It is helpful in describing these characteristics of electricity if one develops a frame of mind where electricity is imagined as a flow from entry to exit. Where the flow widens and spreads, the electricity is "safe" in that it won't create unwanted burns. Where the flow narrows and concentrates, burns will occur.

Electricity must have an entry and exit, otherwise known as two poles, as illustrated in Fig. 3-5. The surgical electrode is known as the active electrode, and the return electrode is known as the ground pad, or dispersive electrode. The burn or cut is created at the active electrode only because it presents a smaller surface area where the flow narrows and concentrates. The dispersive electrode, as the name implies, disperses the electricity over a broader surface area to prevent burns from occurring.

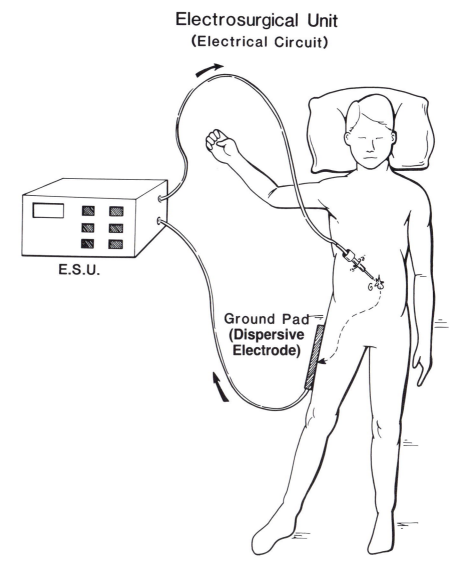

Figure 3-5
For electricity to flow, a complete circuit must exist. Electricity enters the tissue through the active electrode (monopolar) and travels through tissue until it exits via the ground pad. Even though we refer to this arrangement as mono- or unipolar instrumentation, there are in fact two electrodes, the ground pad being the second.

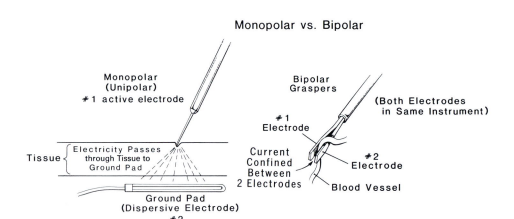

Figure 3-6
Monopolar electricity gives less control than bipolar to where the current is flowing. With monopolar, it must find some pathway all the way back to the ground pad, whereas bipolar current is more confined.

This scenario describes monopolar electrosurgery but makes the point that any electrosurgery requires two poles for electrical conduction to occur.

The two electrical poles may be configured as either monopolar or bipolar instruments—the two basic configurations of electrosurgery. The differences between monopolar (unipolar) and bipolar are illustrated in Fig. 3-6. Intraabdominally, bipolar is almost always safer and more controllable than monopolar because the electricity is confined to the small area between the electrodes.[6]

Remembering that electricity requires two poles to flow, we note that the active electrode becomes one pole and the ground pad becomes the second in monopolar use. This is true even if using a pair of graspers as the active electrode. Though the graspers have two jaws, the current is still monopolar because both jaws act electrically as one electrode.

Bipolar units include both of the electrodes within the same instrument. Each blade of the grasper becomes a separate electrode, and the electricity simply flows from one to the other. Ground pads are usually left attached when using bipolar, but they do not function. It is easier for the staff to attach the ground pad before the patient is draped, rather than trying to place it later if one decides to use monopolar. Currently, bipolar is configured only as various graspers for coagulating structures. Several companies do have plans for bipolar cutting instruments.

When using bipolar to coagulate, you must be careful to ensure that the tissue rests squarely between the electrodes. The electricity must pass through the tissue to work. For example, the tissue may be grasped too high up in the jaws, where insulation covers the electrode. This prevents the electricity from flowing. Another common problem is in squeezing the tissue too tightly and extending the ends of the jaws past the tissue, so that the exposed jaws touch one another at their tip. This creates an electrical short circuit at the tip so that the electricity will bypass the tissue entirely.

Bipolar undoubtedly provides much better control over "stray" electrical current than does monopolar, but one should not be overly complacent. Electricity does arc its way outside of the direct path between the jaws of the grasper, particularly when higher powers are used. Therefore, the minimum power required to achieve coagulation is preferred when coagulating adjacent to critical structures, and a watchful eye should be kept on the lateral coagulation that is occurring.

The electricity used in current ESUs is al-

---

[6] There are also some differences in the driving voltages between monopolar and bipolar. Bipolar units require less voltage because the space is so small between the two electrodes. This, along with the spatial confinement of the electrical flow, makes it fundamentally safer than monopolar.

ternating current (AC) electricity—similar to that from a household outlet but at a higher frequency. Household outlets have two flat prongs (the two poles just like in electrosurgery) with the third rounded prong being a safety ground to prevent unwanted shocks. Direct current (DC) is what a flashlight battery uses to light its bulb—the electricity flows "directly," or only one way. In 110-V household current, AC electricity alternates its direction back and forth.[7] It kind of "shakes" its way through the wires. It changes direction 60 times every sec, so its frequency is 60 hertz (Hz).

Electricity is part of the continuum of electromagnetic waves—in this case with a frequency of 60 Hz. Radio waves are also on the electromagnetic spectrum at higher frequencies 500,000 Hz (500 kilohertz [kHz]), and light is at much higher frequencies still!

Electrosurgical units utilize AC electricity at frequencies of 500 kHz or more. Because this high frequency approximates that of some radio waves, it is termed radio frequency (RF) current. RF current is of such a high frequency that it will not interfere with our own biological circuits. In other words you cannot get shocked or electrocuted from this electricity. To illustrate this graphically, the author will sometimes run 300 W of cutting current into one of his hands, through his chest and heart, and out the other hand to illuminate a light bulb.

When people get "zapped" by an ESU through their gloves, for example, they frequently say it shocked them. It really is not a shock. It is a high current density (like power density) burn, and we shall see later how to decrease this probability. Some consolation—whether an electrical shock or high current density burn—if it hurts, it hurts!

Energy concepts are similar between laser and electrosurgery. Power is simply the rate of energy delivery expressed in watts. This does not say how much energy is delivered, only how quickly any given amount is delivered. Unlike lasers, where higher powers for short times frequently result in better control and tissue effect, electrosurgical units should not be used with excessive powers. Use enough power to accomplish the task effectively. Too low powers simply make the electrodes languish and burn in tissue.

Without delving too deeply into electrical physics, we can review some common electrical relationships to see how these affect one's use of the "cut" and "coag" modes on most ESUs The three parameters we wish to discuss are: voltage (V), current (I), and resistance (R). The relationship between them may be described by the following variations of the same formula, Ohm's law:

$$V = I \times R \quad I = V/R \quad R = V/I$$

Voltage is the driving force behind the electricity. If we go back to our image of the "flow" of electricity, imagine voltage as increasing the height of a water tower. The higher it goes, the more pressure will build, but the actual amount of water (electricity) you get out depends on other things. Higher voltages is what one obtains when using the "coag" mode on an ESU.

Current, measured in amperages or amps, is the total flow of electricity. When you think of someone getting electrocuted from an electrical circuit, amperage is what kills, not the voltage. In terms of our water tower, the larger the outlet pipe, the more water that can flow at any given pressure. Higher current is what one obtains when using the "cut" mode on an ESU.

Resistance indicates the ability of the tissue to conduct electricity—whether it passes easily or with difficulty. Resistive is the opposite of conductive. Copper is highly conductive and passes electricity while rubber resists electricity and makes a good insulator. Likewise ionic solutions like saline are excellent conductors while solutions like distilled water or glycine are poor conductors. Fresh moist tissue is an excellent conductor while burned or desiccated tissue is a poor conductor. Going back to our water flow analogies, if one lives in the Great Lakes, and the city's intake water pipe is heavily clogged with zebra mussels, then the resistance to water flow has increased. The amount of water flow (current) will then decrease. Resistance is determined by tissue characteristics and the surgeon has no direct control over this.

---

[7] Alternating current, rather than direct current, is chosen for household use because AC may be passed through the long runs of transmission lines without the significant power loss that would occur with DC.

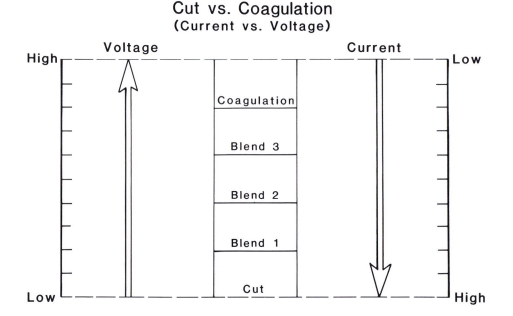

Figure 3-7
The coag mode results in a high voltage, low current output. High voltages make sparks jump larger gaps, and damage to downstream tissues could result if such a spark occurred as the electricity made its way back to the ground pad. Cutting is a low voltage, high current output that can "drive" short sparks through tissue for clean cuts.

Power is described as:

$$W(\text{watts}) = V \times I \;(\text{volts} \times \text{amps})$$

At any given power application, there is a trade between voltage and current (measured in amperage). You can have a high voltage and low current or vice versa, but you can't change both the same direction, or the wattage will change. Therefore, we have a choice of either high voltage/low current or low voltage/high current. This is exactly what the "cut" and "coag" modes choose.[8] Figure 3-7 illustrates the trade-off between voltage and current in these modes.

High current, from the "cut" mode, produces a steady stream of short little sparks from the end of the cutting electrode (Fig. 3-8). These "drive" their way through the tissue to create a very clean cut. A pure cut mode can make such a clean cut that the site bleeds too much. For that reason a blend mode is frequently chosen. It is important that these tiny sparks be allowed to form by letting the electrode ride in a steam envelope. This is done by moving the electrode only gently and not forcing it through the tissue. If it does not cut fast enough, then increase the power some until it does. If the electrode is forced against tissue, losing the envelope, then electrodesiccation begins to occur. The electrode can languish in tissue, causing more lateral damage than the surgeon anticipated.

Voltage is the determinant of how far a spark can jump a gap. When "coag" mode is selected and the electrode held just above or lightly on tissue, numerous long sparks result (Fig. 3-9—fulguration). The spark contains enough energy to "zap" that one place on the surface but not enough energy to continue to drive its way through the tissue. The result is a superficial, but highly burned, eschar on the surface. The single best use of a straight "coag" mode is to dry an oozing, bleeding bed—such as the sur-

---

[8] Because this is not a technical treatise on electrosurgery, a simplified approach is taken here to explain the differences between cut and coag modes in terms of voltage and current. This is not totally technically accurate but serves our purpose in describing reasons why each mode should be chosen. The actual voltages do not really vary on solid state ESUs. Instead, they are simply modulated rapidly on and off to vary the ratio between the peak powers and R.M.S. powers, known as the crest factor. In reference to this modulation, cutting current is sometimes referred to as undampened current, and coag as dampened current. The reader is directed to more technical discussions of the subject if he or she is interested.

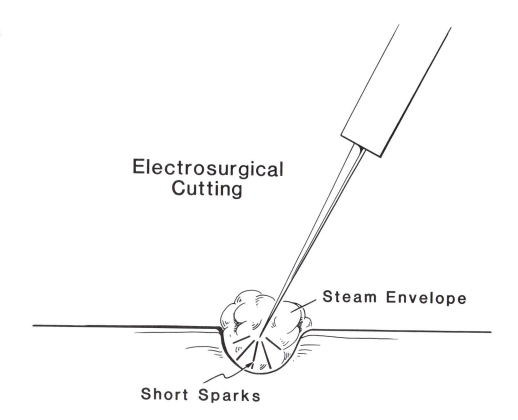

Figure 3-8
When the surgeon is successfully cutting with monopolar instruments, the electrode must "float" within a steam envelope. High current, low voltage sparks "drive" themselves through the steam into tissue, creating high-current density cuts. If the electrode is forced through tissue, the steam envelope is lost and cutting begins to change to electrodesiccation.

face of the liver after dissecting a gallbladder.

An instrument called the argon beam coagulator (ABC) has been introduced within the last couple of years, which does an excellent job of drying large oozing surfaces. This is a conventional ESU but additionally employs the use of argon gas (no it is not a laser, it just blows this gas in the abdomen) blown out the end of the probe to increase the effective sparking length of the "coag." Even with high voltage "coag," a spark will jump only so far from the electrode because air is an insulator. The argon gas provides a conductive gas medium that allows for longer, and much more uniform, sparking. This can result in excellent hemostasis that is very superficial and does not cause deep tissue damage. It can be safely used on bowel. It does require a 10-mm portal.

Use of "coag" on a regular ESU simply to desiccate a blood vessel is a poor choice and potentially dangerous intraabdominally. Desiccation of tissue (i.e., blood vessels) is created by firmly placing the clean electrode in contact with the tissue and using the "cut" setting. Sparks are not formed here since the electrode is in firm contact with tissue, unlike cutting or fulguration, and the heat produced by the electricity simply dries the tissue. A familiar example of this is the practice of touching a monopolar electrode to a hemostat clamped on a vessel (Fig. 3-9—desiccation). Technically, as long as the tissue is firmly grasped, either "cut" or "coag" settings would accomplish the same desiccation at the site. There are several reasons however why the "cut" mode is a safer choice—particularly laparoscopically.

Because desiccation does not rely on any sparking, we do not need the high voltages of "coag" to be effective. Using the "cut" setting drops the overall voltages. This decreases your chances of getting "zapped" through your gloved hand holding the clamp. Without the high voltages, the electricity does not have the "high pressure" needed to get through these

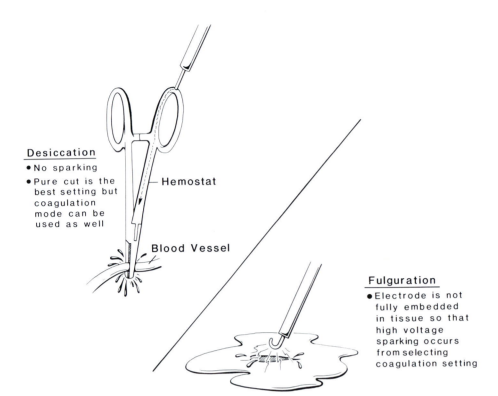

Figure 3-9
When desiccating tissue (i.e., hemostasis), an electrode is firmly embedded in the tissue so that no sparking of the steam envelope occurs. Tissue is desiccated by the heat generated from electrical resistance. Cut or coag modes work equally well, but cut is safer for "downstream" tissues because voltage is lower with cut. Fulguration involves "lightly skimming" the surface with a high voltage coag setting. This generates numerous long sparks to seal a surface. Damage is not deep unless the electrode is firmly embedded in the tissue.

thin areas of your glove. The use of "cut" has also decreased voltages throughout the rest of the anatomy on its way back to the ground pad. If circumstances are right (and this is very difficult to predict), then sparks can form anywhere in the abdomen—such as jumping to bowel and causing an unseen burn. When tissue is well connected over a wide area (such as a pelvic sidewall or the liver itself), then this potential sparking is not such a problem. It shows itself more when structures are lifted or electrically isolated.

This point is made not to say that the use of monopolar is inherently dangerous in the abdomen but only to emphasize that this is a complex and potentially unpredictable process. The high voltage of "coag" could become a tiger if circumstances were right. Why grab a tiger by the tail if you do not need to let him out to begin with?

Another problem with the use of "coag" and associated high voltages is trying to coagulate and desiccate large structures, such as the vessels deep within an infundibular pelvic ligament. As mentioned before, if the electrodes (grasper) were firmly held onto tissue, the desiccation would work well. The problem is that the electrode is frequently not held firmly onto tissue and sparking occurs. Some surgeons even deliberately spark and burn the structure with the "coag" setting, mistakenly thinking that the superficial burned effect is uniformly applied deep within. When such sparking occurs, it electrically isolates the deeper structures. In other words, the superficial burning presents a barrier to the electricity so that deeper structures are preserved—exactly the opposite of what one wanted. The answer is to select the "cut" mode and keep the graspers firmly embedded in tissue. When moving the graspers, first come off the electricity, then regrab and reapply the electricity each time.

Bipolar graspers provide the safest and most controlled method of tissue desiccation. Even

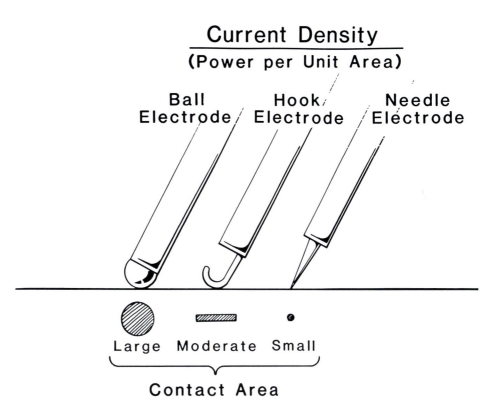

Figure 3-10
At the same power settings, small contact areas produce higher current densities than larger areas. High current densities result in more rapid cutting and tissue vaporization. Too low a current density results in the electrode languishing in and burning tissue. The small surface area of a needle electrode requires less power than a larger hook electrode to cut at the same rate. Too much power causes excessive current densities and can burn out fine wire electrodes like the needle.

though the voltages used with the bipolar are lower than that of monopolar, the "cut" mode should still be used for the reason sited above.

We said in the beginning of this section on electrosurgery that effects were created at the active electrode because the flow of electricity got "bottled up" in this narrow surface contact area. This is the concept of current density and is exactly analogous to power density with lasers. At any given power, the smaller the contact area to which it is confined will produce more intense effects.

Figure 3-10 illustrates how the contact area, and hence current density, might be varied by changing electrodes. The ball electrode presents a relatively large surface area, while the needle electrode presents a very tiny one. A hook is in between.

Since the needle electrode presents a very tiny surface, it can create tremendous current densities. All the electricity is concentrated as it bunches up through the fine tip. This makes it an excellent dissecting and cutting instrument intraabdominally, with very limited lateral effects. Because the tip is so fine, it need not, and should not, be operated at the same power settings as one might with a larger electrode. If you've been using a hook electrode at 50 W, then switch during the case to a needle electrode, the power should also be reduced to prevent burnout of the tip.

Conversely, if you've been cutting just fine with a small electrode, then switch to a larger cutting electrode, the power will probably also have to be increased to compensate for this larger contact area. Otherwise it again languishes and burns in tissue.

We also said in the beginning of this section that the reason a surgical effect was created at the active electrode, and not the dispersive electrode, was that the surface area was very small at the active electrode, resulting in a high current density. The ground pad, or dispersive electrode, dispersed the electricity over a broader area, thereby lowering current density and preventing burns. Some safety problems can occur with this arrangement.

If a grounding pad begins to pull loose from

the patient, it may be left with only a small portion of its original surface contacting the skin. This results in high current densities and can produce very bad burns. Some ESUs have incorporated safety alarms in their units so that if part of a pad pulls loose, a fault will prevent the ESU from operating.

Sometimes electricity can find alternate routes back to ground rather than the intended ground pad. Contact with a portion of metal on the surgical table, or even EKG electrodes, can provide such routes. If the contact area is sufficiently small, and the current that flows is sufficiently high, then a high current density burn can result at these sites. Some manufacturers have incorporated electronic sensing circuits in their units that compares the flow of electricity into and out of the intended two electrodes. If they do not match—because some electricity is leaking to an alternate ground site—then a fault will shut down the unit. Another and sometimes concomitant way of eliminating alternate grounding site burns is to use an isolated power supply for the ESU.[9]

Discussion

Contrary to claims made by some champions of either laser or electrosurgery, these are not mutually exclusive modalities. The choice of when and what high energy modality to use is based largely upon personal preference, after becoming knowledgeable of the true benefits of each device. Those who refer to laser as just an expensive cautery are as wrong as those who say "laser surgery" produces far superior patient results.

The advantages of laser lie in the extreme tissue precision available with various laser devices, when used correctly. This type of precision is not predictable with electrosurgery. Laser fibers are very small—typically from 0.3 to 1.0 mm. This means they can be easily delivered through any port and sometimes inserted even through needle punctures with no need for a separate trocar. The laser fiber can be used for cutting, coagulating, or vaporizing tissue. It is exceptionally convenient to have one tool that does the task of several. It saves time and reduces instrument swapping.

Electrosurgery can provide deep hemostasis in a way in which laser is unable to match. By changing electrodes and settings, it can also provide excellent cutting—so clean in fact that it might bleed too much unless a blend setting is used. An ESU is more readily available than laser and is easier to use for simple applications. By selecting various shaped electrodes—hooks, needles, loops, and so on—an ESU has considerable versatility to fit specific needs.

High energy surgery of any modality can enhance and expand the laparoscopic capabilities of any surgeon.

Bibliography

Absten GT, Joffe SN: *Lasers in Medicine, an Introductory Guide.* London, Chapman and Hall, 1989.

Atkins PW: *The Second Law.* New York, Scientific American Books. Distributed by WH Freeman, 1940.

Driscoll WG, Vaughan W: *Handbook of Optics.* New York, McGraw-Hill, 1978.

Einstein A: Zur quantentheorie der strahlung. *Physiol Z* 18:121–128, 1917.

Fuller TA: *Surgical Lasers: A Clinical Guide.* New York, Macmillan, 1987.

Joffe SN: *Lasers in General Surgery.* Baltimore, Williams & Wilkins, 1988.

Minton JP, Absten GT: Surgical lasers and how they work. *Am Coll Surg Bull* February 1987.

Soderstrom R: Refinements in laparoscopic equipment. *Contemp Obstet/Gynecol* 16:121, 1980.

Soderstrom R: Electrosurgery—Advantages and disadvantages. *Contemp Obstet/Gynecol, Technology* 35, 1991.

US Food and Drug Administration. *Classifications and Guidelines. Subcommittee on Endoscopy.* Federal Register 45:12701, 1980.

---

[9] The technical aspects of isolated power supplies are not addressed here, but this is a way to eliminate stray electrical current going to an alternate ground.

4

Operating Room, Staff, and Administrative Concerns in Laparoscopic Abdominal Surgery

Patricia Hartwig

The introduction of laparoscopic procedures by general surgeons into the conventional operating room has stressed both personnel and resources. Successful integration of these procedures into the operating system calls for an organized team approach.

Unfortunately, most hospital operating rooms and OR staff were not prepared for the demands encountered through these new procedures. This chapter will outline measures that can be implemented to minimize the negative impact and expand on the aspects of these procedures that can enhance an institution.

Credentialing

Credentialing general surgeons to perform laparoscopic procedures poses some difficulty in determining appropriate criteria. Typically, a surgeon will attend a 2-to-3-day laparoscopic course, usually with a hands-on laboratory session, and return to his or her hospital with a desire to begin performing the new laparoscopic procedures as soon as possible. Individual hospitals are left with the task of determining whether the physician should be granted privileges for laparoscopic procedures on the basis of this short, but concentrated, learning session.

Credentialing criteria may vary greatly from institution to institution. An institution may design criteria to inhibit mass implementation of these techniques by their surgeons, while another may opt for a very limited, easily satisfied, list of criteria. There are two basic questions to be answered: (1) What is the appropriate criteria to be met before a surgeon can perform therapeutic video laparoscopy? and (2) What further criteria are warranted in order to perform specific laparoscopic procedures as they are developed?

There are published reviews of these matters, and they mostly deal with the criteria needed to perform laparoscopic cholecystectomy.[1,2] Most suggest that credentialing criteria should

TABLE 4-1 Credentialing Criteria for Therapeutic Video Laparoscopy

A surgeon must
- prove completion of course specific to basic therapeutic video laparoscopic abdominal surgery, including a minimum of 10 h CME hands-on laboratory experience.
- have a physician credentialed in laparoscopy assist him or her on the first 10 cases.
- have the first 20 cases he or she performs be specifically reviewed by quality management.
- alternatively prove that he or she has obtained equivalent training in a residency or equivalent experience at another facility.

TABLE 4-2 Laparoscopic Procedure Specific Credentialing

A surgeon must
- have privileges to perform the procedure in an open incisional manner.
- have privileges to perform therapeutic video laparoscopy.
- perform all "new" procedures under an institutional human research review board (IRB) protocol.

  "New" procedures are not those that are done in a conceptually similar fashion other than using laparoscopic access. Instead, "new" procedures are ones accomplished with a different concept or technique that does not have documented supportive peer review.

indicate the number of contact hours required, including hands-on experience, and the need for a preceptorship to be served with a skilled laparoscopist. The Society of American Gastrointestinal and Endoscopic Surgeons (SAGES) has developed a set of criteria for laparoscopic procedures that calls for training through courses sponsored or recognized by a university or an academic society but does not require participation in a preceptorship.[2]

Because of the emergence of multiple laparoscopic abdominal surgeries, credentialing criteria should not be as procedure specific as they were when the only laparoscopic operation that surgeons were performing was cholecystectomy. Today, appendectomy, inguinal herniorrhaphies, vagotomies, bowel resection, and many other procedures are being performed laparoscopically. To require a specific course for each of these operations is no longer reasonable. Instead, emphasis on credentialing for "therapeutic video laparoscopy" for general surgeons is more appropriate (Table 4-1). It is the technique of laparoscopy that is foreign to the general surgeon. Once laparoscopy is mastered, the ability to translate the technique to other abdominal procedures is not so difficult.

A surgeon who has met the criteria to perform abdominal video therapeutic laparoscopy and who holds privileges to perform a particular procedure in an open setting should then be allowed to do that operation with laparoscopic access. This would hold true only as long as the procedure is done using the same general approach and concept as is used in the open setting (Table 4-2). Appendectomy, cholecystectomy, tumor biopsy, and bowel resection are good examples of this. However, hernia repair and possibly procedures such as posterior truncal vagotomy with anterior seromyotomy are examples of operations done with a new concept and technique quite different from standard open approaches. These procedures may require a higher degree of scrutiny and may more appropriately be done through an institutional human research review board (IRB) protocol.[3] The term *new procedures* is outlined in Table 4-2.

Each institution must struggle with the nuances, acceptability, and community standards for new procedures. An IRB setting is a good arena for these debates with the important common goal of patient safety.

The Team Approach

Laparoscopic general surgery requires the use of a surgical team, expanded beyond what is required for most gynecologic laparoscopy. The operating team should include a surgeon, the operating assistant, an anesthesiologist/anesthetist, 1 to 2 scrub nurses, a circulating nurse, a video specialist, and possibly a laser specialist. In many hospitals, the advanced technical roles of the video specialist and laser specialist are combined in the person of a second circulator, and the role of assistant may be delegated to a second scrub nurse.

In operating rooms with specialized teams, a decision must be made regarding whether to work with the gynecology team, who generally have laparoscopic expertise, or to work with the general surgery team, who may not have laparoscopic experience. Experience suggests that the general surgery team should learn to handle laparoscopic technique. The prior experience of the team members will help determine the amount and type of training needed.

Additional nonsurgical team members should include postanesthesia recovery personnel, postprocedure unit nurses, and home health nurses as needed. These nonsurgical team members need to be aware of the changed postsurgical care requirements of this group of patients. Patients may be discharged directly from the postanesthesia care unit to home or may spend several hours or days on a postsurgery care unit. On occasion, patients may be sent home under the care of a home health nurse or technician.[4]

Team Training

Before performing laparoscopic general surgery procedures clinically, the team should practice in a lab setting or in a mock-up of the operating suite to allow all team members an opportunity to learn their roles. The ideal laboratory situation would allow the use of animal models, on several occasions, until the team is comfortable with its new responsibilities. If appropriate animal models are not available, a laparoscopic training device may be used to simulate the human abdomen (Fig. 4-1).

All equipment to be used in the surgical procedure should be brought into the surgical suite and arranged in a manner to allow ease of movement throughout the room and to provide adequate visualization of the video monitors.

The circulators should be comfortable with the set-up and operation of the camera, light sources, video monitors, insufflators, and laparoscopic equipment. If a laser is to be used, an additional nurse or technician should be provided to operate the laser equipment.

Because the scrub nurse/tech may be required to hold instruments or manipulate the camera during the procedure, in addition to

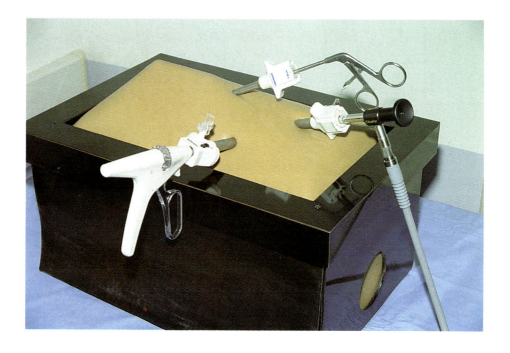

Figure 4-1
A laparoscopic abdominal trainer with a simulated costal margin and rubber surface that can be repeatedly punctured.

Part One Basic Considerations

regular scrub nurse/tech responsibilities, laboratory practice time should be provided to allow practice of these new roles. Opportunities to assemble and use the new disposable instruments and staplers should be provided.

For those individuals taking on expanded or advanced nursing roles, such as the role of a surgical assistant or laser specialist, documentation of the training provided is essential.

Nurses involved in the care of the patients after surgery should be provided with information regarding the new approach to general surgery and the changed post-op presentation of the patient as compared with that of the conventional surgery patient.

Room Set-Up

Because of the large amount of equipment required to support laparoscopic procedures, finding a functional arrangement may be difficult (Figs. 4-2 and 4-3).

Because it is important that both the primary surgeon and the assistant be able to view the monitors, many room arrangements have two monitors placed at each side of the patient's head. A second option is to mount one video monitor above the patient's head. Unfortunately, the anesthesiologist or anesthetist may object to this arrangement because the monitor may inhibit access to the patient in the event

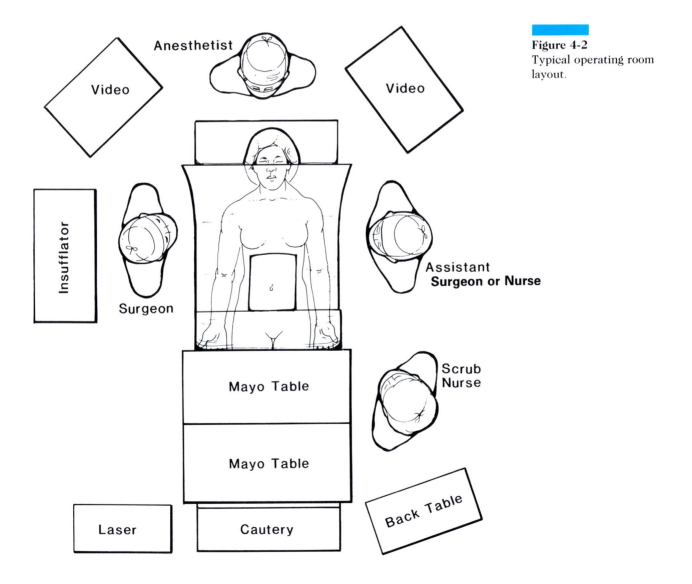

Figure 4-2
Typical operating room layout.

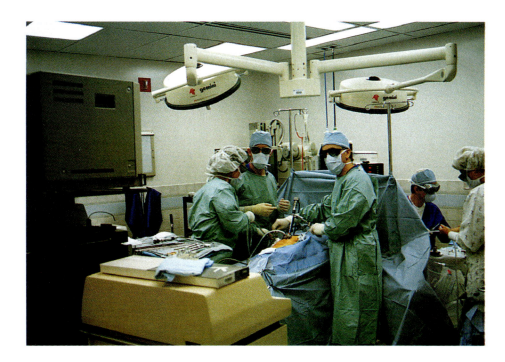

Figure 4-3
Operating room scene during laparoscopic abdominal surgery.

of an emergency. For procedures on groin or pelvic organs, a monitor placed at the foot of the operating table is necessary.

Because of the large amount of laparoscopic instrumentation required for these procedures, and because the scrub nurse may be called upon to maintain the position of an instrument or the camera, two mayo stands may be needed to allow the physician access to the instrumentation.

All other supporting equipment, such as the insufflator, suction, cautery, and laser, should be positioned around the table in a manner to allow the circulators access to the equipment and provide a comfortable working space for those at the operating table.

Instrumentation Issues

Initially, the new laparoscopic procedures were done with laparoscopic equipment purchased mainly for gynecologic use. Hospitals soon found that the stress placed on the equipment by handling heavier tissues and the programmatic stress of trying to schedule use of the equipment by an additional, new set of physicians indicated a need to purchase additional laparoscopic sets.

A complete laparoscopic equipment set including laparoscopic instruments, camera/video set-up, and insufflator will cost approximately $54,000.00. If a laser is purchased, the capital expense may exceed $136,000.00 (1992 prices).

Because laparoscopic general surgery procedures called for placement of trocars and instrumentation in nontraditional sites, surgeons became concerned about the sharpness of existing, reusable trocars and the possibility of inadvertent puncture of intraabdominal structures. The need to grasp heavy tissues for long periods of time called for heavier, sturdier instrumentation than usually supplied in gynecology sets. Although laparoscopic suturing materials were already in use by gynecologists, general surgeons preferred to use staplers.

The manufacturers responded rapidly to these demands by working with physicians to develop and market new laparoscopic equipment, including disposable trocars, disposable and reusable laparoscopic staplers, and specialty instrumentation. Some manufacturers are now marketing completely disposable laparoscopic sets.

When a disposable Verres needle, 4 disposable trocars, and 1 disposable stapler are used in a given procedure, the patient charge is approximately $800.00 more than if no disposable equipment is used.

The disposable equipment is attractive in that the trocars are sharp and made with a retractable, protective shield to decrease the possibility of puncture of intraabdominal structures and are not dependent upon the "human element" to sharpen the instrument between uses. The use of disposable staplers may aid in decreasing the operative time.

Hospitals and physicians must weigh these advantages against the increased cost of disposable equipment and the ecological issues of how and where to dispose of the used equipment.

Economic Issues

Initially, many hospitals assumed that laparoscopic surgical approaches would decrease the cost of treatment to the patient, mainly through decreasing operating time and by sending the patient home the day following surgery or possibly the day of surgery.

Early analysis of patient accounts showed that the cost to the patient generally did not decrease but in many cases increased substantially. This increase was partially due to the equipment used in the procedure but also reflected the increased operative time required to complete the procedure. Even though the postsurgical patient stayed only one night in the hospital, the charge for a one-night hospital stay is small as compared with the charges incurred in the operating suite (Table 4-3).

In many of the early procedures, extra scrub and circulating personnel were requested to assist with the procedures, which also drove up costs.

As surgeons became more proficient and the operating room personnel became more efficient, operating times began to decrease and fewer personnel were required to complete necessary procedures, resulting in reduced charges

TABLE 4-3 Hospital Charges*

Operating room time	40%
OR supplies	20%
Laser supplies	20%
Anesthesia	15%
Room charge recovery	5%

* Modified from Abbott Northwestern Hospital, 1992.

to the patient. However, the mix of charges has remained relatively stable throughout our experience.

Quality Management

The introduction of the new laparoscopic general surgery procedures calls for surveillance through a comprehensive quality management plan. Initially, the surveillance criteria established by an institutional review board (IRB) will serve as the quality management criteria. Once the procedure moves into unrestricted clinical practice, procedural quality should be monitored through the quality management plan for the department of surgery.

Although there are important aspects to monitor within the clinical procedure itself, the measurement of outcomes is just as important in assessing the total quality of the procedure. The hospital, in partnership with the surgeons, should compile and study this data, to determine the effectiveness of not just the procedure but of the systems supporting the procedure.

Marketing

As with most new techniques and technologies, the temptation to market laparoscopic procedures is present. Several marketing strategies have proven successful, including direct mailings to prospective patients, billboards, television and newspaper advertisements, and physician presentations on radio and television talk shows.

While advertising through paid advertisements on television, radio, or in newspapers may create interest, the population seeing and responding to these types of marketing is generally small and unpredictable. Physician presentations on radio and television talk shows, while usually free of charge to the physician or hospital, have somewhat better but short-lived results.

A proven, low-cost marketing strategy is to ask a recent patient with an interesting personal history if he or she would allow placement of a story in the patient's local newspaper. The article could detail the benefits realized by the patient through the procedure. This is an exceptionally good method of marketing, which can give a very honest and accurate description of the procedure.

The payers must not be ignored when developing a marketing plan. A proactive approach to educating the payers may allow for earlier acceptance of the laparoscopic approach in many general surgeries (see Chap. 25).

Many of these new procedures are "patient driven," and as the public becomes better educated regarding treatment options, it tends to "shop" for physicians who are able to provide the latest technology and techniques. This public can be very disappointed if the outcome isn't what was expected. Thus, it is most important that a true picture of these procedures is presented no matter what the medium.

A formal marketing plan should be developed to take into consideration all possible approaches.[5] In this regard it is of major importance to understand that quality care will result in pleased patients who will be the best marketing tool available.

Discussion

An accurate claim can be made that patients undergoing laparoscopic procedures by experienced surgeons in quality facilities will benefit by a decreased recovery time and a faster return to normal levels of activity. For inexperienced surgeons and hospitals to reach and maintain this ideal, it is essential that an organized approach be planned and followed by the entire operating room team when establishing these procedures clinically.

Surgeons must receive adequate training, and hospitals must develop and enforce credentialing standards and safety policies. The entire preoperative, intraoperative, and postoperative nursing staff and ancillary personnel must be included in educational efforts.

Hospitals should invest adequate capital funds to allow for purchase of the appropriate instrumentation, video equipment, and facilities to allow for efficient performance of these procedures. Also, the implementation of a cooperative quality management plan including outcomes measurements is essential to provide safe patient care and to determine the efficacy of the procedure.

A well organized quality program in minimally invasive surgery will soon develop a local and regional image of being the source for superior health care. This is an image that must be earned.

References

1. Hartwig PA: Overview of the administration of laser safety controls. *Laser Nursing* 5(2):59–62, 1991.
2. Society of American Gastrointestinal Endoscopic Surgeons, Guidelines for Granting of Privileges for Laparoscopic General Surgery, January 1992.
3. Easter DW, Moosa AR: Laser and laparoscopic cholecystectomy: a hazardous union? *Arch Surg* 126(9):423, 1991.
4. Bellinger K, Smit LA: *J Post Anesthes Nurs* 6(5):309–310, 1991.
5. Ball KA (ed): *Lasers: The Perioperative Challenge.* St. Louis, Mosby, 1991, pp 218–230.

5

Preoperative Patient Education

W. Jean Reavis

A patient who is confronted with the need for surgery may have a number of concerns and anxieties. The patient not only dreads the likelihood of pain and discomfort, but there are also other concerns, such as cost, safety, and effectiveness of the surgery. With the emergence of an alternative to the conventional way of removing a gallbladder or repairing a hernia, the patient has the choice of a newer technique that holds the prospect of less pain or inconvenience. The patient will want to know two things right away: Is the newer technique safe, and will his or her insurance cover the costs? We have developed a system for educating our patients and making sure these concerns are met.

Much of the preoperative information is addressed when our patients make the initial call to our office to find out about the "new" procedure. Often the first question asked is whether insurance companies are covering the costs. For this information I refer the patients back to their insurance companies to find out if their company covers the procedure they require. Some companies will require the patient to cover a preset percentage of the bill or have a substantial deductible to be met. In these situations the patient will want to know what their "out of pocket" expense will be. In some cases, the deductible and percentage not covered by insurance may still be too much for the patient to pay. This is especially true if the patient has to go to a hospital that is not in his or her insurance provider network.

Time is needed to deal with the insurance question because the technique of surgery scheduled depends upon what the carrier will cover. Although the patient has the option of personally paying for a procedure, hospital charges and physician fees are a considerable expense and may have to be avoided by having the procedure done in the traditional manner.

Other issues that patients want addressed during the initial phone conversation are: (1) admission status, (2) type of anesthesia, (3) length of operation, (4) length of stay, and (5) length of time until they can resume their activities.

The patients need to know if they are going to be admitted overnight or go home the same day so that they can make appropriate arrangements. Many patients are concerned about a general anesthetic and are reassured to know that they will have a consultation with the anesthesiologist before the surgery. Family and friends will want to know the approximate length of the procedure and how long the patient will likely need to stay in the hospital. Finally, all patients want to know about how long they will be "laid up." The length of time away from family or work is crucial information because patients often wish to return as quickly as possible to avoid loss of wages or vacation time. Although senior citizens may be retired, they are very concerned about returning to their daily activities.

The patients are scheduled for a 30 to 45 min consultation with the doctor, and, before the consultation, the patient is offered the opportunity to watch a video pertaining to the specific surgical procedure. This video is about 10 min in length, and it is very helpful in educating the patient as to what will happen during the procedure. Also, the video is helpful to the doctor during the consultation visit because the patient can understand the surgery better. This usually produces a very healthy conversation (Fig. 5–1). Because the availability of the video is mentioned during our phone conversation, those patients who are too squeamish to watch the video themselves often bring a friend or relative along who will watch for them.

At the time of the consultation, the patients are examined and there are five major topics discussed: (1) documentation of medical history, (2) review of pertinent data (patients are asked to bring any ultrasounds, x-rays, or lab data they have had pertaining to this problem), (3) indications for surgery, (4) risks of the proposed surgery, and (5) potential benefits of the laparoscopic approach. A specific effort is made to explain the possible complications of the surgery especially if the procedure is considered investigational.

After the doctor and patient decide upon the laparoscopic procedure, the patient comes to the scheduling nurse to determine a surgery date, to get on the surgery schedule, and to receive necessary information regarding surgery requirements. To accomplish this, we have several forms we fill out to give to our patients. These forms are used to tell the patient whether they are going to be admitted or come home the same day. They also provide information such as date and time of surgery, arrival time at facility where surgery is being done, eating

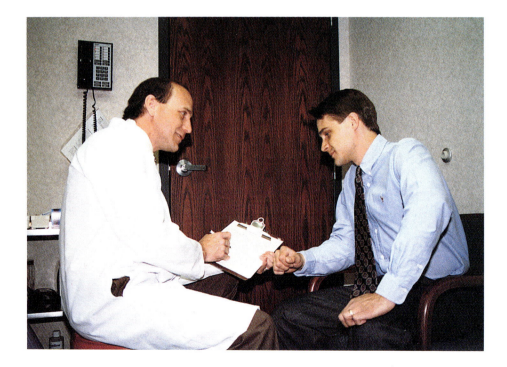

Figure 5-1
The doctor confers with his patient.

instructions and any other presurgery preps required, the need for someone to provide a ride home, and any other instructions the surgical facility may require. This is written information that has already been discussed verbally.

The concept of "informed consent" is important but difficult to define. To document the fact that the patient has been given in-depth information regarding the surgery, including possible risks, complications, or failure to meet expectations, we provide them an "informed consent" form to review. This includes all information that has been reviewed verbally. We ask our patients to sign and date this form, and it becomes part of the patient's chart. If the patient understands and accepts the procedure, the patient is offered a copy of the form for his or her records. The patient understands that this form is independent of the surgical consent form, which is signed at the surgical facility the day of the procedure.

We also provide the patient with a history and physical form to be taken to the primary care/referring physician to be filled out. It is a basic form, and how extensive the physical and lab workup will be usually depends upon the patient's medical history. This information can be faxed or called in to the surgical facility or directly to our office. The history and physical and lab workup is usually required within 5 days or less of surgery depending on the patient's medical history. After the patient is scheduled for surgery, the referring physician is called to inform him or her of the date of surgery and need for a preoperative history and physical examination.

Reprints of articles detailing the different laparoscopic procedures are available to our patients to take home and share with their friends and families. Often it is necessary to educate the family as well as the patient for their peace of mind. Finally, we assure the patient we will certify the procedure with their insurance company if required.

On occasion, a patient will ask to talk with another patient who has already had the same procedure that they are about to experience. This should be encouraged, but it is necessary to find previous patients who would offer their names and telephone numbers as contact people. Patient to patient discussion has proven very beneficial.

The time spent addressing these issues and concerns has resulted in excellent patient-physician relationships. The patient has a better understanding of what to expect and can realistically plan for the surgery.

References

1. Reavis WJ, Schultz LS: Laser laparoscopic cholecystectomy: Initial patient contact (abstract). *Lasers Surg Med* (supplement) 3:24, 1991.

6

Anesthetic Considerations in Laparoscopic Abdominal Surgery

Jonathan T. Gudman
David A. Plut

Laparoscopic surgery has been performed since the early 1950s. Initially, most surgical procedures consisted of simple lower abdominal operations or other relatively short procedures. Most of the anesthesia literature involves short gynecological procedures on healthy young patients. The proliferation of laparoscopic surgical techniques has placed increased demands upon the knowledge and skill of the "laparoscopic anesthesiologist."

The absolute number of laparoscopic surgeons and procedures has increased dramatically, raising the number of potential complications unique to this technique. The desire to perform these procedures in an outpatient setting to some extent dictates the anesthetic technique and places increased scrutiny on side effects such as nausea and vomiting. The adaptation of laparoscopic techniques to longer and more complicated procedures and their use in older and potentially sicker patients and in emergency situations have increased the importance of the unique physiologic stresses of laparoscopic techniques. This chapter attempts to discuss some of these issues from the anesthesiologist's point of view.

Anesthetic Techniques

Laparoscopic surgery has been performed under local, regional, and general anesthesia. The variety of surgical procedures performed, however, places different demands upon the technique chosen.

The literature is replete with reports of gynecological laparoscopic operations performed under local anesthesia. These are simple operations of limited duration usually done on young, healthy, motivated patients.

Laparoscopic procedures of the lower abdomen have also been performed under epidural anesthesia. This has been shown to be a viable alternative to a general anesthetic with no associated ventilatory depression.[3] This is also an alternative for laparoscopic procedures of the upper abdomen, including cholecystectomies. A case has been reported of a cholecystectomy in a patient with a history of cystic fibrosis. An epidural provided excellent anesthesia for this procedure.[5]

At our institution, general anesthesia with endotracheal intubation and mechanical ventilation is the technique of choice. Although intubation has not been advocated by all authors,[17] protection of the airway and control of ventilation without gastric distension provide adequate justification in our opinion. In addition, intubation allows the use of muscle relaxants and has been advocated to allow better insufflation of the abdomen with reduced carbon dioxide pressure. The use of lower pressures could lessen the chance for subcutaneous emphysema, pneumothorax, and gas embolism, which are complications discussed later in this chapter.

As with most general anesthetics, numerous induction and maintenance techniques have been suggested for laparoscopic procedures. Propofol, a new anesthetic induction agent, has been associated with a lower incidence of postoperative nausea. However, there are not currently sufficient studies on the use of propofol to show a statistical significance whether or not it is used as an induction agent, as well as a continuous infusion agent, throughout the procedure.[16] A propofol induction followed by maintenance with the inhalation agent isoflurane has been shown to provide a more stable anesthetic technique.[4] The use of nitrous oxide as an anesthetic agent in laparoscopic procedures is controversial. There are studies that have shown an increase, as well as no difference, in the incidence of postoperative nausea and vomiting with the use of nitrous oxide.[6,7]

Regardless of the anesthetic technique used, vigilance is very important. Despite the fact that laparoscopic surgery has smaller incisions and is less invasive to the patient, there are significant physiologic effects that need to be considered. These can be divided into three categories: cardiovascular, pulmonary, and gastrointestinal effects.

Cardiovascular Effects

Bradycardia from positioning or visceral traction is not uncommon. Sudden cardiovascular collapse has been attributed to severe atypical vagal reactions.[2] Tachycardia can result from inadequate anesthesia, hypovolemia, the reverse Trendelenburg position, and carbon dioxide absorption resulting in hypercarbia.

Circulatory impairment can be produced by a decrease in venous return. In laparoscopic surgery, this is primarily caused by the insufflation of the abdomen with carbon dioxide, producing an increased pressure on the intraabdominal vessels. The use of the reverse Trendelenburg head-up position that is required to move the abdominal contents down in upper abdominal procedures will also cause a decrease in venous return by a gravitational pooling of blood in the lower extremities.[11]

The increase in the tidal volume that is required to compensate for the carbon dioxide absorption from the abdomen produces an increase in the mean pulmonary artery wedge pressure. This can lead to a significant, though tolerable, decrease in stroke volume and cardiac output.[1] If there is no compensatory increase in tidal volume, the hypercarbia that occurs could increase cardiac rate and contractility by its cardiovascular sympathetic effects.

The risk of a carbon dioxide embolism into the venous system should always be considered in the differential diagnosis of cardiovascular collapse in the intraoperative and immediate postoperative period. Other sequelae of a carbon dioxide embolism include noncardiogenic pulmonary edema and neurologic complications from either anoxia or cerebral embolization.

Venous gas embolism can occur whenever the pressure in an open vein is less than the surrounding pressure. In the case of laparoscopic surgery, it can occur whenever the pressure in the vein or the central venous pressure is less than the surrounding abdominal insufflation pressure. If a venous gas embolism occurs, the volume, rate of entrainment, and cardiopulmonary compensatory capacity can influence the outcome. Small amounts entrained at a slow rate usually cause minimal physiologic changes. Larger amounts can produce hypoxemia due to low ventilation perfusion ratios, pulmonary hypertension from gas pulmonary embolization, and mechanical obstruction in the outflow of the right ventricle. Cardiogenic shock can rapidly ensue from right ventricular failure.[19] Treatment includes ventilating with 100% oxygen, trying to prevent further gas entrainment at the surgical site by immediate release of the pneumoperitoneum, and inserting a central venous catheter to try to aspirate any air if possible.

Fortunately, the incidence of venous gas embolism is low. We do not routinely monitor by precordial Doppler or place central venous catheters in these patients. Since the gas embolism is carbon dioxide, the fall in end tidal carbon dioxide may not be dramatic enough to alert the anesthesiologist. Vigilance is critical in this life-threatening complication. As with other etiologies of gas embolism, hyperbaric oxygen has been used in carbon dioxide embolism from laparoscopy.[12]

The video screen allows the anesthesiologist an excellent view of the operative field. Now bleeding can be observed directly by all members of the operative team rather than having the team wait for comments by the surgeon or for the sound of excessive suctioning. The magnification of the camera can make it difficult to assess the amount of blood loss in the operative field. Massive bleeding can occur, requiring open laparotomy, if the trocar pierces any abdominal vessels. The possibility of bleeding into the abdominal wall from a subcostal trocar puncture wound is also of concern. In one patient, this required a transfusion of 3 units of blood. The bleeding, however, stopped spontaneously.[13]

Pulmonary Effects

All laparoscopic procedures are similar regarding the consequences of carbon dioxide insufflation. This in itself can produce pulmonary ateletcasis, a decrease in the functional residual capacity of the lungs, and cause high peak airway pressures. The absorption of carbon dioxide, a highly diffusible gas, through the peritoneum can also cause hypercarbia in the absence of compensatory hyperventilation. Consequently, the continuous monitoring of the end tidal carbon dioxide concentration is necessary throughout the procedure. Controlling hypercarbia requires an increase in the minute ventilation.[10] If the hypercarbia is not controlled, an increased risk of cardiac arrhythmias can result. This effect has been shown to be lessened with the use of isoflurane.[11]

Complications that may occur associated with insufflation of the abdomen with gas are rare, but as more procedures are performed, the incidence will tend to rise. The primary complications may present as subcutaneous emphysema, pneumothorax, or pneumomediastinum. Patients may present with crepitance into the chest, shoulders, and neck with subcutaneous emphysema or with respiratory distress if a pneumothorax develops. A chest x-ray should be obtained on all of these patients. Arterial blood gas analysis may also be helpful to determine if hypercarbia is present.

We have experienced several cases of subcutaneous emphysema that resulted in increased end tidal carbon dioxide concentrations. Increasing the minute ventilation to maintain control of high carbon dioxide levels was required. If the subcutaneous carbon dioxide extends into the neck, then the patient should remain intubated until there is no evidence of airway compromise. Mechanical ventilation will also help normalize the hypercarbia and acidosis that may develop. In our cases, the subcutaneous emphysema resolved rapidly with little crepitance noticeable upon leaving the postanesthesia care unit.

The most common cause of these complications is related to the improper placement of the insufflating needle and high insufflating pressures. The development of a tension pneumothorax is of major concern in this situation. If significant respiratory distress develops, it should be treated as soon as possible by a needle or tube thoracostomy.[9]

Gastrointestinal Effects

Most authorities have recommended that patients undergoing any laparoscopic procedure be intubated with ventilation controlled.[14] Intubation should be considered mandatory if the patient is to be in excessive Trendelenburg position, more than 5 to 10°, or if intraabdominal filling pressures exceeding 15 to 20 mmHg are used. Intubation and airway control will help prevent the potential of acid aspiration. However, the adaptive mechanism of the lower esophageal sphincter causes an equal rise in the pressure of the sphincter as the intraperitoneal pressure is increased, resulting in no change in the pressure gradient.[8] The pressures were measured in patients without a gastric tube that may act as a wick for gastric contents. A nasogastric or orogastric tube should be placed prior to the insufflation of the abdomen in order to decompress the stomach and decrease the risk of puncturing the viscera with the placement of the trocar. With an increase in the intraabdominal pressure from the insufflation, the gastric tube left on low suction will decrease the possibility of passive reflux during the procedure. Decompression of the stomach also allows for better visualization of the right upper quadrant when cholecystectomies are performed. The tube can be removed at the end of the procedure.

Most of the effects that are observed are well compensated in otherwise healthy patients. As more patients being seen for laparoscopic procedures are older and sicker, they may not be able to do as well. Patients that have significant cardiac and pulmonary disease do not handle the increase in carbon dioxide clearance as do healthy patients.[18] These patients would require closer monitoring and management to be certain of a good result.

Pain Control

Patients often complain of pain following laparoscopic surgeries. A common complaint of patients is pain in the shoulders or between the shoulder blades. This is due to referred pain from irritation of the diaphragm from the pneumoperitoneum. The usual treatment has been with opioids, which may cause further nausea and vomiting following surgery. Nonsteroidal antiinflammatory medications such as ibuprofen PO prior to surgery have been shown to be useful in providing postoperative analgesia.[15] Ketorolac IM may also provide similar analgesia. Injection of the local anesthetic bupivicaine around the puncture sites is helpful to reduce pain in the immediate postoperative period.

Discussion

The sudden emergence of laparoscopic abdominal surgery for upper abdominal procedures by general surgeons has challenged the anesthesiologist to adapt many of the standard anesthetic choices. As more laparoscopic procedures are performed and seen as routine, the demand for outpatient care will also increase. The literature on outpatient anesthesia is growing and will surely be applicable to this surgical technique. Newer inhalation anesthetics will allow for a more rapid induction and recovery from anesthesia due to their low blood solubility. Shorter acting muscle relaxants may also help as the procedures become quicker. New problems have accompanied the new techniques. As each problem is identified, it is solved in turn. This joining of efforts from different disciplines has resulted in a remarkable improvement in the character of abdominal surgical procedures.

References

1. Andel H et al: Cardiopulmonary effects of laparoscopic cholecystectomy. *Anesth Analg* 74(2S):S8, 1992.
2. Brantly JC, Riley PM: Cardiovascular collapse during laparoscopy: A report of two cases. *Am J Obstet Gynecol* 159:735–737, 1988.
3. Ciofolo MJ et al: Ventilatory effects of laparoscopy under epidural anesthesia. *Anesth Analg* 70:357–361, 1990.
4. deGrood PM et al: Anaesthesia for laparoscopy. *Anaesthesia* 42(8):815–823, 1987.

5. Edelman DS: Laparscopic cholecystectomy under continuous epidural anesthesia in patients with cystic fibrosis. *Am J Dis Child* 145(7):723–724, 1991.

6. Felts JA, Poler SM, Spitznagel EL: Nitrous oxide, nausea, and vomiting after outpatient gynecologic surgery. *J Clin Anesth* 2(3):168–171, 1990.

7. Hovorka J, Korttila K, Erkola O: Nitrous oxide does not increase nausea and vomiting following gynecological laparoscopy. *Can J Anaesth* 36(2):145–148, 1989.

8. Jones MJ, Mitchell RW, Hindocha N: Effect of increased intraabdominal pressure during laparoscopy on the lower esophageal sphincter. *Anesth Analg* 68:63–65, 1989.

9. Kent RB: Subcutaneous emphysema and hypercarbia following laparoscopic cholecystectomy. *Arch Surg* 126:1154–1156, 1991.

10. Liu SY et al: Prospective analysis of cardiopulmonary responses to laparoscopic cholecystectomy. *J Laparoendosc Surg* 1(5):241–246, 1991.

11. Marco AP, Yeo CJ, Rock P: Anesthesia for the patient undergoing laparoscopic cholecystectomy. *Anesthesiology* 73:1268–1270, 1990.

12. McGrath BJ et al: Carbon dioxide embolism treated with hyperbaric oxygen. *Can J Anaesth* 36(5):586–589, 1989.

13. Meador JH, Nowzaradan Y, Matzelle W: Laparoscopic cholecystectomy: Report of 82 cases. *South Med J* 84(2):186–189, 1991.

14. Roberts CJ, Goodman NW: Gastro-oesophageal reflux during elective laparoscopy. *Anaesthesia* 45(12):1009–1011, 1990.

15. Rosenblum M et al: Ibuprofen provides longer lasting analgesia then fentanyl after laparoscopic surgery. *Anesth Analg* 73:255–259, 1991.

16. Stanton JM: Anesthesia for laparoscopic cholecystectomy. *Anaesthesia* 46(4):317, 1991.

17. Natof HT: Complications, in Wetchler BV (ed): *Anesthesia for Ambulatory Surgery*. Philadelphia, Lippincott, 1985, p 348.

18. Wittgen CM, Andrus CH, Fitzgerald SD: Analysis of hemodynamic and ventilatory effects of laparoscopic cholecystectomy. *Arch Surg* 126:997–1001, 1991.

19. Yacoub OF et al: Carbon dioxide embolism during laparoscopy. *Anesthesiology* 57:533–535, 1982.

7

Complications of Laparoscopy

Edward M. Beadle

Introduction

Operative laparoscopy has proliferated almost exponentially in the last 10 years. Gynecology and now general surgery and urology have extended the technique to replace major open procedures. The trade-off for this advanced technology may be complications that are due to limited visualization, delayed thermal effects of cautery and lasers, and the systemic effects of pneumoperitoneum.

Complications may be early or delayed. Early complications during the procedure can be corrected if recognized via laparoscopy or laparotomy. Delayed complications can be divided into those that occur shortly after the procedure such as bleeding or late complications such as bowel injury or infection.

The mortality rates for laparoscopic gynecologic procedures are very low with most series reporting less than 0.1 percent.[1,3,5] A compilation of 145,000 gynecologic procedures demonstrated a rate of 0.01 percent. There is a very low rate of cardiovascular complications; however, statistics for older persons undergoing gastrointestinal procedures may be significantly higher.

The incidence of morbidity (Table 7-1) ranges from 2 to 5 percent for minor to major complications.

Complications are frequently related to operator training or experience.[6,7] Adequate training encompasses basic information with respect to equipment and techniques, observation of a teaching surgeon, and preceptorship with an experienced surgeon.

Video review of previous cases as well as intraoperative monitoring allows teacher and student to see the same field simultaneously. Even with observation most complications occur in early basic procedures. The complication rate is highest in the first 100 procedures and decreases remarkably after 200 cases. Experience should be continuous to ensure developing good repetitive safe habits and build experience with each clinical procedure.

A basic tenet of surgery is *primum non nocere* (first do no harm). Failure to complete a procedure laparoscopically should not be considered a complication. Good surgical judgment and an appreciation of the limitations of the equipment, procedure, and surgeon are the basics for the making of a good surgical endoscopist.

TABLE 7-1 Incidence of Laparoscopic Complications

Complications	Rate
1. Pneumoperitoneum	0.7%
2. Bleeding	0.6%
3. Perforating Injuries	0.4%
4. Infection	0.1%
5. Intestinal Injury	0.05%
6. Cardiac Arrest	0.03%

Source Modified from J. Phillips, AAGL Proceedings.[2]

TABLE 7-2 Absolute Contraindications to Laparoscopy

1. Hypovolemic shock.
2. Intestinal obstruction with extensive bowel distension.
3. Large pelvic or abdominal mass.
4. Severe cardiac decompensation.

Physiology of Laparoscopy

The performance of laparoscopy has profound effects on hemodynamics and respiration but is well tolerated in healthy young patients. Emergent, older, or acutely medically impaired patients may not tolerate changes as well.

Hemodynamically, postural changes as well as the pressures of pneumoperitoneum decrease stroke volume and cardiac output through decreased venous return.[10] If adequate preload is available, these effects are not profound. The induction of anesthesia is well recognized to cause arrhythmias, but most are felt to be benign extrasystoles.[11]

Postural changes and pneumoperitoneum effect elevates the diaphragm decreasing vital capacity. Muscle relaxants allow "ballooning out" of the abdomen to lessen the pressure. Oxygen and CO_2 homeostasis can be managed easily by the anesthesia staff.[12]

The choice of anesthetic is limited to general anesthesia for all these reasons. There are reports of laparoscopy under local anesthesia, but the procedures are short and essentially uncomplicated. Endotracheal intubation and muscle relaxation are mandatory for positioning and adequate intraabdominal visualization as part of advanced endoscopy procedures.

Contraindications

Perhaps more significant than the myriad of indications for surgical endoscopy are the contraindications. They may be broken down to absolute (Table 7-2) and relative (Table 7-3) contraindications. Time and experience have altered the list with some absolute contraindications now considered relative or even indications for certain procedures.

Hypovolemic shock is an absolute contraindication due to unstable blood pressure or poor preload. Patients with this condition cannot tolerate the hemodynamic stresses of positioning or insufflation. Intraabdominal bleeding may be evacuated by the experienced surgeon, but the origin of bleeding may be difficult to identify and remedy laparoscopically.

Intestinal obstruction with marked bowel distension presents a prohibitive risk of perforation as well as minimal potential for visualization.

The presence of a large pelvic or abdominal mass at or above the umbilicus is contraindicated because of poor visualization and possible eruption of the mass prior to pathologic identification.

Severe cardiac decompensation is also a contraindication because insufflation and positioning may throw the decompensated heart into irreversible arrhythmia and failure.

Septic peritonitis and the presence of an intraabdominal abscess were previously felt to be absolute contraindications due to the risk of perforating dilated bowel or spreading infection systemically. It is now commonplace to perform laparoscopy to confirm and treat the diagnosis of pelvic inflammatory disease with debridement and lavage of large abscesses. This same concept is being extended to the treatment of the ruptured appendix with appendiceal abscess.[8]

Multiple previous surgical procedures still present risks of perforation of an adherent loop

Chapter 7 Complications of Laparoscopy

TABLE 7-3 Relative Contraindications to Laparoscopy

1. Septic peritonitis.
2. Multiple previous surgical procedures.
3. Obesity.
4. Diaphragmatic hernia.
5. Chronic pulmonary disease.
6. Intolerance to positioning.

of bowel. Preoperative bowel preparation and the use of new disposable external obturator sheaths and trocars will minimize these risks.

Obesity, diaphragmatic hernia, and chronic pulmonary disease do not absolutely preclude laparoscopy but require extra consideration by the surgeon and anesthesiologists prior to performing.

Intolerance to positioning due to neurologic, cardiac, or ophthalmologic disease may preclude adequate visualization necessary in operative laparoscopy.

Equipment Failure

Proper visualization with adequate mobilization of internal organs is vital for proper performance of operative laparoscopy. It is incumbent upon the surgeon to review all of his or her equipment prior to initiation of a procedure. Endoscopy units should have adequate duplication of equipment to prevent any procedure from being terminated because of lack of secondary equipment. Telescopes and light cables should be periodically inspected for common mishandling, disrupting lenses, or fracturing fiberoptic cables.

The insufflator is the ongoing monitor of pneumoperitoneum in that the gauges show gas available, amount of gas insufflated, and intraabdominal pressure. The Verres needle and line should be tested prior to insertion and again when placed into the peritoneal cavity. Differential pressure should be less than 10 mmHg. For operative endoscopy, new electronically controlled insufflators are preferable to the older devices because much larger volumes are being used as a result of smoke evacuation and length of procedure. These new fast fill, high flow rate insufflators have changed simple laparoscopy and offer greater safety in that they have pressure governors to prevent overinflation.

The Verres needle must be sharp and have good spring action of the internal obturator. If improperly cleaned, the Verres needle can cause injury to internal organs on placement. The disposable needles available have the advantage of sharpness due to single use, as well as adequate spring-loaded obturators.

The placement of the trocar and sleeve through the umbilicus is the most critical moment of laparoscopy because of potential laceration of internal organs and blood vessels. There have been recent reports extolling the safety of direct trocar placement prior to formation of a pneumoperitoneum. Placement of large trocars prior to formation of a potential space can be hazardous, and this procedure should be attempted only by very experienced laparoscopists.

The trocar should be recently sharpened to prevent undue resistance to placement. It should be held firmly to prevent backsliding into the sheath during insertion through the fascia. The spring-loaded valve must function smoothly and quickly to prevent gas loss when changing laparoscopes.

The new disposable trocars and sheaths have the advantage of spring-loaded external obturator sheaths and single-use sharpness (Fig. 7-1). They have adapters that allow different size instruments and flap valves so that they can be used with one hand. One negative is the cost per unit that may preclude the use of multiple trocars in an era of cost containment in medicine.

Unipolar and bipolar electrogenerators are available in many forceps and needle configurations. Unipolar current must return to the ground electrode through the entire body, thereby risking arcing to unwanted structures if the route was more direct. By contrast, the bipolar system develops current only between the jaws of the forceps. This offers much greater safety due to lower voltage and decreased surrounding thermal damage to tissue.

All equipment must be compatible because

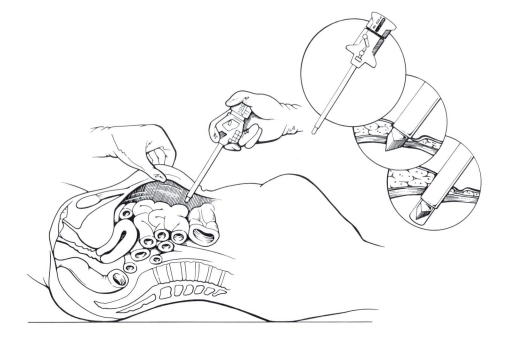

Figure 7-1
Disposable trocar and sheath with spring-loaded safety shields.

many instruments and generators come from various companies. All insulated surfaces should be inspected prior to each case to minimize inadvertent burns. Electrocautery malfunction is most likely due to poor cable connection or operator error.

Visualization has been stressed as a key to advanced laparoscopy. It also allows the surgeons and assistants to monitor procedures rather than blindly stand by throughout the case. The same principles of equipment inspection and maintenance are paramount in this highly technical phase of surgery.

The complexity of lasers has mandated separate teams of technicians to monitor their use. Laser safety is very important to any advanced endoscopic application. The free beam of light that performs many miraculous procedures may just as easily stray to other tissues if delivered by faulty equipment.

Procedure Failure

Procedure failure is most likely related to the inability to attain a pneumoperitoneum initially.[9] Extraperitoneal placement of gas is a common complication and is usually due to inexperience, improper equipment, or poor patient selection. Testing intraperitoneal placement with fluid in a syringe is mandatory prior to gas insufflation. Undue resistance from previous scars mandate using disposable sharp insufflating needles as well as trocars and sheaths. Extraperitoneal gas should be exhausted prior to reinsertion if incorrect placement has been identified.

Previous adhesion formation presents the most difficult roadblock to trocar placement or instrument excursion. Manipulation to take down adhesions may be required if the procedure is to proceed. Vascular interruption within the adhesion or the omentum is a common occurrence and should be identified and cauterized prior to further surgery because ongoing blood loss may obscure the operative field.

Obesity presents a challenge to the laparoscopist. Not only is the abdominal cavity more remote, necessitating a longer Verres needle, but the distance between accessory ports may cause constant instrument collision. Initial Verres needle placement should be within the umbilicus where all layers of the abdominal wall are fused and thinnest. Higher pressures are encountered on insufflation because the added weight of the anterior abdominal wall must be lifted. Positioning of the patient may be limited because of hemodynamic and respiratory considerations, thereby limiting adequate visualization of the operative site.

Bleeding Complications

Bleeding is the most prevalent complication after minor anesthetic and pneumoperitoneum problems. Anterior abdominal wall injury from blind puncture is common and usually self-limited. Transillumination of the anterior abdominal wall and visualization by the laparoscope may greatly reduce vessel injury. Superficial epigastric bleeding responds to pressure, but inferior epigastric arterial injury usually requires suturing. Ongoing loss during the case may obscure the operative field as well as cause abdominal wall hematomas. Similarly, the superior epigastric vessels may be injured with upper abdominal procedures such as cholecystectomy and highly selective vagotomy.

Retroperitoneal bleeding results from inadvertent puncture of major vessels below the posterior parietal peritoneum.[4,14] The usual causes include perpendicular Verres needle placement at the umbilicus or straying laterally to the pelvic side wall (Fig. 7-2). These injuries are often hard to visualize, and extensive bleeding may occur prior to recognition. Extreme care varies in patients and adolescents, and the use of newer disposable trocars with obturator safety sheaths may minimize these problems.

Mesenteric bleeding may occur with any dissection or lysis of adhesions. Careful visualization prior to cutting and the use of hook rather than straight scissors may minimize overcutting. Vasopressin injection or aqua dissection may clearly delineate cleavage planes, facilitating adequate cutting. Adequate traction on tissue is mandatory for visualization and avoidance of vascular injury.

Careful observation of any bleeding injury and judicious use of clips and endosuturing may prevent the need for laparotomy. If one is not positive that hemostasis is assured or vascular instability without cause is noted, laparotomy may be necessary.

Gastrointestinal Injuries

Bowel injury may occur at every step of laparoscopy, from placement of the Verres needle to definitive surgery.[13] Proper instrumentation and technique are mandatory to lessen this risk. Patients with multiple previous surgical pro-

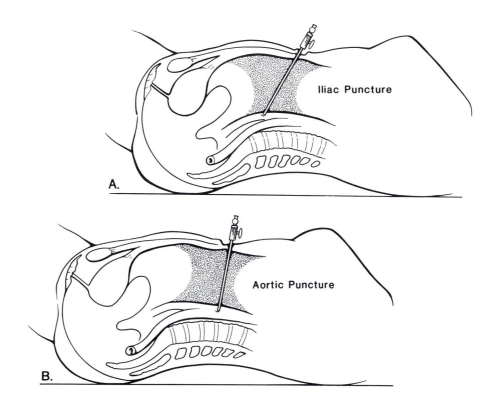

Figure 7-2
A. Incorrect perpendicular Verres needle placement. **B.** Incorrect lateral Verres needle placement.

cedures or history of peritonitis are good candidates for open laparoscopy. A direct periumbilical cut-down and placement of special sheaths sutured in place may allow safe insufflation.

The Verres needle puncture of bowel is usually evident by either mesenteric bleeding or emphysema. If a small bowel leak is evident, therapy must follow, but most needle puncture injuries can be observed during the case and followed postoperatively without laparotomy. Large bowel puncture is usually easily diagnosed because of fluid leakage or bleeding. The instrument or sheath should be left in place to identify the site for repair at laparotomy and to minimize spill. An alternative method would be to place a clip at the site to facilitate identification at laparotomy.

Careful dissection requires adequate atraumatic grasping forceps and avoidance of undue traction. Blunt probe dissection or aqua dissection with pressurized suction irrigators may delineate safe planes. Forceps or scissor opening to delineate planes prior to cutting is very important. Coagulation or clipping vessels prior to cutting rather than observing bleeding is a very good rule. Vessel retraction and loss of visualization may prevent any chance of achieving hemostasis at a later time.

Laser and electrocautery injuries may occur from either defective equipment, spark gap energy sources creating an arcing effect, a unipolar capacitance effect from sheaths or from operator error. Most injuries unfortunately are not recognized initially and present with late postoperative perforation symptoms.[17] Patients present with abdominal pain, nausea, and fever on the second or third postoperative day. Peritonitis is evident and immediate exploration is mandatory.

If thermal injuries are recognized, the most expedient and safe treatment is laparotomy with either resection of the injured segment or oversewing. Laparoscopic suturing with adequate imbrication of the damaged area has been reported but is adequate only in the hands of very experienced laparoscopists. Healthy respect for and understanding of all energy sources employed and direct visualization of the bowel at all times during endoscopic surgery will minimize, but not completely remove, the risk of gastrointestinal (GI) complication.

Bowel obstruction following laparoscopic surgery can be due to adhesions or abdominal wall herniation at a puncture site.[18] If a mass is palpable at a puncture site, then herniation is easily diagnosed. A Richter's hernia in which only one wall is incarcerated will probably not be palpable. Repair of an incarcerated puncture site hernia can be done under local anesthesia and intravenous sedation. The fascial defect is exposed and the intestine reduced. The defect usually is larger than expected, being two or three times the size of the cannula used, and several sutures will be required.

Genitourinary Complications

Injury to the bladder is rare if all patients are catheterized prior to placement of the insufflating needle, trocars, and sheaths.[15,16] Longer endoscopic procedures require ongoing catheterization as in laparotomy.

Ureteric injury may occur from inadvertent retroperitoneal puncture or laser electrocautery treatment of peritoneal lesions or adhesions. Obviously, such injury is worsened by lack of discovery initially. Management consists of urologic consultation, endoscopy, ureteral catheter placement, and possibly reanastomosis.

Prevention of ureteric injury stems from awareness of anatomy and active effort to observe it either transperitoneally or via an open retroperitoneum. Additional safety may be obtained by injecting saline under peritoneal lesions prior to laser vaporization.

Infection

Infection is a very rare complication of laparoscopy even with very complicated and lengthy cases. Overall, the incidence has been reported to be less than 1.4 per 1000 cases in a large gynecologic series. Rates for appendectomy and cholecystectomy appear to be less than for standard laparotomy approach. Although still considered by most to be a sterile procedure, there is certainly a break in technique with the use of video cameras and laser couplers handled by technicians outside the field.

The most common infection is cystitis due to catheterization. Wound infections and small abscess formations are rare. Peritonitis is related to bowel injury or poor treatment of an appendiceal stump at the time of removal. Adequate techniques and removal of the appendix or other infected tissue through large cannula sheaths will minimize abdominal wall exposure to bacteria and thereby lessen wound infection. Copious irrigation also lessens the chance of infection and complicated abscess removal procedures.

Prevention of infection by initial sterilization of equipment followed by disinfection between cases has been shown to be adequate in large endoscopic centers. Surgeons should make every attempt to minimize contact with nonsterile equipment followed by handling operating instruments. Frequent glove changes may minimize bacterial contamination. Prophylactic antibiotics is not recommended unless transient bacteremia is expected or a very prolonged procedure is contemplated.

Postoperative Complications

Postoperative shoulder strap pain from CO_2 irritation of the diaphragm is universal and should be discussed preoperatively with the patient. Incisional pain and sore throat from intubation are also common. Surgeons should remember that extensive operative procedures, although performed through small incisions, may carry the same inherent amount of pain as the same major procedure. Postoperative analgesia and often hospital observation are prudent for any procedure lasting longer than 2 to 2 ½ h.

Pain usually subsides within 26 to 48 h, and failure to follow this pattern should alert the surgeon to look exhaustively for urinary or gastrointestinal injury.

Neurologic sequelae are rare because few nerve roots have been affected by intraabdominal surgery. Incorrect positioning or prolonged deep Trendelenburg positioning may cause shoulder pain. Likewise, adequate padding and protection of upper extremities are mandatory if the laparoscope or other instruments are pressed against them for prolonged periods of time.

Groin herniation after laparoscopy has been reported. Intestinal incarceration in such a hernia during a laparoscopic procedure could potentially cause severe pain and evidence of a bowel obstruction within 24 h. Consequently, it should always be part of the differential diagnosis for pain, nausea, and vomiting after laparoscopy.

Discussion

Complications in laparoscopy have been found to be rare, but most published rates arise from populations of young gynecologic patients with limited procedures. As more general surgical series are published covering appendectomy, cholecystectomy, and hernia repair, more meaningful rates will appear.

It is incumbent upon every laparoscopist to know his and her equipment and test it preoperatively as well as to follow strict repetitive protocols for insufflation and trocar placement. Laparoscopy is not an arena for shortcuts.

Adequate initial training and active preceptorship programs will lessen the well-known pattern of complications in a surgeon's initial cases.

Good laparoscopists understand the limitations of their equipment, their support staff, and most importantly their own surgical abilities. Not every case can be accomplished via laparoscopy, and it is incumbent upon the surgeon to have every patient prepared for major surgery should technical difficulties or complications arise. An informed consent will lessen any later medicolegal repercussions.

If any potential complications arise, it is better to stop the case and exhaustively search for them rather than expectantly ignore the problem. Intraabdominal anatomy may change rapidly with bowel reposition, and delay of inspection of potential injury may result in losing the opportunity. Preventing or avoiding complications is the best way to obviate the need for laparotomy. If a complication is encountered, consultation with other surgeons may be helpful. If a laparotomy is needed, it should not be viewed as a failure but instead as sound surgical judgment.

References

1. Phillips JM: Complications in laparoscopy. *Int J Gynecol Obstet* 15:157–162, 1977.
2. Phillips JM, Hulka JF, Keith GL: Laparoscopic procedures AAGL membership survey for 1975. *J Reprod Med* 18:227–238, 1977.
3. Levinson CJ, Hulka JF, Richardson DT: *Laparoscopy: Complications in Obstetric and Gynecologic Surgery*. Hagerstown, MD, Harper & Row, 1981, pp 281–298.
4. Katz M, Beck P, Tater R: Major vessel injury during laparoscopy. *Am J Obstet Gynecol* 135:544–545, 1979.
5. Newton M: Complications of abdominal operations, in Newton M, Newton ER (eds): *Complications of Gynecologic and Obstetric Management*. Philadelphia, Saunders, 1988, pp 143–174.
6. Kane MG, Kreijs GJ: Complications of diagnostic laparoscopy in Dallas; A seven-year prospective study. *Gastrointest Endosc* 30:237–240, 1984.
7. Borton M: *Laparoscopic Complications: Prevention and Management*. Toronto, Decker, 1986.
8. Gotzf Pier A, Bacher C: Modified laparoscopic appendectomy in surgery: A report of 388 operations. *Surg Endosc* 2:46–49, 1990.
9. Pentecost MP, Curtis DM: Laparoscopy, in Ridley JH: *Gynecologic Surgery: Errors. Safeguards. Salvage*. Baltimore, Williams & Wilkins, 1981, pp 135–158.
10. Carmichael M: Laparoscopy: Cardiac considerations. *Fertil Steril* 22:59–70, 1971.
11. Scott DB, Julian DG: Observations on cardiac arrhythmias during laparoscopy. *Br Med J* 1:411–413, 1972.
12. Smith I et al: Cardiovascular effects of peritoneal insufflation of carbon dioxide for laparoscopy. *Br Med J* 3:410–411, 1971.
13. Endler GC, Moghissi KS: Gastric perforation during pelvic laparoscopy. *Obstet Gynecol* 47:40–42, 1976.
14. Baadsgaard FE, Bille S, Egelblad J: Major vascular injury during gynecological laparoscopy: Report of two cases and review of published cases. *Acta Obstet Gynecol* 68:283–285, 1989.
15. Deshmukh AS: Laparoscopic bladder injury. *Urology* 18:306–307, 1982.
16. Georgy RM, Fetterman H, Chefet MD: Complications of laparoscopy: Two cases of perforated urinary bladder. *Am J Obstet Gynecol* 120:1121–1122, 1974.
17. Soderstrom RM, Levy BS: Bowel injuries during laparoscopy: Causes and medicolegal questions. *Cont Obstet Gynecol* 27:41–45, 1986.
18. Cristalli B, Cayol A, Landowski P: Hernias of the groin: A new complication of celioscopy. *J de Gynecologie, Obstetrique et Biologie de la Reproduction* 20(2):221–222, 1991.

8

Ergonomics and Laparoscopic General Surgery

Michael Patkin
Luis Isabel

The rapid uptake of laparoscopic techniques by general surgeons since 1989 has been too fast to allow design of equipment and to develop techniques that seek normal human capacities while still offering the powerful advantages of this new technology.

This early mismatch between technology and normal human capacity suggests an important opportunity for the application of *ergonomics,* which is the scientific study of people at work or in other structured activity. Ergonomics has been used to analyze and improve many types of work in the past fifty years;[1] it was applied to microsurgical instrument design in the 1970s.[2]

Ergonomics in general is applied to equipment design, workplace layout, environmental conditions such as lighting, and the process of acquiring skill. It has the aims of improving productivity, accuracy, safety, and satisfaction at work. Its possible applications to laparoscopy include improved eye-hand coordination, clarity of the visual image and of tactile feedback during dissection, improved design of equipment for handling, and other applications still to be explored.

The problem of eye-hand coordination and paradoxical movements using a video system is a good example.

Eye-Hand Coordination and Paradoxical Movement

If laparoscopic forceps placed in the abdominal cavity are moved in one direction by the hand of the operator, and the image shown on a video monitor is displayed normally, the working end of the forceps is seen to move in the opposite direction. The same applies to up-and-down movements.

Adapted from a paper of the same title presented at the Annual Scientific Meeting, Royal Australasian College of Surgeons, South Australian Branch, Adelaide, August 1991.

Often a new operator can get used to this new direction of movement in a few minutes. It is the kind of movement that occurs with any first-order lever, such as an oar or a rudder on a boat. Both horizontal and vertical movements are affected in the same way (Fig. 8-1*A*). To-and-fro movements in the third dimension, the "z-axis," are still seen in the expected way. This combination can be described as "first-order paradoxical movement."

Consider the case, however, where the instrument and the viewing telescope are now directed opposite to the operator's line of sight to the video monitor. This occurs if equipment is arranged in a normal way for a cholecystectomy, but the operator sets out first to divide some adhesions in the lower abdomen, for example, to the underside of an old appendectomy scar.

In this case, a left-to-right movement by the operator's hand is seen as a left-to-right movement on the video monitor. The sideways movement seen by the eye is not opposite to the hand movement but in the same direction, while up-and-down movements are still reversed (Fig. 8-1*B*). To reverse one axis of movement but not the other, like work viewed through a mirror, is much more difficult and even impossible in the short term. This combination can be considered as "second-order paradoxical movement." Control of movement becomes much easier if the monitor is shifted to the other end of the body (Fig. 8-1*C*), restoring the more familiar first-order paradoxical movement. The same problem is found when the gallbladder is removed at the umbilicus.

Problems of displaced vision coordination of this kind were studied extensively by Kohler (1939).[3] He and other experimental subjects wore reversing prisms on spectacles for days and weeks at a time, giving rise to troublesome effects and aftereffects. "Days and even weeks were spent in correcting movements disturbed by the reversal, some of which were repeated incorrectly hundreds of times. The subject tried to correct such movements, not because of false conscious perception, but because he couldn't endure false movements" (Smith, 1962).[3] In cases where left and right were reversed, someone trying to walk along a straight path would lurch from side to side like someone drunk (Fig. 8-2).

Strategies for controlling paradoxical movement include deliberately thinking about movements as they are carried out. This has limitations because mental blocks occur, especially if the situation is a dangerous one. Moving in the opposite direction to the apparently correct one is another solution, and even though this slows movements down, the early experimenters noted that this was the simplest solution and helped in such general movements as walking and finding doors. However "quick localizing movements were the most difficult to cor-

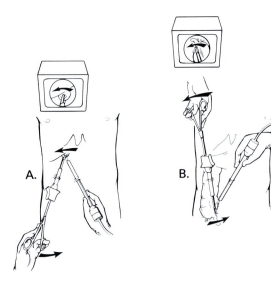
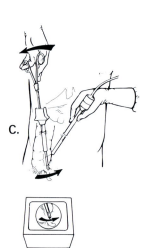

Figure 8-1
A. First-order paradoxical movement. The hand moves in the opposite direction to the instrument on the screen in both horizontal and vertical axes. **B.** Second-order paradoxical movement. The hand moves in the same direction horizontally but the opposite direction vertically as the instrument on the screen. Similar to a mirror image. **C.** First-order paradoxical movement is restored by placing eye, hand, and monitor in line.

Chapter 8 Ergonomics and Laparoscopic General Surgery

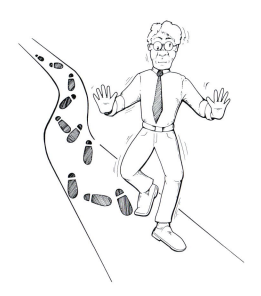

Figure 8-2
Walking with reversing prisms (after Kohler).

rect. Such paradoxical movements during surgery must be much slower, deliberate, and stepwise but are still frustrating and error-prone."

While gynecologists have used laparoscopy extensively in the past 20 years, this extensive use has not led to the study of such problems because traditional laparoscopy has been a one person activity with direct view through a rigid endoscope, rather than the dissociated view through a video system; the types of manipulation have generally been simpler ones, such as the mere lifting or prodding of structures or application of diathermy or clips; and these manipulations have been confined to the lower abdomen, avoiding the problems of paradoxical movement.

Visual Aspects of Laparoscopic Surgery

Loss of stereoscopic vision is of special interest, at least until stereoscopic video is available. Sometimes depth perception is sacrificed deliberately in favor of magnification; for example, a watchmaker, using a simple monocular loupe, or a microscopist. However, lack of normal depth perception during laparoscopic maneuvers impairs eye-hand coordination, slows down dissection, and makes it less accurate.

Equally important to depth perception is the dynamic view achieved by head movement, which is also lost when looking at a video screen. Several other factors are:

1. *Comparison with the observer's normal mental model*: The gallbladder usually protrudes from the undersurface of the liver, so it will be closer to the observer when seen from this aspect. The gallbladder and other rounded structures have the central part closer than its edges. The common bile duct is seen foreshortened from a laparoscope through the umbilicus and will appear to run slightly upward into the liver.

2. *Lighting intensity*: Closer structures appear brighter with the present concentric lighting around the laparoscope rather than through a separate port. There is a molded effect of shading that would be increased if the light source were not in the same line as vision.

3. *Relative size*: The geometric shape, relative size of instruments, and converging straight lines are important cues. However, relative size of tissue structures, such as the neck and body of the gallbladder and various vessels and ducts, can be misleading when seen in isolation, especially during the early stage of a dissection.

4. *Overlap and relative movement*: Many of the movements of an instrument are exploratory, with successive trials and correction of error, and often at a much slower rate than with everyday manipulations.

5. *Convergence*: Using extraocular muscles and the ciliary muscle to focus on the real object, rather than on the virtual reality of the monitor.

Interventions to improve visual acuity have already been considered for microsurgery.[2,4] Magnification, the most obvious, allows much finer and more accurate dissection and manipulation to take place, with less tissue trauma. Occasionally there is confusion between "the forest and the trees," and it is possible to dissect the wrong structure, albeit with great accuracy and delicacy. Within broad limits, visual acuity increases with lighting intensity, until impaired by glare, which occurs in laparoscopy from intruding structures such as the pale omentum obscuring the lower part of gallbladder and from instruments too close to the laparoscope, especially if they have a reflective surface. Contrast of lighting and color improves visual discrimination of structures. A tiny speck of green staining by bile is valuable confirmation of the cystic duct. Venous blood on the liver bed is much more difficult to localize. Replay of videos of this stage of dissection shows that the bleeding source is generally higher and much tinier than the operator imagines.

Hand Movements and Their Control during Laparoscopy

Unlike freehand movement in general surgery, movements of laparoscopic instruments are constrained by the fulcrum at the abdominal wall at the point of entry of each port. The slight movements here are not significant. Paradoxical movements were discussed at the start of this chapter.

By contrast with microsurgery, hand tremor is much less of a problem because each instrument is stabilized at the fulcrum where it enters the abdomen. Control of in-and-out movement is more of a problem, especially if there is friction from soiling between the instrument and its port. The jerkiness this causes obviously interferes with control and smooth dissection and may cause "oops" damage to vital structures. Prevention of this problem depends on care in engineering and maintenance of equipment, especially cleaning, and possibly the use of sterile aqueous lubricants specially designed for surgical instruments to avoid a build-up of residue. The skill and care of staff who clean these instruments is critical and needs more attention. Design improvements are needed.

Tactile Feedback

Normal surgery depends a great deal on delicacy to avoid breaking some structures while applying stronger forces to break others under careful control. The "hook and cook" technique to break successive fibers may be done with obvious force, probably up to 1 kg (10 n) at times. Prodding or lifting the liver must be done with rather less force to avoid injuring it.

The fulcrum of the abdominal wall shifts slightly as instruments are moved in and out. This alters the power of the lever and further confounds tactile feedback, as do the multiple linkages and often poorly designed handles of laparoscopic instruments.

Skill Acquisition

Traditionally the acquisition of manipulative skills in surgery has been through apprenticeship and experience, largely unstructured. More recent years have seen formal training through workshops on bone fixation and bowel anastomosis.[5] Even in these instances, formal analysis in ergonomic terms has been rare, though it has been carried out in microsurgery[2,4,6] as well as in some aspects of general surgery.[1]

Video recording, replay, and analysis are ob-

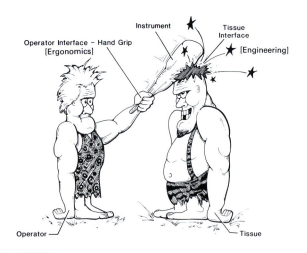

Figure 8-3
Surgical interfaces, between operator and instrument and between instrument and tissue.

vious tools for the study of surgical technique and its advancement. This can be done quite cheaply by adding a $300 videocassette recorder to the camera-monitor system during laparoscopy, though more expensive systems with a crisper freeze-frame facility have obvious advantages. There is no reason to restrict such recording to the intraabdominal aspects of a procedure, and it will be possible to study the hand movements during insertion of the Verres needle into the abdominal cavity, as well as other hand movements outside the abdomen during laparoscopic manipulation.

Broadening the Systems Approach

Effective work depends not only on controlled human movement and technology but also on an understanding of the properties of the material being worked on and its interface to equipment, the subject of engineering rather than ergonomics (Fig. 8-3). Such properties include whether or not tissue splits better in one direction and basic "theorems of dissection," such as the need to incise at right angles to lines of tension, an aspect of operating geometry (Fig. 8-4).

A systems approach includes study of such questions as security of grip of tissue. If grasping forceps repeatedly slip off the gallbladder during dissection, this delays and interrupts smooth dissection. What should the design of teeth or other jaw lining be to grip a gallbladder securely without slipping off and without perforating? Laparoscopic cholecystectomy was initially performed using instruments designed for gynecological procedures.

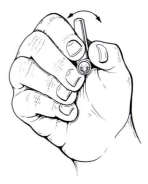

Figure 8-5
Use of pinch grip to facilitate instrument rotatability.

Some maneuvers consist of rotating instruments along their long axis; for example, twirling the handle of a diathermy hook to widen the window behind the cystic artery or duct. Sometimes grippers need to be rotated either for a better angle of attack on the tissue or else to wind the neck of the gallbladder onto the jaw to increase the security of grip. In this case, the normal two finger rings on the forceps grip restrict rotation of the instrument to the limited range of rotation of the forearm. Study of the handle design for microsurgical instruments showed the usefulness of "rotatability" of two handles each forming half a cylinder.[1] Such instruments can be twirled in the fingertips while still shut (Fig. 8-5). Similar principles may apply to laparoscopic instruments and have been applied to at least one model of laparoscopic needle holder.

Further Developments

The laparoscopic surgical arena offers a wide new opportunity for the inventiveness of general surgeons previously frustrated by the maturity of surgical instrument design developed over many decades. Numerous advances can be expected both major and incremental. Older,

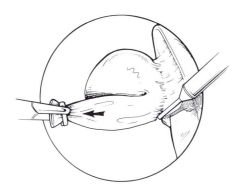

Figure 8-4
The "dotted line" of tissue tension.

conventional instruments may be recalled into duty, as in the use of tonsil forceps or sponge holding forceps to remove stones from the gallbladder before its final extraction through a 1-cm incision or a grooved director for enlarging this incision more safely.

Advances from the application of ergonomics to laparoscopy aim primarily at maximizing the abilities of operators by studying their interface, both physical and mental, to this new technology. Its methods will include conscious awareness and analysis of technical factors, video recording and analysis of technique, collaboration with ergonomists and engineers, and making use of their knowledge and methods while prototyping new techniques, instruments, and other technology.

Developments in robotics and artificial intelligence are occurring very rapidly and will allow surgical technology that is beyond imagination today. These and other advances, as yet not imagined, can only occur in a climate of inquiry, encouragement, at least a modest dedication of human and material resources, and continuing discussion. The benefits of laparoscopic cholecystectomy, already established so dramatically for patients leaving the hospital in comfort one day after surgery or even the day of surgery, have opened our eyes to the huge benefits to be extended in other fields of surgery. The prospects are bright and wonderful.

References

1. Patkin M: Ergonomic aspects of surgical dexterity. *Med J Aust* 2:775–777, 1967.
2. Patkin M: Ergonomics applied to microsurgery. *Aust N Z J Surg* 47(3):320–329, 1977.
3. Kohler I. Quoted by Smith KU, Smith WM: Perception and motion, in Vernon, MD (ed): *Experiments in Visual Perception*. Penguin, 1966. Excerpted from Smith KU, Smith WM: *Perception and Motion*. Philadelphia, Saunders, 1962, chap 5.
4. Patkin M: Ergonomics and the operating microscope. *Adv Ophthalmol* 37:53–63, 1978.
5. Kirk RM: Report on day course in basic surgical techniques. *College and Faculty Bulletin Supplement to Ann RCS*, 22, March 1991.
6. Patkin M: Selection and care of microsurgical instruments. *Adv Ophthalmol*. Basel, Karger, 1978, vol 37, pp 23–33.

PART TWO

Laparoscopic Abdominal Surgery

9

Initial Survey of the Peritoneal Cavity, Diagnostic Laparoscopy, Lysis of Adhesions, and Tumor Biopsies

John N. Graber

Laparoscopy offers some special advantages, but the one advantage that does not require any significant effort or risk during an elective procedure is the opportunity to explore the abdominal cavity and note any pathology. As part of every laparoscopic case, the findings of a brief survey should be recorded and reviewed with the patient. Within some limits, a patient should not have to find out that she has symptomatic ovarian cancer 3 months after an uneventful laparoscopic cholecystectomy. This type of lesion, as well as others, would likely be identified if the ovaries and the remainder of the abdominal cavity are routinely examined during laparoscopic procedures.

For open incisional surgeries, such as cholecystectomy and appendectomy, incisions have been developed that expose only the specific target organ. Consequently, surgeons have not had a liberal approach to abdominal exploration for all cases. It requires discipline to add this part of the surgery to laparoscopic procedures. A good survey should follow a serial inspection of the abdominal organs and takes only 2 to 3 min.

As a rule, unexpected pathologies, such as cancers, that are found during an unrelated operation do not need to be treated immediately. Laparoscopy is different from incisional surgery in that completing the planned procedure and waking the patient to discuss the findings do not result in a dramatic increase in pain, incision, or even time to recover. Consequently, if treatment of the condition discovered is at all involved, it is reasonable to plan a second operation after reviewing the matter with the patient.

Diagnostic laparoscopy is performed for the purpose of diagnosing or ruling out specific abdominal pathologies or to obtain a biopsy or culture to determine the extent of disease. Laparoscopy is an excellent tool for the evaluation of abdominal disorders.[1] A contingency plan of operative therapy should be reviewed with the patient in light of the preoperative symptoms before the surgery. To be done properly, a diagnostic laparoscopy should follow a serial inspection of the entire abdominal cavity.

Pelvic and Inguinal Organs

Because the cannulas are usually inserted into the pelvis, the first intraabdominal view is often of the pelvic organs. The bladder, sigmoid colon, and inguinal anatomy should be observed in all patients. In the female the uterus, fallopian tubes, and ovaries are also seen.

The bladder is easily seen laparoscopically, usually as a deflated hollow below the pubic bone. There are few problems to be encountered by the laparoscopist when examining the bladder. Transmural cancers or urachal cysts could be seen.

Diverticulosis and chronic diverticulitis may be evident as scarring and lack of mobility of the sigmoid colon. Active or acute diverticulitis would most likely be symptomatic before surgery and will be evident by the erythematous and inflamed colon. Colon cancer, colitis, and ileitis can be identified laparoscopically.

Groin herniation is easily identified and is discussed elsewhere in this text (Chap. 20). Enlarged lymph nodes can be seen along the iliac arteries and veins. Biopsy can be accomplished and is also detailed elsewhere in the text (Chap. 22).

The intraabdominal reproductive organs of the female are easily seen, and many pathological entities can be identified.[2] In most cases, therapy is not warranted, but specific notation of the degree and site of involvement is helpful.

Uterine myomata or fibroids are the most frequent tumors found in the female pelvis, with a reported incidence of from 4 to 11 percent. Most often fibroids are multiple and occur with highest frequency in the fifth decade but may occasionally reach a large size by age 30. They can be submucosal or intramural and not be visible externally aside from an enlarged and misshapened uterus. A subserosal fibroid appears as a red/brown mass that may be pedunculated or broad based and protrudes from the uterine surface. Conversion to a malignant form is very rare and if asymptomatic can be observed safely without further intervention. The size and position of the fibroid should be noted and reviewed with the patient.

Transmural uterine cancers will look different than myomata, having a whitish gray color and a variegated surface. There may be extension into other adjacent organs. Gynecologists or gynecologic oncologists usually manage these lesions, and immediate consultation is best. If gynecological consultation is not immediately available, then completion of the planned procedure and postoperative consultation with review of the videotape is warranted.

Fallopian tube disease is also rather common and includes congenital anomalies, various degrees of infection and inflammation, and tubal pregnancies. A general surgeon may encounter these pathologies during a laparoscopic exam for right lower quadrant abdominal pain. (See also Chap. 10 and Fig. 10-1.) Parametritis and acute salpingitis are important tubal disorders because of their frequency and their serious consequences. The infection can advance to pyosalpinx or hydrosalpinx, in which case the tube becomes large, fluctuant, and dramatically inflamed. In the chronic stage, it can be associated with extensive adhesions matting the entire pelvis. Most often these disorders are treated successfully with antibiotics, and resection or drainage is not needed. In their most fulminant form a tubo-ovarian abscess can form. These abscesses can be successfully treated using laparoscopic technique that includes drainage and copious irrigation of the abscess cavity with antibiotic saline solution and placement of a drain.[3]

Ovarian diseases are often asymptomatic, but they can produce symptoms that may simulate general surgical disorders. The most common findings are nonneoplastic cysts that are physiologic variations of the normal ovulatory cycle. Cystic follicle hematomas, corpus luteal hematomas, or especially ruptured hemorrhagic corpus luteal cysts may present as acute appendicitis.

A cystic hematoma that has not ruptured will appear maroon or dark blue and generally can be observed. A ruptured cyst is best identified by close examination of the ovary. This is greatly assisted by placing a uterine sound tenaculum transvaginally before the surgery is begun (see Chap. 10). By manipulating the tenaculum, you can retract the uterus, allowing easier access to the ovary. A ruptured cyst should be explored for ongoing bleeding and controlled with cautery or suture ligature. Extensive irrigation of the pelvis with antibiotic saline is warranted.

Ovarian cysts can become quite large and symptomatic. They usually can be diagnosed preoperatively by ultrasound or physical examination. They can be treated by removal of the external wall, using laparoscopic technique that is beyond the scope of this text.

Endometriosis is the growth of aberrant or ectopic endometrium that retains the histologic characteristics and biologic responses of uterine mucosa. It is not cancerous and is dependant upon hormonal stimulation. Periodically these tissue proliferate, bleed, become locally invasive, fibrotic, and constrictive. The lesion can spread by direct invasion, lymphatic, or hematogenous mechanisms. Active endometriosis is dependent upon functioning ovaries. This disorder is most common from 30 to 40 years of age.

Although endometriosis is often asymptomatic, it can cause sacral backache, dyspareunia, abnormal uterine bleeding, or gastrointestinal symptoms, depending upon which organs are involved. Pain usually begins premenstrually and resolves shortly after the menstrual flow.

The laparoscopic appearance of endometriosis is usually that of small, scattered, scarred puckerings or irregular, brown "tobacco-stained" areas anywhere on the pelvic peritoneum (Fig. 9-1).[3,4] Dark blue or brown hemorrhagic blebs can be seen on the surface of other intraabdominal organs. Ovarian implants can appear as large "chocolate cysts" that may become adherent to the uterine ligaments. An attempt to free the ovary often results in tearing the cyst capsule and spilling large quantities of thick, chocolate-colored fluid that may disseminate the disease.

A biopsy of an easily accessible lesion can be done, but management is usually through hormone manipulation or oophorectomy. Documentation and referral to a gynecologist is appropriate.

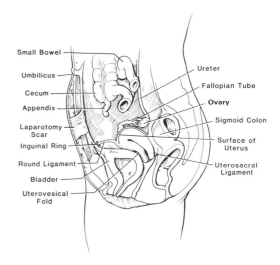

Figure 9-1
Typical sites of intraabdominal implants of endometriosis.

Ovarian tumors include cystadenomas, teratomas, feminizing and masculinizing neoplasms, and carcinomas, as well as others. They may be cystic, cystic and solid, or solid masses. Surface excrescences, penetration of the capsule, multiple dense adhesions, infiltration into surrounding structures, and ascites are suggestive of malignancy. Local peritoneal implantation, omental nodules, and retroperitoneal lymphadenopathy are typical sites of metastatic extension. Completion of the planned operation and documentation of the findings with subsequent referral are appropriate.

Upper Abdominal Survey and Tumor Biopsy

Upper abdominal pathologies may be more familiar to general surgeons than gynecological entities; however, a survey of the upper abdomen is often neglected because of the focus on the primary procedure. Lesions can be identified on the diaphragm, liver, stomach, spleen, and small intestine.

Congenital diaphragmatic hernias could be identified at laparoscopy.[5] In fact, the pneumoperitoneum may result in forcing abdominal contents into the chest. Hiatal hernia repair may become a routine laparoscopic procedure in the future, but at present further investigation needs to be done.

Liver lesions that may be seen at laparoscopy include nonneoplastic hepatocellular diseases (e.g., cirrhosis), simple cysts, hamartomas, hemangiomas, primary hepatocellular carcinomas, cholangiocarcinomas, and metastatic neoplasms.

Liver cysts can be very large and can cause abdominal pain. Their highest incidence is after age 60. If they are asymptomatic, they can be observed; however, they can become so large as to cause difficulty breathing. They can be managed very well and safely with laparoscopic technique usually resulting in permanent cure and relief of symptoms (Fig. 9-2). Outcomes with polycystic disease may not be quite as good, but the patient's symptoms are usually improved.

Using cautery or laser, we can unroof the cyst at the liver margin. The capsule should be sent for pathological examination. The surface of large cysts is usually 40 or 50 percent extrahepatic, whereas smaller cysts may be grossly intrahepatic, with less than 10 or 20 percent visible. Their management is the same, but the risk may be higher for the cyst to recur with an intrahepatic cyst if the wall reforms postoperatively. This can be prevented by inserting a pedicle of omentum into the cavity. It can be held in place with clips. Technically, it is best to start the dissection at the most posterior or inferior part of the cyst margin and move anteriorly because bleeding and drainage will obscure the anatomy at this site if it is done last.[6] With polycystic disease, an effort should be made to drain the largest of the cysts but not necessarily all of them. Intraoperative ultrasound may be helpful in this regard.

Other lesions such as carcinomas can be biopsied by direct needle technique. In the setting of metastatic liver involvement from otherwise unobstructing pancreatic cancers or hepatoma in both lobes, a biopsy of the liver lesion may be all that is needed.[7] A laparoscopically

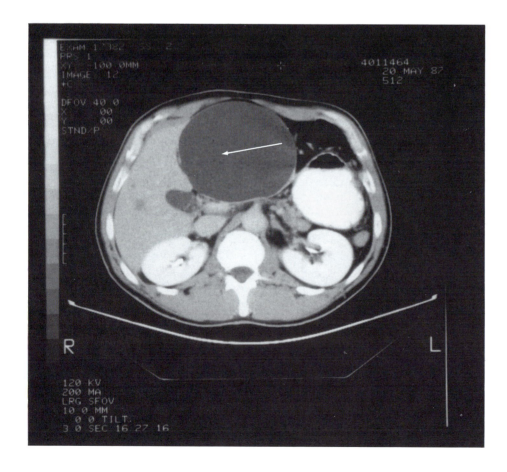

Figure 9-2
Benign liver cysts (arrow) can be unroofed using laparoscopic technique. Omentum should be placed in the cavity to prevent reoccurrence.

created stapled cholecystojejunostomy and/or gastrojejunostomy could be accomplished in the setting of obstruction. Techniques of passing a laparoscope through the lesser omentum to allow complete evaluation of the pancreas have been described.[8]

Diagnosis and culture of liver abscesses or other infectious processes can be done effectively, using laparoscopic technique.[13] Cultures can be obtained by aspirating collections or by gathering exudates or fluid with a cupped biopsy forceps.

Stomach lesions can be identified; however, their management will typically require a laparotomy. Perforated gastric and duodenal ulcers have been treated laparoscopically by oversewing the defect and using extensive abdominal lavage.[9]

For pathological diagnosis of lymphomas, in general, more tissue than a needle biopsy may be required in order to obtain the desired tissue typing and markers. For non-Hodgkin's lymphoma, an intact lymph node or a substantial biopsy is usually satisfactory. For Hodgkin's lymphoma, a splenectomy may be required for the initial staging. If so, it is not clear that a laparoscopic approach is best.

Splenectomies for idiopathic thrombocytopenic purpura (ITP) or hairy-cell leukemia have been accomplished.[10] The technique of the hilar dissection must be impeccable to avoid serious bleeding. The removal of the spleen is accomplished by placing it in a bag and morcelating it with a finger or a mechanical device.

Technique of Intraabdominal Biopsies

Needle biopsies can usually be done easily and without causing harm. Newer spring-loaded biopsy devices make laparoscopic biopsies more efficient because they can be done with one hand (Fig. 9-3A, B, and C). After cocking the device, you can pass the needle through a cannula or percutaneously. When its tip is touching the surface of the lesion, it can be fired by pressing the release lever, and the needle core is projected through the lesion and automatically followed by the cutting sheath. The instrument is then withdrawn, and the specimen saved before another core is taken. Usually two good cores are sufficient. Of course, this device can be used to biopsy any solid mass or organ. Bleeding is usually minimal and can be controlled by pressure and cautery at the surface of the puncture site. When a biopsy is all that is desired, often the only cannula required is for the umbilical camera port.

For taking larger specimens, as may be needed for lymphomas, cautery or laser cutting devices are necessary. Hemostasis is the major obstacle. We have found that contact Nd:YAG laser works well to cut out a piece of a large tumor without destroying the specimen and yet provide adequate hemostasis. Because the location of these lesions may be retroperitoneal or mesenteric, exposure is often difficult (Fig. 9-4A and B). It may be helpful to roll the patient to one side or the other, depending upon the tumor location identified by computerized tomography (CT). A sandbag placed under the flank can make visualization much easier. The greater risk in this type of biopsy is injury to adjacent bowel when attempting to provide hemostasis with cautery or laser. Wide exposure will help prevent this. The mass needs to be controlled by grasping it and we have found the 10 mm pelviscopic claw to be large enough to grasp the lesions satisfactorily to keep them above and away from intestine. A bleeding lymphomatous lump that slips under loops of intestine is a very difficult problem and must be avoided by obtaining solid control of the lesion before the biopsy is attempted.

Diagnostic Laparoscopy

The safety and efficacy of diagnostic laparoscopy has been reported for evaluation of abdominal pain,[11] abdominal neoplasms,[7] and abdominal disorders in the intensive care patient.[12] Laparoscopic examination revealed the etiology of acute and chronic abdominal pain in 98 percent of patients in one study.[11] In the majority of these patients, a local anesthetic was used with a low-volume and low-pressure pneumoperitoneum.

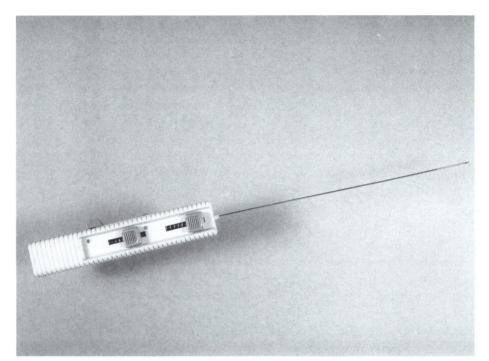

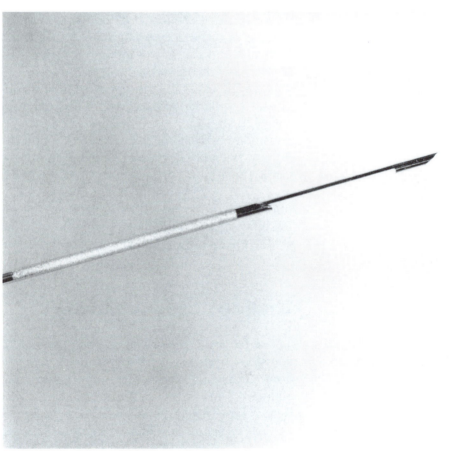

Figure 9-3
A and **B.** Spring-loaded needle biopsy device (Microvasive, Inc.).

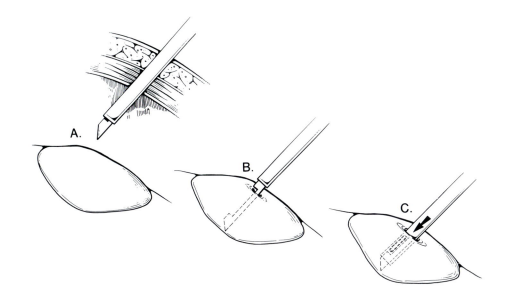

Figure 9-3
C. (*a*) The device is positioned next to the lesion. By compressing the lever, (*b*) you can fire the central biopsy core through the tissue which is immediately followed by the cutting sheath (*c*) so that the biopsy can be accomplished with only one hand.

Abdominal neoplasms are not always detectable with physical exam or radiological investigation. Other neoplasms may be identified but lack satisfactory staging or biopsy results. Again, laparoscopy has been reported to identify previously undetected cancers, rule out cancer, or accurately establish the stage of a known cancer in 98 percent of cases.[7]

For evaluation of intensive care patients, a laparoscopic exam was shown to avoid an unnecessary laparotomy or to indicate a laparotomy in a patient who would otherwise been observed in 50 percent of cases.[10,11] In the remaining 50 percent of patients, prior management decisions were confirmed.

Trauma patients can benefit from a diagnostic laparoscopy by potentially avoiding an otherwise unnecessary laparotomy for penetrating wounds that have not entered the peritoneal cavity or bleeding that spontaneously has abated by the time of the procedure.

Lysis of Adhesions

Adhesions are encountered routinely in laparoscopic surgery. Rather than being a contraindication, they are considered by some to be an indication for laparoscopic intervention.[1] Usually, adhesions are a nuisance encountered when attempting to perform an unrelated surgery (Fig. 9-5*A* and *B*). In general, lysis of adhesions should be kept to a minimum in order to allow completion of the planned procedure.

Traction and countertraction is paramount for taking down adhesive bands. The pneumoperitoneum supplies most of the traction by elevating the abdominal wall because the only adhesions that typically interfere with other surgeries are those to previous incisions. Potential problems that can arise from lysis of adhesions are noted in Table 9-1. Postdissection inspection of the visceral and abdominal wall sides of the divided tissue is absolutely mandatory to avoid complications.

Adhesions of the liver to the lateral abdominal wall and diaphragm are seen in patients who have had previous hepatitis or in some cases of gonorrhea (Fitz-Hugh-Curtis syndrome). Lysis of these adhesions is not difficult (Fig. 9-6), but extreme care to avoid perforation of the diaphragm is warranted. If the diaphragm is perforated, the pressure of the pneumoperi-

TABLE 9-1   Lysis of Adhesions

Potential Problems

- Intestinal Injury (Cautery or laser burn) (Known or unknown)
- Bleeding (Often unappreciated)
- Creation of potential internal herniation
- Postoperative abdominal-wall pain

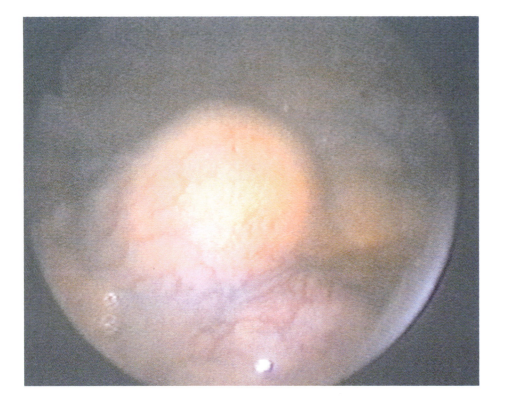

**Figure 9-4
A.** Biopsy of a retroperitoneal lymphoma may require more tissue than the needle device will obtain.

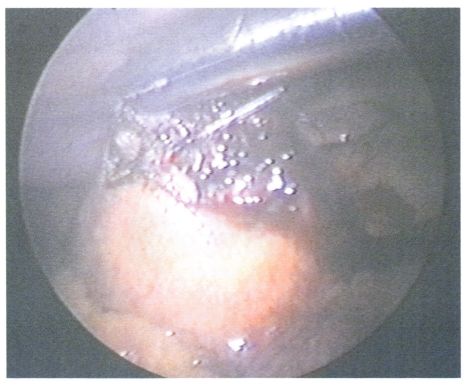

**Figure 9-4
B.** In this case a large 10-mm biopsy forceps is used.

Figure 9-5
A. Mild adhesions to the neck of the gallbladder.

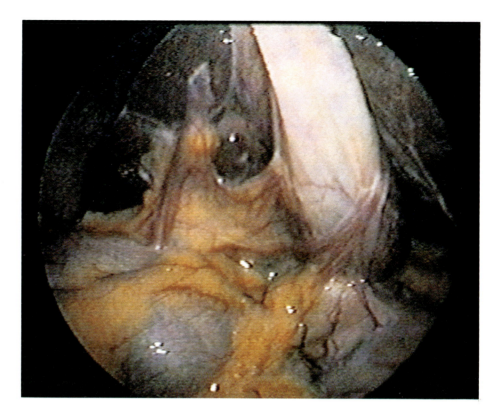

Figure 9-5
B. Severe adhesions covering the entire gallbladder.

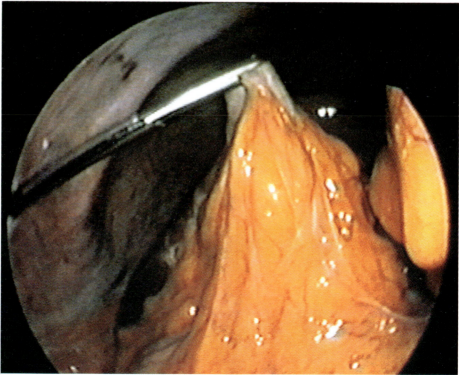

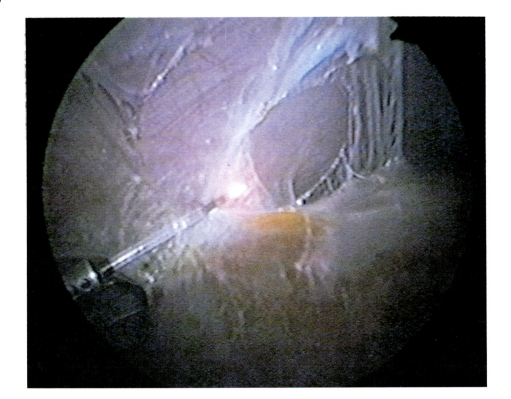

Figure 9-6
Lysis of adhesions from the liver to the lateral abdominal wall and diaphragm from previous hepatitis.

toneum will cause rapid collapse of the right lung and theoretically a tension pneumothorax. This injury may not be appreciated via the laparoscope if the hole is small. Treatment should be immediate abdominal decompression and placement of a chest tube. If the operation is otherwise completed and a laparotomy is not needed, no repair should be necessary unless the defect is extraordinarily large.

Bowel obstruction is often caused by an adhesive band. Finding this band laparoscopically can be difficult. We have not been able to accomplish this seemingly simple feat despite multiple attempts. In all cases, we have had to resort to open laparotomy to identify the source of obstruction adequately.

Discussion

The ability of the laparoscope to offer an extensive exploration of the intraabdominal contents for otherwise localized surgeries cannot be neglected. The potential information can have tremendous repercussions.

Biopsies and lysis of adhesions can be done safely if accomplished with appropriate technique and planning. The volume of tissue obtained in a biopsy and the extent of lysis of adhesions are determined by an understanding of what is required to accomplish the preoperative goal. Similarly, the preoperative goal of improved quality of patient care through less invasiveness can be met by using the laparoscopic approach to these time-honored surgical problems.

References

1. Easter DW et al: The utility of diagnostic laparoscopy for abdominal disorders. *Arch Surg* 127:379–383, 1992.

2. Cline DL: Managing gynecologic problems found at laparoscopy. *Surg Laparosc Endosc* 2(1):82–84, 1992.

3. Semm K: *Operative Manual for Endoscopic Abdominal Surgery*. Chicago, YearBook Medical Publishers, 1987.

4. Netter FH, Oppenheimer E: *Reproductive System, in the CIBA Collection of Medical Illustrations*. Summit, NJ, CIBA, 1974, vol 2.

5. Campos LI, Sipes EK: Laparoscopic repair of diaphragmatic hernia. *J Laparoendosc Surg* 1(6):369–373, 1991.

6. Way LW, Wetter A: Laparoscopic treatment of liver cysts. Presentation and Abstract. Washington, DC, SAGES Scientific Session, April 1992.

7. Easter DW et al: Laparoscopy for the evaluation of abdominal neoplasms. Presentation and Abstract. Washington, DC, SAGES Scientific Session, April 1992.

8. Warshaw AL, Fernandez-del Castillo C: Laparoscopy in preoperative diagnosis and staging for gastrointestinal cancers, in Zucker KA: *Surgical Laparoscopy*. St. Louis, Quality Medical Publishing, 1991.

9. Nathanson LK, Easter DW, Cushieri A: Laparoscopic repair/peritoneal toilet of perforated duodenal ulcer. *Surg Endosc* 4:232–233, 1990.

10. Tulman S, Reynhout J: Laparoscopic splenectomy. Video Presentation and Abstract. Washington, DC, SAGES Scientific Session, April 1992.

11. Salky B, Bauer J: The use of laparoscopy in the evaluation of abdominal pain. Presentation and Abstract. Washington, DC, SAGES Scientific Session, April 1992.

12. Bender JS, Talamini MA: Diagnostic laparoscopy in critically ill intensive care unit patients. Presentation and Abstract. Washington, DC, SAGES Scientific Session, April 1992.

13. Phillips EH et al: Laparoscopic-guided biopsy for diagnosis of *hepatic candidiasis*. *J Laparoendosc Surg* 2(1):33–38, 1992.

10

Laparoscopic Appendectomy

Joseph J. Pietrafitta

Appendectomies have been performed for a number of years laparoscopically.[1–4,9] Until recently, in the United States, most of the laparoscopic appendectomies that have been performed have been incidental appendectomies. The majority have been performed by the gynecologist during other laparoscopic (pelviscopic) procedures. It was not until the advent of laparoscopic cholecystectomy that the general surgeon felt that laparoscopic appendectomy was a feasible alternative to the open technique.[7] In addition, the performance of laparoscopic cholecystectomy gave the surgeon the skills as well as the confidence to perform appendectomies and other advanced laparoscopic procedures.

Laparoscopy opens a door to the surgeon with respect to the diagnosis and treatment of appendicitis. It is now possible to evaluate the patient, using laparoscopic techniques without specifically proceeding with an appendectomy as is generally done through an incision in the right lower quadrant.[5,9] With respect to appendicitis, laparoscopy will represent the ultimate diagnostic technique. When the patient is admitted to the hospital with the tentative diagnosis of appendicitis, it may be preferable in many instances to perform laparoscopy in order to establish a definitive diagnosis. In addition to diagnosing and treating appendicitis early, laparoscopy will allow surgeons to diagnose a number of other conditions including Crohn's disease and gynecologic problems that may be responsible for the patients' presenting symptoms.

There are a variety of techniques that have been employed. Many of these have been made possible through technological advancements in endoscopic suturing and stapling.[6] We will review the basic technique of the straightforward laparoscopic appendectomy, step-by-step, including the individual technical variations that are available to perform each step. In addition, we will discuss the more difficult laparoscopic appendectomy.

In the female patient, there is always the possibility that gynecological pathology exists. Consequently, it is imperative to be prepared in the event that a gynecologic problem is found (see also Chap. 9). After induction of anesthesia, the patient should be placed in the lithotomy position. A bimanual pelvic examination should then be carried out followed by catheterization and emptying of the bladder. Then a uterine sound with a single-tooth cervical tenaculum is placed for uterine manipulation should it be necessary. This allows the uterus to be brought out of the pelvis and manipulated from side to side in order to expose the other pelvic organs completely (Fig. 10-1). The cervical tenaculum has a malleable sound that is approximately 5 cm long. The sound is introduced through the cervical os into the uterine cavity. Cervical dilatation is not necessary to place the sound. The single tooth is clamped onto the anterior lip of the cervix. The patient is then taken out of the lithotomy position and placed supine. If gynecologic pathology is found, the patient is placed back into the lithotomy position and manipulation of the uterus can be accomplished during the operation. At the completion of the procedure, the uterine sound/cervical tenaculum is removed. The patient should be told postoperatively that she might experience some vaginal bleeding and that this does not necessarily represent her menstrual period.

The first step in any laparoscopic procedure is creation of the pneumoperitoneum, followed by trocar placement. In general, a three-puncture technique has been employed. After the pneumoperitoneum is accomplished, the first trocar is placed. It is placed at the umbilicus and should be 10 mm in size. Once the initial trocar is inserted, a 45° viewing, 10-mm laparoscope is introduced. The patient is then placed in the Trendelenburg position in order to aid in displacing the bowel from the lower abdomen and pelvis. After the laparoscope is placed, the abdomen is examined. The diagnosis may be readily apparent at this time. If the diagnosis is not apparent, then a second trocar is placed. This is generally 5 mm in size and is placed on the right side of the abdomen at the level of the umbilicus lateral to the rectus muscle. A blunt probe is then introduced through this trocar to manipulate the bowel and aid in making a definitive diagnosis. Uterine manipulation is also employed at this time if necessary. This ability, to examine the abdominal cavity and the pelvis completely, is certainly not available when a standard appendectomy incision is made (Fig. 10-2).

After the abdomen and pelvis have been examined and a decision has been made to remove the appendix, a third trocar is placed. The pattern of trocar placement varies according to the preference of the surgeon. A common pattern of placement is three trocars directly across the abdomen at the level of the umbilicus (Fig. 10-3A). A minor variation is to place the left lateral trocar in the left lower quadrant below the level of the umbilicus. If the appendiceal extractor is to be used for removal of the specimen, then

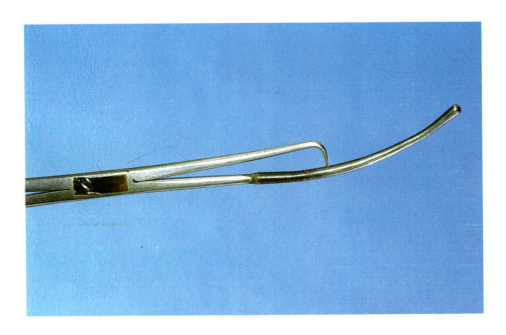

Figure 10-1
Uterine sound with single-tooth cervical tenaculum for uterine manipulation.

Chapter 10 Laparoscopic Appendectomy

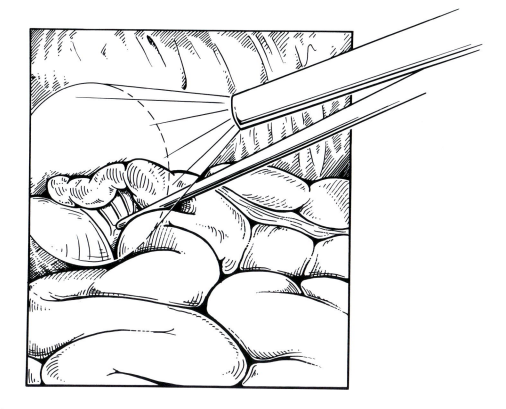

Figure 10-2
A blunt probe has been introduced through the accessory trocar. The right lower quadrant is examined and the appendix is identified.

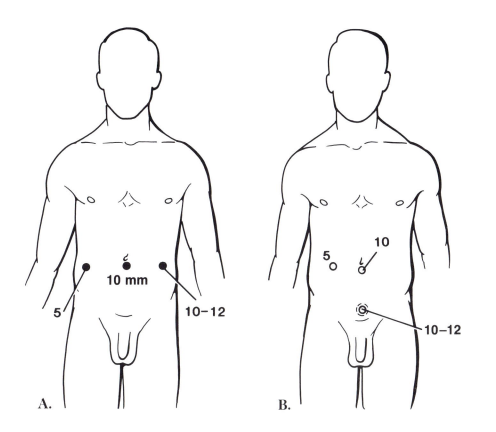

Figure 10-3
Patterns of trocar placement for appendectomy. Note that regardless of the pattern, none is placed directly over the appendix. **A.** Three trocars placed across the abdomen at the level of the umbilicus.
B. Trocars placed in an L shape with none on the left side of the abdomen. The larger trocar (11 or 12 mm) is generally placed either on the left side of the abdomen at the level of the umbilicus or in the suprapubic area.

the third trocar must be 11 mm in size. If a linear stapler is to be used for transection of either the mesoappendix or the appendix, then that trocar should be 12 mm in size to allow introduction of the stapling device.

Another common pattern of trocar placement involves placement of one of the trocars in the suprapubic position rather than on the left side of the abdomen at the level of the umbilicus in order to surround the operative site more symetrically and be closer to it. In addition, this placement allows one of the trocars to be hidden in the hairline in the suprapubic area (Fig. 10-3B).

A decision on the size of the third trocar and the instruments that will be used through it will depend upon the type and location of the inflamed appendix that is found and how it will be handled. If the base of the appendix is not involved with the pathologic process and it is to be secured with endoscopic loop sutures, an 11-mm trocar can be placed for the appendiceal extractor. If the base of the appendix is involved or if there is adherent small bowel and the linear stapler will be advantageous, a 12-mm trocar is placed to accommodate the stapler.

Before removing the appendix, the surgeon should look for any fluid or purulent material either in the right lower quadrant or in the pelvis. If any is found, it should be removed prior to commencing with the appendectomy. This is done in order to prevent spreading of this material throughout the peritoneal cavity. The fluid is first aspirated and the area is then gently irrigated (Fig. 10-4A and B).

The first step in appendiceal removal is designed to prevent rupturing of an unruptured appendix intraabdominally. Rupturing of the appendix can be seen with repeated manipulation. After the appendix has been identified, it is grasped and elevated toward the anterior abdominal wall. It is then encircled with an endoscopic loop suture that is introduced through the third trocar (see also Fig. 1-17). The loop is cut, but a long segment of suture (4 to 6 in.) is left intraabdominally. The suture is then grasped with a needle holder near the appendix, and the appendix is again ele-

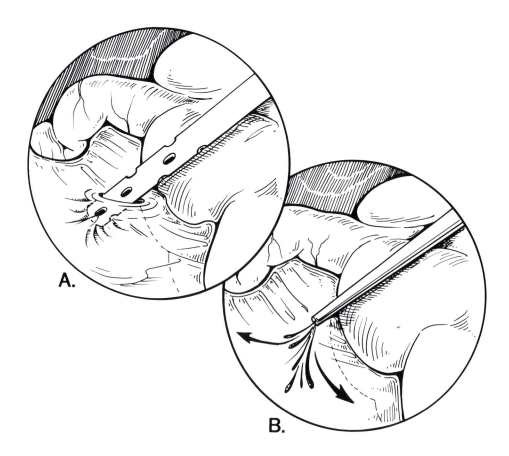

Figure 10-4
A. Pelvic fluid aspirated with a suction irrigation cannula. **B.** The area is gently irrigated after the material has been removed.

Chapter 10 Laparoscopic Appendectomy

Figure 10-5
A. An endoscopic loop suture is placed through an accessory trocar. The loop is placed around the appendix and tied down. **B.** The suture is grasped with a needle holder and the excess suture is cut off leaving a 4- to 6-in. intraabdominal segment. The appendix is elevated, placing traction on the mesoappendix.

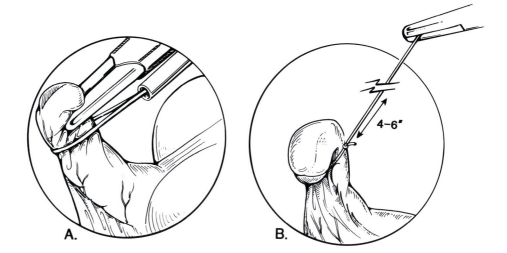

vated toward the abdominal wall (Fig. 10-5A and B).

Once the mesoappendix has been placed on stretch, it can then be transected. A number of methods are available. The mesoappendix can be secured with clips and then cut with a scissors or contact laser (Fig. 10-6A), the mesoappendix can be transected with a vascular stapling device that will secure and transect at the same time (Fig. 10-6B), or the mesoappendix can simply be transected with a monopolar electrocautery device (scissors, hook cautery, etc.)

or electrocoagulated with the bipolar forceps and then cut (Fig. 10-6C).

After the mesoappendix has been taken to the base of the appendix, the appendix must be transected. This can also be performed in several ways. The most commonly used method is to apply three endoscopic suture loops sequentially at the base of the appendix. These can be made of heavy chromic catgut or polyglactin 910 (Vicryl) suture. Two are left on the stump of the appendix, and the third is removed with the specimen (Fig. 10-7). The other method

Figure 10-6
A. Mesoappendix secured with ligating clips and then cut with a scissors.
B. Mesoappendix taken with a linear stapler.
C. Mesoappendix electrocoagulated and then cut or cut directly with electrocautery scissors.

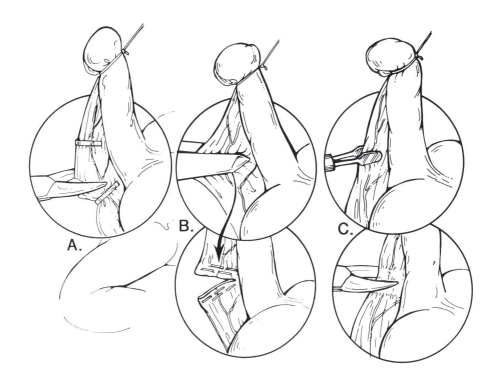

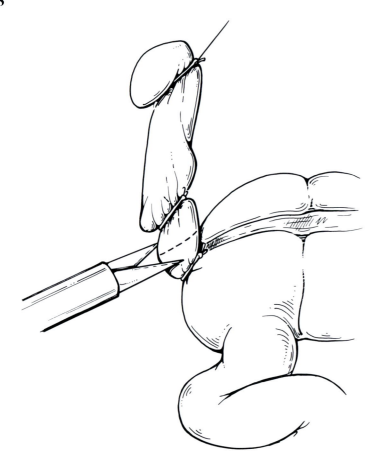

Figure 10-7
Three endoscopic loops have been placed on the appendix. The appendix is transected between the 2 distal loops.

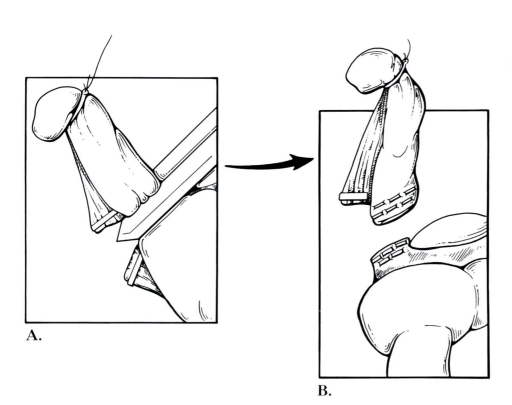

Figure 10-8
A. Linear stapler applied to the appendix.
B. Stapler fired. Appendix amputated from the cecum.

Figure 10-9
A and **B.** Both mesoappendix and appendix taken with the vascular linear stapler.

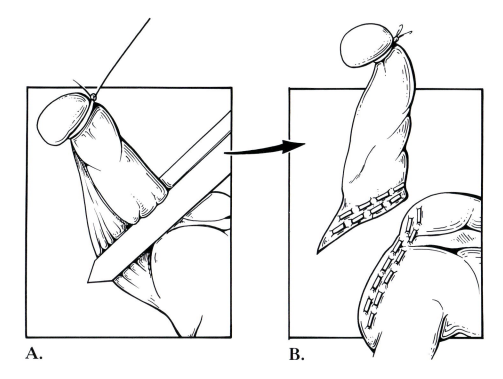

would be to transect the appendix with a linear stapler (Fig. 10-8A and B).

It should be mentioned that one application of the linear stapler can occasionally be used to transect both the mesoappendix and the appendix. In this case, however, it is mandatory to use a vascular stapler, that is, a stapler with a 3.0-mm staple height, in order to assure that the mesoappendiceal transection is hemostatic (Fig. 10-9A and B).

There is one case when the linear stapler is of unquestionable value. That is when the ap-

Figure 10-10
The cecum is transected **(A, B, C)** removing the appendix and its involved base with a portion of the cecum **(D)**.

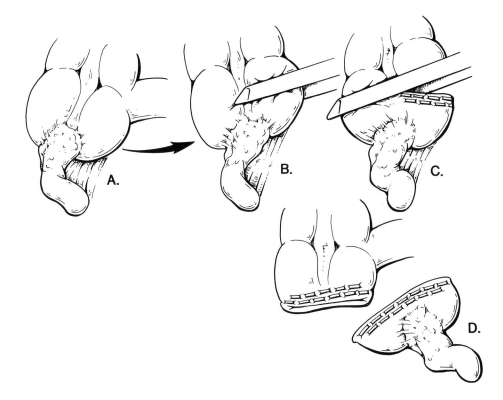

pendiceal stump is involved with the acute process and there is not enough room to place endoscopic suture loops. In this situation, the linear stapler can be used to transect the base of the cecum below the appendiceal stump in an area of healthy tissue (Fig. 10-10A, B, C, and D).

Once the appendix has been amputated, it must be removed from the abdominal cavity. This can be accomplished in a number of ways. How the appendix is removed depends to a great degree on the size of the appendix. The small appendix, that is, 10 mm or less in diameter, can be extracted directly through a trocar. This can be done, with or without using an endoscopic bag (see also Fig. 1-20A and B), remembering to open the valve as the appendix is being removed. If an endoscopic bag is not used, the trocar will be contaminated as the appendix is being withdrawn (Fig. 10-11A). Using a 10-mm extractor sleeve introduced through an 11-mm trocar will also prevent contamination of the

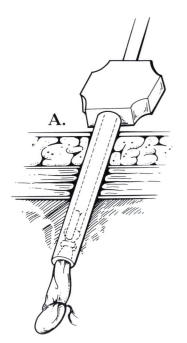

Figure 10-11
A. The appendix can be extracted directly through the trocar or withdrawn into an extractor sleeve (**B**), and the entire sleeve removed.

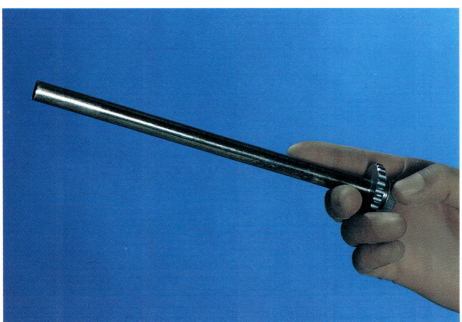

Figure 10-11
C. The appendix can be placed into an endoscopic bag.
D. The bag is withdrawn through the enlarged trocar incision after the trocar has been removed.

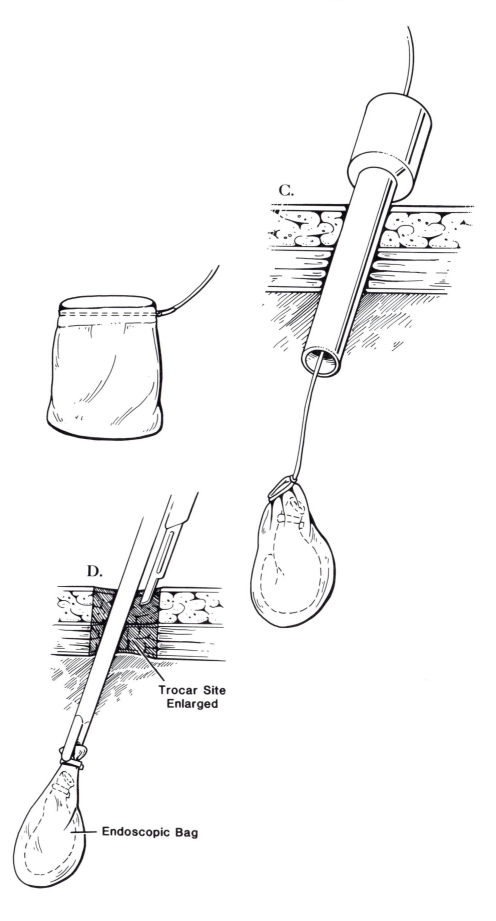

trocar (Fig. 10-11*B*, *C*, and *D*). If the appendix is too large to be removed in this manner, it can be extracted using an endoscopic bag that is placed into the abdominal cavity through a trocar. After the appendix is placed into the endoscopic bag, the trocar is removed. The trocar fascial defect is enlarged, and the bag is removed through the incision (Fig. 10-11*D*).

After the appendix has been amputated, the area should be inspected for any signs of bleeding as well as for the security of the appendiceal closure. If the appendix is to be removed either through a trocar or a sleeve, it should be removed at this point. The area is then copiously irrigated prior to decompression of the pneumoperitoneum and removal of the trocars. If the appendix is to be removed through an enlarged trocar site, this should be done after abdominal irrigation is carried out and the operation is completed because the pneumoperitoneum will be decompressed once the trocar is removed. If there is difficulty removing the appendix or if the surgeon wants to inspect the peritoneal cavity further, the incision that is used to extract the appendix can be closed and the pneumoperitoneum reinflated. Two trocar sites will still be available for inspection, manipulation, and irrigation. After the trocars are removed, the incisions are all closed. The 11- and 12-mm trocar sites should have the fascia closed with a single suture to prevent visceral herniation.

The Difficult Appendix

Retrocecal Appendicitis

The laparoscopic surgeon must also be able to handle the appendix that is not totally intraperitoneal. Retrocecal appendicitis should not be a reason to abandon the laparoscopic procedure and perform the operation open. There is little that distinguishes the two forms of appendicitis other than the fact that the retrocecal appendix is covered by a peritoneal leaf (Fig. 10-12).

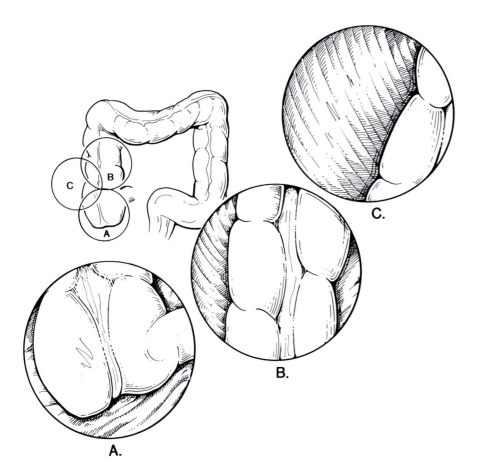

Figure 10-12
Cecum (**A**), ascending colon (**B**), and lateral peritoneum (**C**) visualized, but the appendix is not seen.

Once an intraperitoneal location cannot be identified, the retrocecal appendix must first be brought into an intraperitoneal location. The cecum and proximal ascending colon are grasped and retracted toward the midline (Fig. 10-13A). The lateral peritoneum is then incised with continued traction on the colon. This mobilization is usually accomplished by working in a bloodless plane (Fig. 10-13B). The dissection is then continued bluntly, as we look with a 45° telescope into the retroperitoneal area. The appendix will usually come into view very quickly (Fig. 10-13C). The subsequent steps are then the same as have been outlined for the routine intraperitoneal appendix.

Ruptured Appendicitis with Periappendiceal, Pericecal, or Retrocecal Abscess

The patient with ruptured appendicitis with either a periappendiceal, pericecal, or retrocecal abscess presents an increased challenge to the laparoscopic surgeon.[8] This is undoubtedly the most difficult type of appendectomy to perform laparoscopically. After the telescope is placed and a determination is made that there is indeed a ruptured appendix with an abscess, a decision must be made by the surgeon as to whether or not he or she has the technical expertise to perform the procedure laparoscopically. The surgeon must also decide whether or not the patient is best served by continuing with laparoscopic techniques. If the surgeon proceeds after answering those two questions, he or she must not be disturbed by bleeding or by the need to use rather gross dissection techniques to mobilize the appendix. It should be remembered that when an open appendectomy is performed in this situation, the entire dissection and mobilization of the appendix are performed not only bluntly but also blindly.

Employing laparoscopic techniques will not make ruptured appendicitis any less virulent. It will be necessary to admit the patient and deliver supportive care, including antibiotics, allowing the acute infectious process to subside.

The first step in the operation is to identify the cecum and ileum, which in turn identifies the location of the appendix. If necessary, the cecum and a portion of the right colon are mobilized to allow visualization of the abscess (Fig. 10-14A, B, and C). The abscess must then be opened. If it is a well-formed abscess, it should be incised using laser or cautery (Fig. 10-15). If the cavity is less well formed with structures that are loosely attached to each other, the dissection can be performed very easily using blunt dissectors, especially Kittner dissectors (Fig. 10-16).

Once the appendix is identified and removed, the wall of the abscess must be debrided as extensively as possible and the area copiously

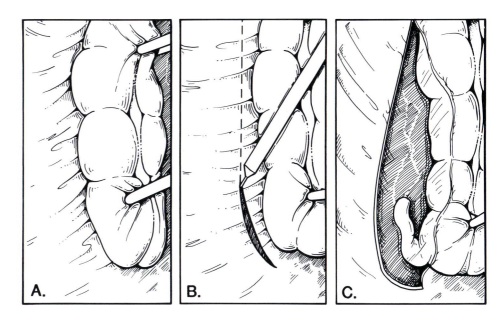

Figure 10-13
A. Cecum and ascending colon retracted toward the midline. Tension placed on the lateral peritoneum. **B.** Lateral peritoneum incised. **C.** Appendix visualized after peritoneum incised.

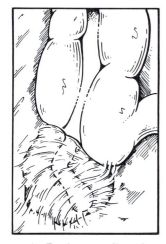 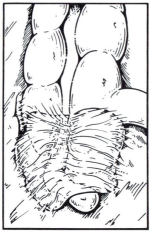 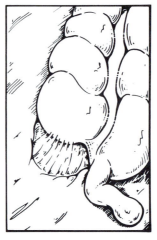

A. Periappendiceal   **B.** Pericecal   **C.** Retrocecal

Figure 10-14
Visualization of cecum and ileum that identifies location of appendix and surrounding abscess. The abscess can be in several locations.
A. Periappendiceal.
B. Pericecal.
C. Retrocecal.

irrigated (Fig. 10-17A and B). The debridement and irrigation can be performed much more completely laparoscopically than when using open techniques. The position the patient is kept in for irrigation varies; however, the surgeon should try to avoid steep Trendelenburg position in order to prevent excessive fluid from accumulating in the upper abdomen.

After the appendix has been removed, the stump secured, and the abscess debrided and irrigated, it may be necessary to place a drain. Drain placement through an existing trocar is the simplest method. The locations, however, of the trocars that are placed for laparoscopic appendectomy are generally not good for drains. A simple technique is to decide on an

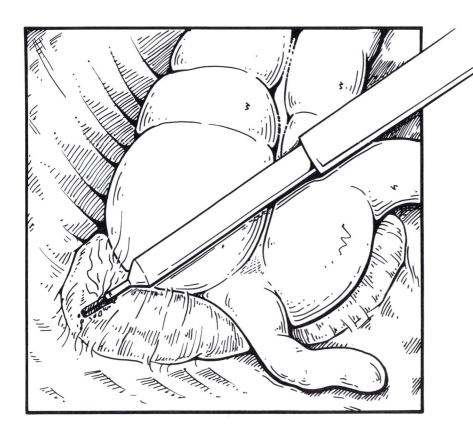

Figure 10-15
Abscess cavity being incised with the Nd:YAG contact laser or needle electrocautery.

Figure 10-16
Blunt Kittner dissection with traction on the ileum, using a grasper in order to separate cecum, ileum, and appendix.

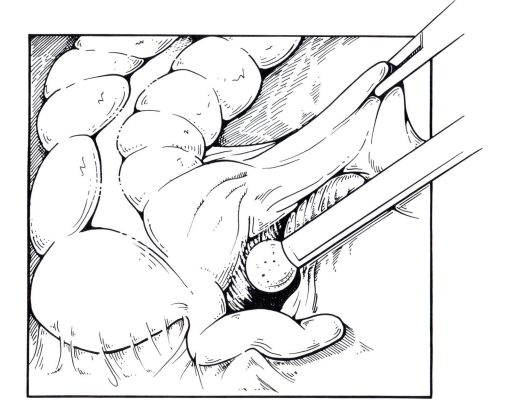

exit site for a drain and then puncture through into the peritoneal cavity at this location using a 5-mm trocar (10 mm if a larger drain is to be placed). The drain is then introduced down the largest trocar (suprapubic or lateral to umbilicus on the left) proximal end first. It is grasped with an instrument placed through the trocar at the drain exit site, and the trocar and end of the drain are removed through the puncture once the drain has been positioned intraperitoneally.

Advantages of Laparoscopic Appendectomy

There are a number of criticisms concerning laparoscopic appendectomy. First of all, the time required to perform the procedure has been said to be a problem. Laparoscopic appendectomy for most cases of acute appendicitis can, however, be performed quite quickly.

Figure 10-17
A. Wall of abscess extensively debrided.
B. Area copiously irrigated before drain placement.

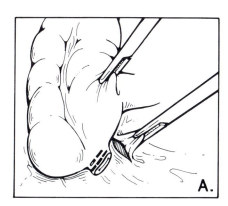
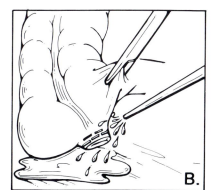

Most of the procedures can be completed in 30 to 45 min. The second major objection to this laparoscopic procedure regards the size of the incision. Open appendectomy can be performed through a very small incision. The incision in open appendectomy, however, is only the tip of the iceberg. When an open appendectomy is performed, there is a large amount of tissue trauma. The surgeon will mobilize the appendix by bluntly dissecting through this small incision. This technique also results in a certain degree of bleeding, which is inevitable. In addition, bowel is grasped and withdrawn into the incision in an attempt to locate the appendix. This process may induce a certain degree of ileus. With respect to laparoscopic appendectomy, these matters are often minimized. The appendix can be visualized and then removed with less surrounding trauma or bleeding.

The direct advantages of laparoscopic appendectomy are many. The trocars that are placed minimize incision size and therefore cosmesis is generally improved. The postoperative ileus that is usually seen with open appendectomy can be dramatically less with laparoscopic appendectomy. Oral intake can often be resumed soon after surgery.

Because of the absence of an ileus following uncomplicated laparoscopic removal of an early appendicitis, patients can be operated upon in an outpatient setting, thus saving hospital costs.

TABLE 10-1 Potential Advantages of Laparoscopic Appendectomy

Combination of diagnostic and therapeutic techniques
Small incisions
Improved cosmesis
Ability to treat other pathology through same incisions
Decreased tissue trauma
Decreased postoperative ileus
Rapid recovery
Procedure may be performed as an outpatient
Decreased postoperative pain
Reduced need for pain medication
Decreased risk of hernia formation
Decreased adhesion formation
Subsequent decreased risk of small bowel obstruction

TABLE 10-2 Potential Disadvantages of Laparoscopic Appendectomy

General laparoscopic complications
Increased operative time
Increased cost
Possibly multiple wound infections

Postoperative discomfort is less and pain medication requirements are therefore minimized. There is little need to restrict postoperative activity. Adhesion formation is likely to be decreased, thereby decreasing the risk of subsequent small bowel obstruction (see Tables 10-1 and 10-2).

The clear advantage gained by the increased diagnostic capabilities of laparoscopy can be employed to intercede earlier in the management of patients presenting with lower abdominal symptoms. In the 10 to 20 percent of patients in whom a normal appendix is encountered, the appendix can be removed rather easily and a better survey of the abdominal cavity performed than can be done via a small right lower quadrant incision. In the remaining patients who have acute appendicitis, early laparoscopy may result in treatment before rupture, preventing the more severe associated complications.

Further studies will delineate other true differences between the standard incisional appendectomy and the laparoscopic approach.

References

1. Semm K: Endoscopic appendectomy. *Endoscopy* 15:59–64, 1983.

2. Leahy PF: Technique of laparoscopic appendicectomy. *Br J Surg* 76(6):616–619, 1989.

3. Browne DS: Laparoscopic-guided appendicectomy. A study of 100 consecutive cases. *Aust N Z J Obstet Gynaecol* 30(3):231–233, 1991.

4. Gotz F, Pier A, Bacher C: Modified laparoscopic appendectomy in surgery. A report of 388 operations. *Surg Endosc* 4(1):6–9, 1990.

5. Graham A, Henley C, Mobley J: Laparoscopic evaluation of acute abdominal pain. *J Laparoendosc Surg* 1(3):165–168, 1991.

6. Daniell JF et al: The use of an automatic stapling device for laparoscopic appendectomy. *Obstet Gynecol* 78(4):721–723, 1991.

7. Nowzaradan Y et al: Laparoscopic appendectomy for acute appendicitis: Indications and current use. *J Laparoendosc Surg* 1(5):247–257, 1991.

8. Schultz LS et al: Retrograde laparoscopic appendectomy: Report of a case. *J Laparoendosc Surg* 1(2):111–114, 1991.

9. Chen S, Wilson T, Kent C: Laparoscopically assisted appendicectomy. Proceedings, Annual Registrars Paper Day, N.S.W. State Committee, Royal Australasian College of Surgeons. 6:17, 1987.

Bibliography

Schreiber JH: Laparoscopic appendectomy in pregnancy. *Surg Endosc* 4(2):100–102, 1990.

11

Laparoscopic Cholecystectomy

Leonard S. Schultz

In 1987, the French surgeon Philippe Mouret performed the first laparoscopic cholecystectomy. Dr. J. Perissat in Bordeaux and Dr. F. Dubois in Paris popularized the operation using electrocautery technology.[1-3] The first reports of the procedure in the United States were from our group (Schultz et al.)[4] and Dr. E. J. Reddick[5,6] in April 1989 at the American Society of Laser Medicine and Surgery. Dr. J. B. McKernan and Dr. W. B. Saye were also instrumental in the development of the procedure[7] and were probably the first physicians to perform a clinical case in this country.

Dr. E. J. Reddick and Dr. D. O. Olsen went on to popularize this procedure in the United States.[6,8] Unlike our French counterparts, Dr. Reddick's and our group used laser technology, which was popular in the United States since the mid-1980s.[9-12]

Within one year of the introduction of laparoscopic cholecystectomy to the United States, other surgeons entered the field, relying on electrocautery methods.[13-15] Although it has been our practice to have the surgeon stay on the right side of the patient, the more popular position for the surgeon in the United States has been on the patient's left, as described by Reddick and Olsen. The most successful results have occurred where operative teams have developed.[16] Usually two surgeons consistently work together to carry out the procedure. In the past 2 years, techniques have improved and a clear understanding and an appreciation for the differences in visualization of the gallbladder as seen laparoscopically have emerged. As a result, complication rates and operating times have diminished and the possibility of routine outpatient cholecystectomy has more recently become a clinical reality.

Back in 1988, the media and scholastic pressures on surgeons from medical groups claiming to have a better method of treatment for cholecystitis and cholelithiasis made the gallbladder the obvious organ for laparoscopic treatment. In fact, the ultrasonic shock wave lithotripsy became a rather popular, albeit partially effective, method of treatment for those individuals who desired to avoid a surgical incision and its consequences.[17]

In 1988, we carried out laboratory evaluations of laparoscopic cholecystectomy in the canine model. During this time, we developed a technique of cystic duct occlusion that involved use of a compressive clip that was for-

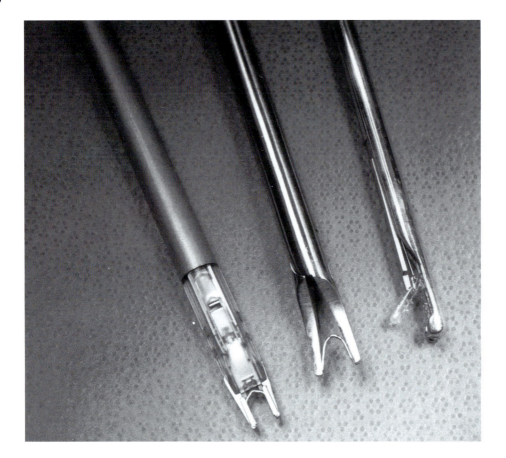

Figure 11-1
Initially, the cystic duct was secured with the Hulka clip seen on the right side of the photograph. Newer occlusion devices include the single reusable and multiple disposable clip appliers.

merly used for laparoscopic tubal ligation (Fig. 11-1). Five of these animals were maintained postoperatively for up to 4 months. They were sacrificed at 1, 2, 3, and 4 months. Results showed that the procedure could be done safely and effectively.

A separate technique for management of the deep intrahepatic gallbladder (Fig. 11-2) was also developed in the canine model. In these cases, the anterior wall of the gallbladder was removed and then a free beam fiber of the neodymium: yttrium-aluminum-garnet (Nd:YAG) laser at various doses of power was used to ablate the remaining posterior wall. The appropriate dosimetry was determined so as not to penetrate too deeply into the liver substance.

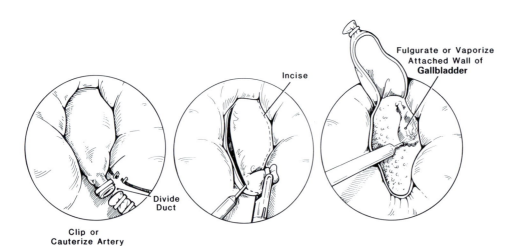

Figure 11-2
After the surgeon secures the cystic duct and artery, the front wall is excised and removed along with stone debris and bile. The residual mucosa is ablated.

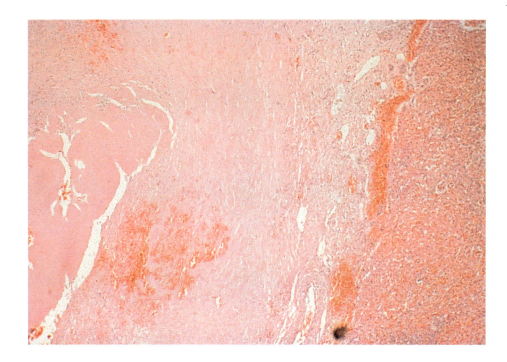

Figure 11-3
Gallbladder mucosa and adjacent liver 3 months after laser ablation. Typical hyalinization reaction following lasing seen to the left; normal liver parenchyma to the right side of the photomicrograph.

Multiple trials in the canine model indicated that doses of 50 to 60 W of power with the fiber held 1 cm from the tissue in individual pulses of 0.5 s resulted in complete ablation of the mucosa with depth of penetration into the liver of no more than 3 to 4 mm (Fig. 11-3). When this method was first transferred to the operating room, the usual sequence was to carry out routine laparoscopic cholecystectomy and then subject the extracted gallbladder to the effects of the laser immediately following removal to assess the ability of this laser to ablate the mucosa completely.

To determine whether gallstones that might have spilled into the peritoneal cavity could serve as a nidus for infection, a separate series of studies were done in the rabbit model. Human gallstones were harvested and 5 of them were placed in the right subhepatic space through a small subcostal incision. Animals were allowed to recover for a period of 1 month and then autopsied. Studies indicated that a gelatinous film was formed around the gallstones and that they remained on the right side of the abdomen. No evidence of injury to any abdominal tissue nor evidence of infection was noted. Pathologic examination of the gallstones indicated the presence of foreign body giant cells within the gelatinous coating (Fig. 11-4). It was presumed, but of course never proven, that the same process occurred in human beings when gallstone material was left within the abdomen. This study has been repeated recently with similar results.[18]

With these three aspects of the experimental protocols completed, i.e., the technique and instrumentation, the management of intrahepatic gallbladders, and consequence of residual stone debris understood, attention was drawn to clinical trials.

Initial Clinical Cases

As general surgeons, the authors were relatively unskilled in laparoscopy and found it both necessary and wise to team up with an experienced group of gynecologists who were skilled in therapeutic laparoscopic techniques. As a combined effort, a clinical protocol, entitled "Laser Laparoscopic Cholecystectomy," was submitted to the Institutional Review Board of Abbott Northwestern Hospital in Minneapolis, Minnesota, and was approved for 100 patients. We proceeded with our first clinical case on April 6, 1989. That surgery took 3 h to perform. The

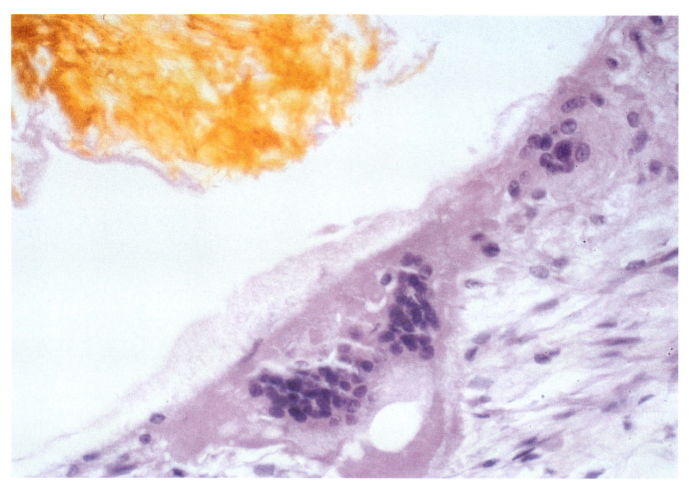

Figure 11-4
The foreign body giant cell is seen at the 5-o'clock position within a fibrous tissue reaction. The yellow gallstone can be seen to the left of the photomicrograph.

patient had moderate postoperative nausea and shoulder strap pain, took meperidine hydrochloride intramuscularly and acetaminophen with ½ grain of codeine, was in the hospital for 3 days but returned to work in 11 days. A member of the same gynecologic group assisted us in the first 80 patients; thereafter, the group's inclusion in our clinical work dropped dramatically. Currently, one of our general surgical group works singly with a skilled operating room technician to carry out the procedure. The results, complications, and changes in operative technique arising from the first 300 patients formed the basis of this chapter.

Outcome data from the first 300 patients have been reviewed. The age range of the patients was from 18 to 86 years, with the average age being 47.5 years. One notes that the majority of patients seen in this elective series involved patients who were employed and/or had families to care for at home.

In the initial 100 patients, there were 61 females and 39 males. The patients were taken in sequence and were entered into an Institutional Review Board (IRB) protocol. It was made quite clear to them that a standard method of surgery was available to them if they wished and that there may be increased risks and potential complications with the newer technique of laparoscopic surgery. With this full knowledge and understanding, they were allowed into the study. Separate consent forms, independent of operative permissions, were presented to the patients and these were signed and kept as part of the office file when patients entered into the study. A modification of these initial consent forms are still reviewed and signed with each of our patients.

Operative Technique

The clinical technique is not that different from the initial laboratory methods. The overall operating room (OR) setup is depicted in Fig. 11-5. The surgeon stays on the right-hand side of the patient and four ports of entry into the abdominal cavity are utilized (Fig. 11-6). After the patient receives general inhalation anesthesia, a nasogastric tube is inserted for gastric decompression and removed at the end of the case. The patients are given an antibiotic, 20 mg of metoclopramide hydrochloride (Reglan) and 1 mg of midazolam hydrochloride (Versed) intravenously (IV) as an antiemetic protocol and 60 mg of ketorolac tromethamine (Toradol) intramuscularly (IM) for postoperative pain relief.

After a standard prep of the abdominal cavity, the surgeon starts the operation on the left side of the patient and makes a small incision cephalad to the umbilicus for insertion of the Verres needle through which CO_2 is insufflated to induce standard pneumoperitoneum. Occasionally, this location may vary depending upon whether or not there is a scar present in the upper abdomen. If there is, then the needle can be placed below the umbilicus. In the setting of a long midline scar, the Verres needle can be placed lateral to the rectus sheath in the right or left lower quadrants. Current use of the Hasson cannula placed under direct vision is appropriate in difficult cases.

After placement of the standard 10-mm can-

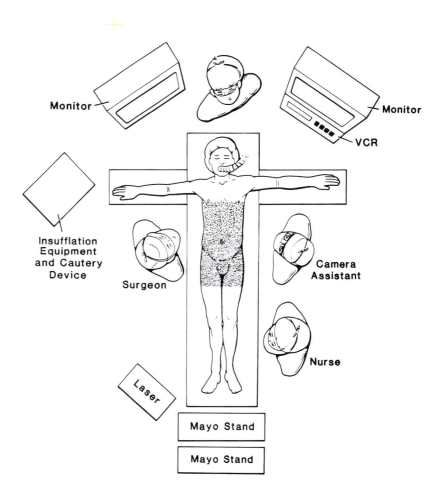

Figure 11-5
Operating room setup.

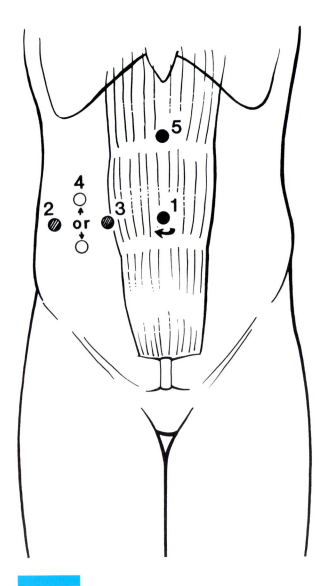

Figure 11-6
Trocar Placement.
Numerals refer to chronological order of insertion.
Trocar No.1: 10-mm trocar used exclusively for the laparoscope and attached camera.
Torcar No.2: 5-mm trocar placed about 3 cm from the costal margin in the anterior axillary line. Instruments used here include bipolar cautery, scissors, dissecting, and toothed graspers.
Trocar No.3: 10- to 11-mm trocar placed lateral to the rectus sheath. Used for pelviscopic claw for upward retraction of the gallbladder neck.
Trocar No.4: 10- to 11-mm trocar placed midway between but not in the same line as 2 or 3 to avoid "fencing." Placed closer to the costal margin if the patient is obese. Instruments used include clip appliers, suction irrigator, laser fiber, and/or bipolar forceps cautery.
Trocar No.5: See page 130.

nula, a 45° angle laparoscope is introduced and the abdominal and pelvic contents are visualized on dual monitors placed at either side of the head of the operating table. After a general inspection is completed, the surgeon gives control of the laparoscope to the assistant. A 5-mm cannula is inserted in the right anterior axillary line about three finger breadths away from the costal margin. We have learned that in order to avoid postoperative costochondritis, one must be careful to avoid placing any cannula close to the costal margin. Pain resulting from cannula pressure against the rib margin has lasted as long as 3 months.

With the patient in a neutral position, a bi-toothed grasping forceps is passed through the 5-mm cannula and is used to retract the fundus of the gallbladder up to the anterior abdominal wall. It is our practice to carry out a cholecystcholangiogram as the initial part of the procedure. This technique is detailed in Chap. 12. The x-rays are taken with the surgeon standing behind a protective lead shield attached to an IV stand and covered with a sterile drape (Fig. 11-7). After the x-rays are taken, excess dye is then aspirated so as to collapse the gallbladder and make it easier for the pelviscopic tenaculum to grab the gallbladder for retraction (Fig. 11-8).

A 10- to 11-mm cannula is then placed to the right of the umbilicus and somewhat cephalad, lateral to the rectus muscle. Care must be taken to avoid entry into the rectus sheath because any bleeding within the sheath can cause spasm that results in marked pain for the patient and prolonged hospitalization. A pelviscopic tenaculum is passed through the cannula and is used to grab the neck of the gallbladder and retract it up toward the right shoulder. This retraction, in conjunction with the 45° angle "scope," provides sufficient visualization for dissection of the gallbladder. The patient is now placed in the reverse Trendelenburg position.

Through the lateral 5-mm cannula, bipolar forceps cautery is then used to cauterize the serosa over the neck of the gallbladder, followed by the use of a scissors to divide the serosa (Fig. 11-9). The cut is then extended down along the free edge of the cystic duct, avoiding the medial

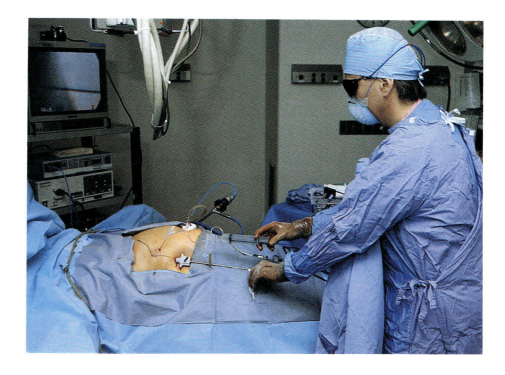

Figure 11-7
Only the surgeon need be present to perform routine cholecyst-cholangiography.

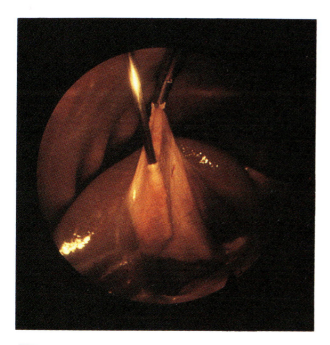

Figure 11-8
Excess dye has been removed to decompress the gallbladder in preparation for retraction by the 10-mm pelviscopic "claw."

side of the duct and therefore avoiding the cystic artery. The orientation of the hepatoduodenal ligament is in a diagonal direction with the gallbladder up toward the "northwest" part of the video monitor and the common bile duct down toward the "southeast" corner of the video monitor. This diagonal orientation throws the cystic duct lateral, out toward the surgeon while the cystic artery remains medial and somewhat hidden from view. This is not a disadvantage, however, because initial concern is with the cystic duct that is dissected free from the neck of the gallbladder down toward the common bile duct where exact identification of the cystic duct and common bile duct junction is made (Fig. 11-9 A and B). This dissection is made considerably easier with the recent addition of the laparoscopic Kittner and right-angled microdissector (Fig. 11-10).

The dissection of the cystic duct deserves special mention because of potential misidentification with the common bile duct. Three points of technique are worth emphasizing. First, try to determine the presence or absence of a cystic duct by doing a cholecystcholangiogram early in the procedure and looking at it

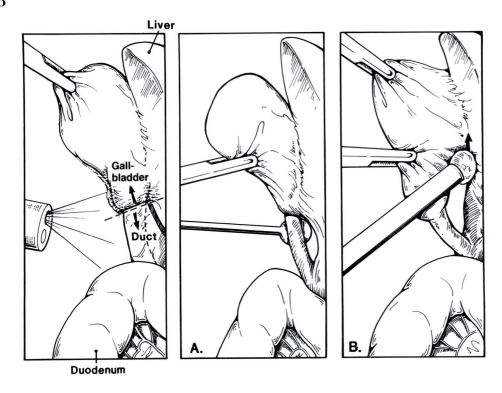

Figure 11-9
Dissection is always begun on the neck of the gallbladder with cauterization of the serosa. If you cannot easily identify the neck, look to where the posterior gallbladder serosa attaches to the liver and imagine a line perpendicular and cephalad to this site to approximate the starting point. **A** and **B**. The Kittner should be used to delineate tissue on the hepatic side of the gallbladder–cystic duct junction, while the right-angled microdissector is ideal for separating the cystic duct from adjacent tissue.

carefully. If no cystic duct is seen, as will be the case with obstruction due to an impacted stone, proceed with care to obtain absolute identification of the cystic duct. If the duct is present but very short, be prepared to start the dissection well up on the gallbladder and anticipate the need of a loop knot to secure adequate closure of the cystic duct stump. Second,

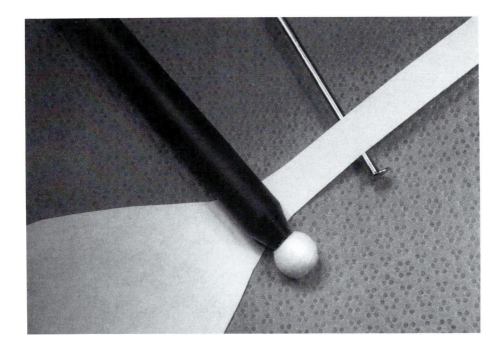

Figure 11-10
10-mm Kittner and right-angle dissector used for cystic duct dissection.

provide lateral traction to the infundibulum with a bi-toothed grasper passed through the most lateral port and dissect the cystic duct through the last of four cannulas now placed between the 5- and 10-mm cannula in the right upper quadrant. Certainly, this traction that opens the space between the medial side of the duct and the liver allows thorough visualization of the medial side of the neck of the gallbladder where a hepatic duct may be found in the case of an absent or of a congenitally short cystic duct. The cystic artery may also be visualized better in this manner.

Third, it may be best to secure and divide the duct before dissecting out the artery. Such a sequence prevents inadvertent proximal arterial bleeding because, with the duct first divided, the artery can be cauterized or clipped as it enters the gallbladder away from the hepatic artery and other structures.

After thorough cystic duct dissection, a clip applicator is passed through the second most lateral cannula and is used to place 2 to 3 clips on the proximal cystic duct and 1 on the gallbladder side of the duct. The device is then removed and the trocar opening is covered with a 5-mm reducer. Through this is inserted a series of instruments, including a scissors to cut the duct and a bipolar forceps cautery to coagulate the cystic artery adjacent to the gallbladder (Fig. 11-11*A, B,* and *C*). By coagulating the artery up on the gallbladder, there is less chance of losing the cystic artery into the hilum of the liver following its division where retrieval of the artery is almost impossible. Even if control of the artery were lost, there would still be an adequate length to retrieve it easily. Our preferred choice of dealing with the artery is to cauterize it with the bipolar cautery taking at least 3 widths of the paddles and continuing cauterization at maximum power until a flat black char occurs indicating desiccation and cauterization of the distal artery (Fig. 11-12). Once secured, the artery is cut and the dissection of the gallbladder is carried out from below upward.

The use of lasers or cautery has been reported for this part of the operation (Fig. 11-13). It is important to use the graspers so that traction is applied to the gallbladder-liver plane regardless of the dissection device used. It is necessary to rearrange the position of the graspers several times to accomplish this as the gallbladder is removed. Although it is usually possible to stay

Figure 11-11
Following placement of individual clips on the cystic duct **(A),** the cystic duct is divided **(B)** and traction on the neck of the gallbladder away from the liver is applied. This more clearly exposes the cystic artery **(C).** Securing the cystic artery immediately adjacent to the gallbladder allows adequate length for retrieval of the artery should bleeding develop. This can be done with bipolar cautery or clips.

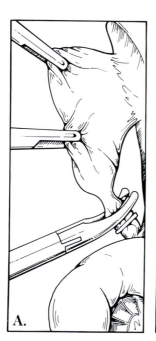
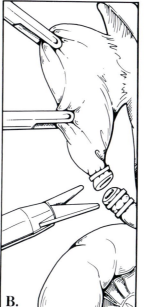
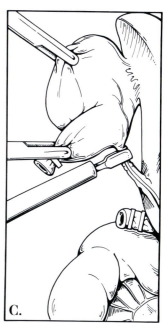

A.   B.   C.

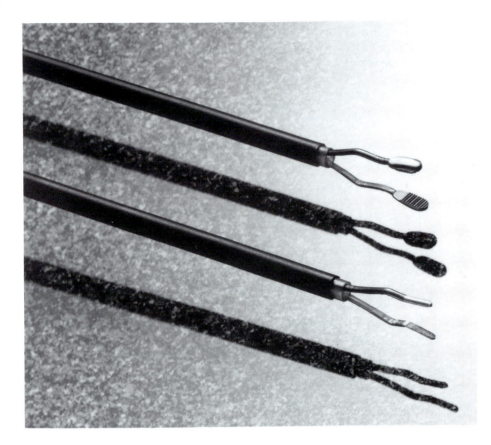

Figure 11-12
Examples of currently available disposable bipolar forceps (Everest Medical).

within the plane of dissection and experience little bleeding, significant blood loss from the liver bed can be encountered. Often this can be controlled within moments by compression using the 10-mm blunt-ended pelviscopic "scoop" or with a newly introduced 10-mm laparoscopic Kittner. Excellent suction irrigation devices and an angled laparoscope are invaluable in such a situation. Persistent oozing along the cut serosal edge is handled well with bipolar cautery. For controlling bleeding that occurs in the bed of the liver, monopolar cautery is excellent.

Recently, we have used the holmium:yttrium-aluminum-garnet (Ho:YAG) laser to dissect the gallbladder off the liver. This laser's

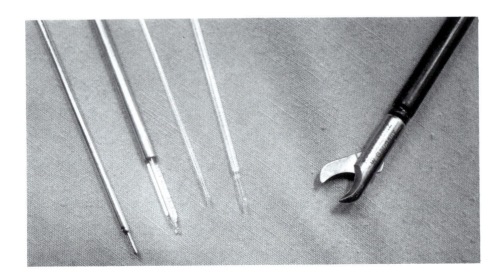

Figure 11-13
Devices used for separation of the gallbladder from the liver bed. Laser fibers to the left and electrosurgical device (monopolar) to the right. (See also Fig. 1-14.)

Chapter 11 Laparoscopic Cholecystectomy

Before you completely remove the gallbladder from the liver, the liver bed and the cystic duct are rechecked for any evidence of bile leakage or bleeding (Fig. 11-14). The placement of the clips is observed to be sure they have not been dislodged. Once this is completed, the gallbladder is removed from its last serosal attachment.

In more than 85 percent of cases, the gallbladder grasped at its neck with a tenaculum will come out rather nicely through the widest trocar (Fig. 11-15). On occasion, however, large or multiple stones or excess bile will require some alternative method for removal of the gallbladder.[19]

You can open the gallbladder internally and use a pelviscopic scoop to take out a large stone, crush it into 2 or 3 smaller pieces, and then remove each separately (Fig. 11-16). On occasion, you can scoop up multiple small stones in a similar manner and then remove the gallbladder tissue with a tenaculum. The purpose of this method is to try to avoid an incision. Another technique, developed by Dr. Reddick, is to bring the gallbladder partially into a trocar and then lead it out of the abdominal cavity and then clamp the gallbladder, which is essentially half in and half out of the abdominal wall. A Randall stone or ring forceps is then used to remove stones from the intraabdominal portion of the gallbladder until the volume is small enough to be removed through the fascia (Fig. 11-17). Occasionally, one of these two methods will fail, requiring the surgeon to make a larger abdominal wall incision, preferably at the umbilical site, to remove the gallbladder and then suture the fascia closed. Although each method of removal can result in either abdominal or puncture site infection, the important thing is to remember to irrigate prior to concluding the procedure.

After removal of the gallbladder and its contents, copiously irrigate the right upper quadrant with 1 to 2 liters of saline. The patient should be placed in Trendelenburg position and rotated toward the right side to allow the irrigant to pool in the right lateral sulcus between the liver and the chest wall and the diaphragm. Under direct vision, the suction-irrigation device is placed into the right upper quadrant lateral

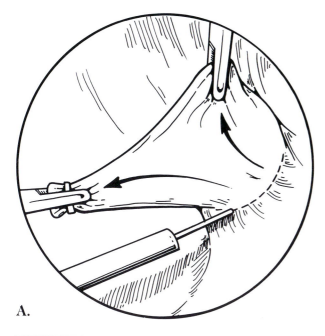

A.

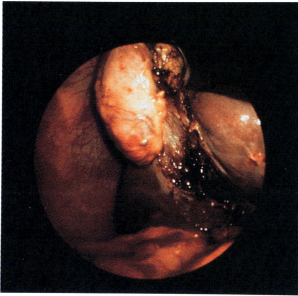

B.

Figure 11-14
A and **B.** Nd:YAG "contact" laser fiber at 20 W being used to incise the serosa. Note two separate directions of traction on the gallbladder. Photo **(B)** shows gallbladder almost completely removed. Now is when one should inspect the subhepatic space for the last time.

wavelength is absorbed almost completely by the high water content found in the surgical planes separating the two tissues. The result is a dry bed and a rapid dissection.

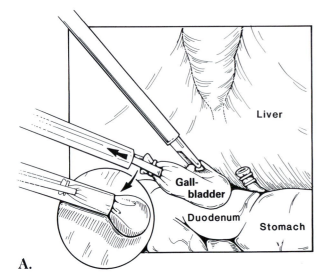

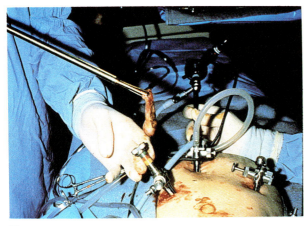

Figure 11-15
A and **B.** To prevent losing the gallbladder among coils of small intestine, keep the open end of the trocar adjacent to the liver edge and the tissue in continuous sight until complete removal from the abdominal cavity. The slide (**B**) shows the gallbladder after emergence from the trocar.

to the liver, taking care not to push it into the lower internal rib margins (Fig. 11-18). Such inadvertent rib trauma can induce significant posterior-lateral sharp pleuriticlike pain that can mimic pulmonary embolism or renal problems that can last for months. To prevent this, press the rigid suction irrigation cannula gently against the right side of the liver to avoid any pressure on the internal surface of the ribs.

Once the saline irrigant is clear of any blood or bile tracings, the suction irrigation device is removed, the anesthesiologist holds the patient in inspiration while the cannula valves are held open, and the surgeon and assistant compress the abdomen to remove as much CO_2 gas as possible. When there is no further egress of gas noted, the trocars are removed. The patient is replaced in a neutral position and the skin of the puncture site is approximated with a single subcuticular absorbable suture and strip tape. Minimal dressings are placed and the N/G tube is removed.

An alternative placement of cannulas, described by Reddick,[8] calls for inserting a subxiphoid cannula, another in the right anterior axillary line, and a third in the right midclavicular line in addition to the umbilical port. The surgeon stands on the patient's left side with an assistant surgeon on the right. The operation then proceeds in a generally similar fashion with the dissection carried out primarily through the subxiphoid port.

Drains

As a rule, drains are not placed following laparoscopic cholecystectomy, although liberal use of these drains was made early in the series. In fact, 17 drains were placed in as many patients, but no particular effect on the ultimate outcome of the patient was noted. The 1 patient in whom a serious postoperative right subhepatic infection developed had a drain placed and removed the following day.

Indications for Surgery

The advent of laparoscopic techniques has not changed the normal customary indications for surgery. The patients were operated upon if they had continuing symptoms despite low-fat diet management with objective evidence of gallbladder disease, notably cholelithiasis (Table 11-1). The occurrence of an acute attack some 6 to 12 months ago but without continuing

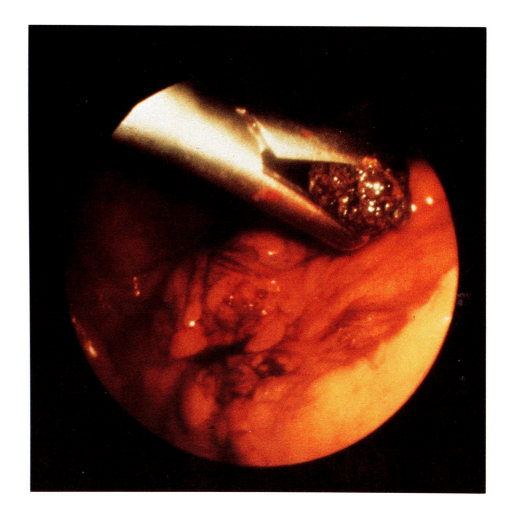

Figure 11-16
One should be conscientious regarding removal of small fragments but not fanatic. The "scoop" serves this purpose well. Copious irrigation until returns are clear is mandatory.

symptoms on diet management did not constitute adequate indications for surgery. Although initial patients did not include anyone who had previous upper abdominal surgery, this is no longer considered a contraindication; nor do we consider acute symptomatology a contraindication to laparoscopy. Morbid exogenous obesity in excess of 300 lb may prevent successful surgery because current instrumentation is not long enough to traverse the abdominal wall and allow surgical manipulation. Such factors as a history of lower extremity phlebitis or use of anticoagulants require special consideration but are not contraindications.

Follow-up has indicated that 6 percent of our patients present to the operating room with acute cholecystitis secondary to cystic duct obstruction (Table 11-2). Persistence in increasing technical skills has allowed these types of cases to be successfully completed in later patients without conversion to laparotomy. This was not true in the first few patients, where 4 of the first 5 acute cholecystitis patients were in fact opened after unsuccessful attempts at dissection of the cystic duct–common duct areas (Table 11-3).

Previous surgery is not a contraindication to laparoscopic cholecystectomy, although, on occasion, you have to be patient and careful in lysing intraabdominal adhesions. The most commonly encountered adhesions are those from previous appendectomy. In this case, the scope can be rotated to the patient's left and then passed underneath the falciform ligament to the right upper quadrant.

Patients who present with jaundice preoperatively should undergo endoscopic retrograde cholangiopancreatography (ERCP) shortly af-

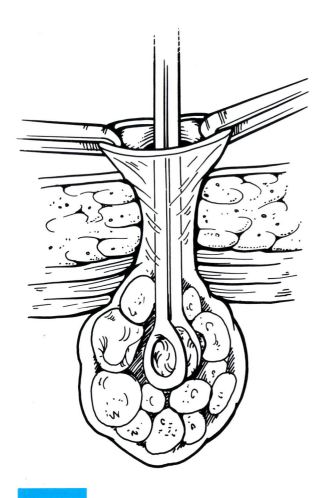

Figure 11-17
On occasion, a finger inserted through an adjacent puncture site can aid gallstone removal by stabilizing the gallbladder. Usually ring forceps will suffice as indicated in this diagram.

ter initial workup, and if the patient does well, we proceed with laparoscopic cholecystectomy the next day presuming the cause of jaundice is common bile duct stones. Alternatively, in those who present with gallstone pancreatitis, we will attempt to cool down the acute inflammatory process and have them return in 3 weeks for elective laparoscopic cholecystectomy. We have, of course, performed laparoscopic cholecystectomy in the presence of minimally elevated urine amylase and have usually found this not to be particularly difficult in the technical sense. However, we adhere to the concept that doing gallbladder surgery in a relatively uninflamed field will provide an additional margin of safety.

Results

Observation of early groups of patients indicated that they were often ready for discharge within 24 h or less after their surgery. For this reason, toward the conclusion of the IRB study of the first 100 cases, patients were usually discharged after a brief overnight stay. Experience with larger numbers of patients has indicated that reasonable operative times and antinausea and improved analgesia protocols have allowed discharge from the operating facility within a few hours after the conclusion of the surgery. This has been confirmed by others.[20,21]

Approximately 30 percent of patients had right shoulder strap pain in association with subdiaphragmatic irritation from retained CO_2 pneumoperitoneum, with pain referred via the phrenic nerve to the shoulder (Table 11-4). This pain was usually transient although it has been known to last 2 to 3 weeks in some patients. Usually it is perceived by the patient as a soreness rather than as a true sharp pain.

Abdominal wall pain was rather rare to see except if trocars were passed through the rectus sheath, which occurred in only two cases that resulted in marked postoperative muscle spasm, requiring muscle relaxants for relief. Now every caution is taken to be sure that the rectus sheath is not traversed to prevent postoperative bleeding within a closed space. Care should be taken with the most lateral trocar to prevent it from putting pressure on the right costal margin.

Nausea was a considerable problem early in the series and necessitated development of an antinausea protocol in order to facilitate early feedings. Initial use of antiemetics such as intramuscular prochlorperazine or trimethobenzamide hydrochloride were not adequate. Oncological and anesthesia consultations were sought in development of a drug protocol. Lorazepam caused agitation in postoperative patients. A scopolamine patch proved unsuitable for elderly patients because it was capable of inducing moderate to severe hallucinations and generally disturbed psyche in the postoperative period. The combination of midazolam hydrochloride 1 mg IV and metoclopramide hy-

Chapter 11 Laparoscopic Cholecystectomy

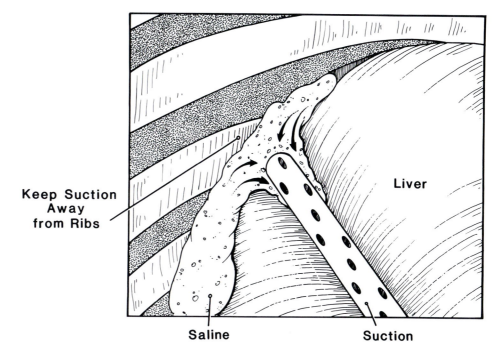

Figure 11-18
Avoid touching the internal rib surfaces with a hard suction tip to prevent postoperative chondritis in the posterolateral chest wall.

drochloride 20 mg IV following induction has served as an excellent antinausea combination, reducing the incidence of nausea from 21 percent in our first 100 patients down to 5 percent in the last third of the 300 patients examined (Table 11-5).

Following dismissal from the hospital after an approximate 24-h admission or from the day

TABLE 11-1 Comparison of Pre- and Postoperative Diagnosis

Preop dx.	
Chronic cholecystitis	100%
Cholelithiasis	99%
Postop dx.	
Chronic cholecystitis	99%
Acute cholecystitis	5.7%

Review of initial 300 patients undergoing laser laparoscopic cholecystectomy. Clinical Diagnosis.

TABLE 11-2 Pathology of Specimen Removed during Laparoscopic Cholecystectomy

Chronic cholecystitis	99%
Acute cholecystitis	5.7%
Cholesterolosis	10%
Cholelithiasis	93%

Review of initial 300 patients undergoing laser laparoscopic cholecystectomy. Pathology.

TABLE 11-3 Conversion Rate to Open Cholecystectomy

Consecutive Case Number	Number
1–100	6
101–200	1
201–300	2
Incidence 3%	

Review of initial 300 patients undergoing laser laparoscopic cholecystectomy. Conversion to open conventional cholecystectomy.

TABLE 11-4 Postoperative Pain—Location

Description	No. of Patients	Percent
Shoulder strap	92	30.1
Puncture site	58	19.3
Rt subcostal site/RUQ	27	9.0
Rt rib	15	5.0
Nonlocalized abdomen	10	3.3
Back	4	1.3

Review of initial 300 patients undergoing laser laparoscopic cholecystectomy. Postoperative pain location.

TABLE 11-5 Incidence of Postoperative Nausea

Consecutive Case Numbers	Percent Experiencing Postop Nausea 12 h
1–100	21
101–200	18
201–300	5

Review of initial 300 patients undergoing laser laparoscopic cholecystectomy. Incidence of nausea (%).

surgery unit, additional outcome data indicated the return of these patients to gainful employment or unrestricted activity within 5 to 6 days (Table 11-6). This rather prompt recovery in contrast to the standard 3- to 6-week convalescence for open cholecystectomy indicates the predictability of patient behavior when the abdominal incision is eliminated.

Complications

Complications of laparoscopic cholecystectomy are reviewed in Chap. 17. It is clear that the only matter more important than diagnosis and management of complications is their prevention. All surgeons need to know what the potential problems are and how to avoid them.

Future

The introduction of laparoscopic cholecystectomy to the general surgical community has ushered in an era of minimally invasive surgery

TABLE 11-6 Postoperative Interval Until Return to Functional Activity (Days)

Consecutive Case Numbers	Return to Activities of Daily Living	Return to Employment without Restriction
1–100	2.9	5.4
101–200	3.2	5.3
201–300	3.2	5.8

Review of initial 300 patients undergoing laser laparoscopic cholecystectomy. Return to activities of daily living (days). Return to gainful employment (days).

for the other surgical disciplines. Today, the uses of laparoscopic technology for hysterectomy and nephrectomy have become realities as have its uses for gastric ulcer and resective bowel surgery. The shortened postoperative convalescence and reduced morbidity with an almost immediate return to unrestricted activity and employment have been revolutionary. The positive economic impact that these phenomena have had and will continue to have is astounding. Of further importance is the fact that simplification of many of these operative procedures has now made it possible to think of their being routinely performed in more cost-efficient environments such as ambulatory surgical centers and in private offices properly equipped for major operative procedures.

An example of this type of technological advance was recently introduced by us in April 1991[22] and was named "laser laparolithic cholecystectomy." The technique, demonstrated in Fig. 11-19, uses a rotor device held within a plastic protective cage that, upon activation, produces a vortex that draws gallstones to the blade, resulting in their emulsification. Acute and chronic laboratory work in the canine and porcine models indicates complete destruction of stones within 10 to 15 s without any evidence of trauma to adjacent tissue.[23] Following removal of debris, the front wall is excised and removed for pathologic examination and the remaining mucosa ablated with free beam Ho:YAG or Nd:YAG lasers. No clinically significant liver injury has been noted.

Early trials in patients indicate reduction of operating time (total operating time now being 30 min or less), elimination of bleeding because the gallbladder need not be dissected from the liver bed, and avoidance of spillage of biliary contents from the gallbladder as it is passed through the abdominal wall. No complications have occurred in patients followed for up to 1 year. Such methodology allowing for a change in venue for a major surgery will undoubtedly have a significant impact on hospital revenues that is yet to be felt. These changes, while both profound and revolutionary, are no more than the normal evolution in the proper and ethical application of modern technology for the benefit of the patient and for society.

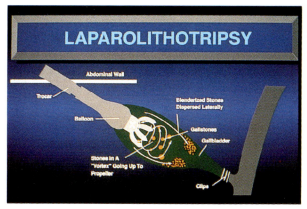

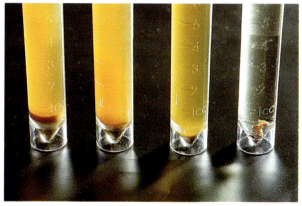

Figure 11-19
A. Diagram demonstrating the mechanism of 10 s of gallstone lithotripsy with the "laparolith." **B.** Note the test tube with untreated, intact stones, while the other three contain gallbladder aspirate following 10 s of laparolithic emulsification of stones.

References

1. Perissat J, Collet D, Belliard R: Laparoscopic treatment, intracorporeal lithotripsy followed by cholecystostomy or cholecystectomy—a personal technique. *Endoscopy* 21:373–374, 1989.

2. Perissat J, Collet D, Belliard R: Gallstones: Laparoscopic treatment—cholecystectomy, cholecystostomy, and lithotripsy. *Surg Endosc* 4:1–5, 1990.

3. Dubois F, Card P: Coelioscopic cholecystectomy: A preliminary report of 36 cases. *Ann Surg* 211:60–62, 1990.

4. Schultz L, Graber J, Hickok D: Laser laparoscopic cholecystectomy, a laboratory study (abstract). Presented American Society for Laser Medicine and Surgery, Arlington, VA, April 1989.

5. Reddick EJ: Laparoscopic laser cholecystectomy. *Clin Laser Monthly* 6(10):400–401, 1988.

6. Reddick EJ et al: Laparoscopic laser cholecystectomy. *Laser Med Surg News Advances* 2:38–40, 1989.

7. McKernan JB, Lawas HJ: Laparoscopic cholecystectomy. *Surg Rounds* 737–746, September 1991.

8. Reddick EJ, Olsen DO: Laparoscopic laser cholecystectomy: A comparison with minilap cholecystectomy. *Surg Endosc* 3:131–133, 1989.

9. Schultz LS et al: The use of lasers in general surgery: A preliminary assessment. *Minn Med* 70:439–442, 1987.

10. Schultz LS et al: Lasers in the treatment of intra-abdominal malignancy. *Laser Med Surg News Advances* 5:15–20, 1987.

11. Rubio PS, Rowe G, Feste JR: Endoscopic laser cholecystectomy. *Houston Med J* 5:125–126, 1989.

12. Lanzafame RJ: Applications of lasers in laparoscopic cholecystectomy. *J Laparoendosc Surg* 1:33–36, 1990.

13. Zucker KA et al: Laparoscopic guided cholecystectomy. *Am J Surg* 161:36–44, 1991.

14. Voyles CR et al: Electrocautery is superior to laser for laparoscopic cholecystectomy (editorial). *Am J Surg* 160–457, 1990.

15. Gadacz TR et al: Laparoscopic cholecystectomy. *Surg Clin North Am* 70:1249–1262, 1990.

16. Phillips E et al: Laparoscopic cholecystectomy: Instrumentation and technique. *J Laparoendosc Surg* 1:3–15, 1990.

17. Vergunst H, Tempstra OT: Extracorporeal shockwave lithotripsy of gallstones: Possibilities and limitations. *Ann Surg* 210:565–574, 1989.

18. Welch N et al: Gallstones in the peritoneal cavity: A clinical and experimental study. *Surg Laparosc Endosc* 1:246–247, 1991.

19. Welch NT et al: Laparoscopic capture of "escaped" gallstones. *Surg Laparosc Endosc* 1:42–44, 1991.

20. Reddick EJ, Olsen DO: Outpatient laparoscopic laser cholecystectomy. *Am J Surg* 160:485–489, 1990.

21. Spaw AT, Reddick EJ, Olsen DO: Laparoscopic laser cholecystectomy: Analysis of 500 procedures. *Surg Laparosc Endosc* 1:2–7, 1991.

22. Schultz LS et al: A simplified method of laparoscopic cholecystectomy (abstract). *Lasers Surg Med* (supplement) 3:24, 1991.

23. Schultz LS et al: Laser laparolithic cholecystectomy II: Laboratory and clinical studies with the Ho:YAG laser (abstract). *Lasers Surg Med* (supplement) 4, 1992.

Acknowledgments

The author would like to acknowledge the contributions of the following gynecologists who helped develop the clinical protocols and provided the expertise needed to allow our surgical group to become competent laparoscopists. We are indebted to them for their efforts.

Charles Haislet, M.D.
David Hill, M.D.
Russell Wavrin, M.D.
Elisa Wright, M.D.

12

Laparoscopic Cholangiography

Joseph J. Pietrafitta

When laparoscopic cholecystectomy was first performed, cholangiography was felt to be an integral part of the procedure.[1-5] As more expertise has been gained by surgeons performing laparoscopic cholecystectomy, many surgeons have begun to apply the same rules in deciding whether or not a cholangiogram should be performed as have been applied in open surgery.[6] There are, however, important differences between the open and laparoscopically performed cholecystectomy that should be considered with regard to obtaining a cholangiogram. When a cholecystectomy is performed laparoscopically, it is not possible for the surgeon to palpate any portion of the biliary tract anatomy. In addition, the view of the anatomy is two-dimensional, making it difficult to appreciate turns in ductal structures. These two "problems" with the technology may increase the possibility of retained stones and injuries to the major ductal structures during laparoscopic cholecystectomy. When this is coupled with operator inexperience, the potential for complications is increased. Consequently, it is important for a surgeon to understand and be able to use the methods of cholangiography that are available and to be aware of their potential benefits and possible problems in the setting of laparoscopic cholecystectomy.

There are two techniques of cholangiography that can be performed during laparoscopic cholecystectomy. The first is cholecystcholangiography,[7] that is, performance of a cholangiogram through the gallbladder. The second is performance of the cholangiogram through the cystic duct. Cholecystcholangiography will be described first.

Cholecystcholangiography

The technique of cholecystcholangiography is very simple. After the umbilical trocar is placed, a site is chosen for placement of the first secondary trocar. This site should be at the level of the gallbladder and lateral usually in the lateral axillary line. The gallbladder is then grasped with a locking toothed forceps. The gallbladder is retracted laterally and lifted up to the abdominal wall (see Fig. 12-1).

After the gallbladder is brought into apposition with the abdominal wall, by means of external digital compression, a point is chosen to puncture the gallbladder percutaneously (see

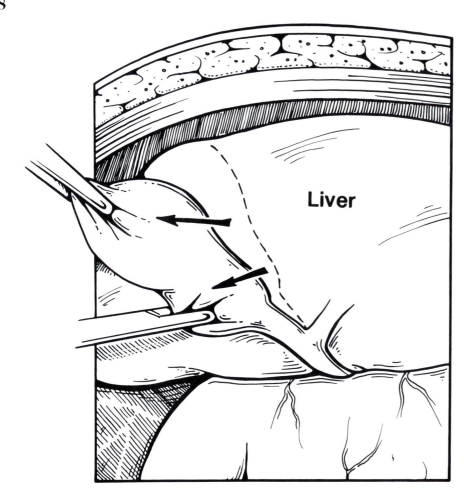

Figure 12-1
The gallbladder is grasped, retracted laterally, and lifted up to the abdominal wall.

Fig. 12-2). If there are adhesions to the gallbladder that will interfere with mobilization of the gallbladder to perform the cholangiogram, a third trocar should be placed in order to lyse the adhesions prior to performing the study.

With the gallbladder held laterally and up to the abdominal wall, the abdominal wall is punctured with a needle of at least 17 gauge. The needle is then introduced into the gallbladder. The needle should puncture the gallbladder near the grasper, which acts as a traction point, preventing excessive gallbladder wall motion. When the needle is introduced into the gallbladder, an attempt should be made to create a tract or tunnel subserosally. This will prevent leakage during the injection. The bile is aspirated and the volume is measured (see Fig. 12-3). An attempt is made to decompress the gallbladder totally (see Fig. 12-4). A syringe of 50% strength contrast material is then attached to the needle with an IV tubing extension set. The gallbladder is then refilled, that is, an amount of contrast material equal in volume to the amount of bile that was aspirated is injected. This refilling of the gallbladder is viewed laparoscopically. At this point, the study is completed radiographically.

Fluoroscopy would be of great value to maximize the quality of the cholangiogram. If it is not available, a standard film approach following the injection of contrast material will give acceptable studies 80 percent of the time.[7] This standard film approach is as follows. After the gallbladder is refilled, an additional 15 cc of contrast material is injected. The first film is taken at the end of the injection. For the second film, an additional 15 cc of contrast material is injected for a total of 30 cc greater than the

Chapter 12 Laparoscopic Cholangiography

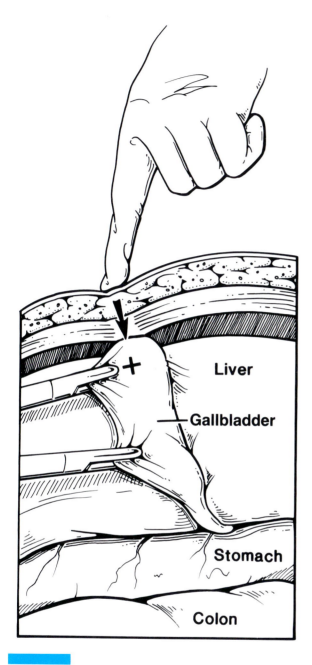

Figure 12-2
The puncture site is chosen by external digital compression.

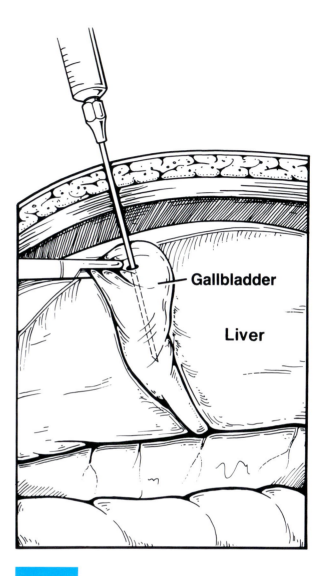

Figure 12-3
The gallbladder is punctured and as much bile as possible is aspirated. The needle puncture is placed close to the grasper. A subserosal tunnel is also seen.

volume of bile that was aspirated. The gallbladder can be seen to be tensely distended (see Fig. 12-5).

An adequate study will be seen in over 80 percent of the cholangiograms that are performed using this technique. *Adequate* is defined as good visualization of the cystic duct/ common hepatic duct junction and common bile duct, with tapering of the common bile duct at the ampulla. In a system that was developed to grade the quality of the studies,[7] this would represent a 3, 4, or 5. Grades 0, 1, or 2 would be considered unacceptable (see Fig. 12-6).

Performing cholecystcholangiography will serve two functions. First, it will demonstrate the cystic duct/common hepatic duct junction

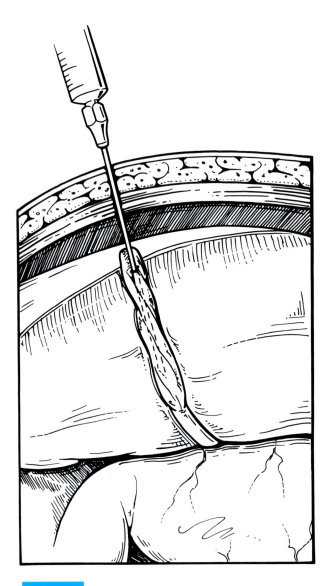

Figure 12-4
The gallbladder is totally decompressed.

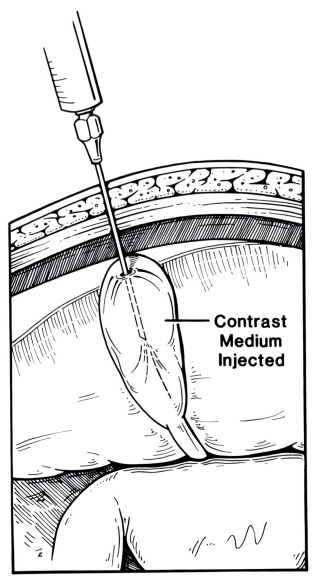

Figure 12-5
Injection of contrast solution is performed. The volume of contrast injected is equal to 30 cc more than the volume of bile that was originally aspirated. Tenseness of gallbladder wall is noted.

before dissection of this area is undertaken. Secondly, it will rule out the presence of stones in the common bile duct. An example of a normal grade 5 study is shown in Fig. 12-7. In order to get a more precise definition of the anatomy, a clip can be placed on the serosa at the neck of the gallbladder before the x-ray is obtained. This will allow for more precise delineation of the anatomy before the dissection is begun. Performance of the cholangiogram will also allow visualization of abnormal anatomy that places the patient at risk for injury (see Fig. 12-8).

After the cholangiogram is completed, the gallbladder is reaspirated to empty it completely. The needle is withdrawn. In general, there is negligible drainage from the gallbladder through the needle tract. At this point, the dissection of the cystic duct is begun.

Several points should be made. If there are

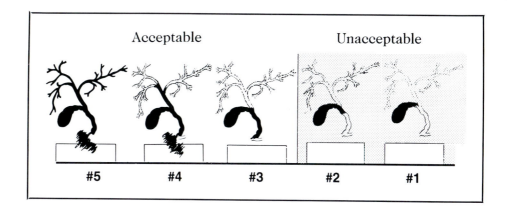

Figure 12-6
Grading system for evaluating the quality of cholecystcholangiography. Grades 3, 4, and 5 are considered acceptable studies.

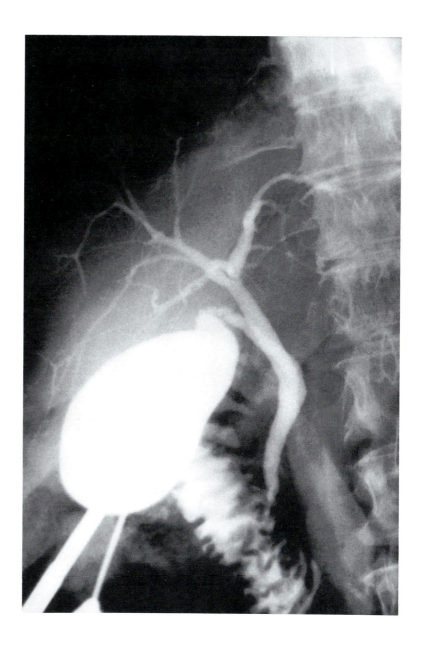

Figure 12-7
Example of a grade 5 cholecystcholangiogram.

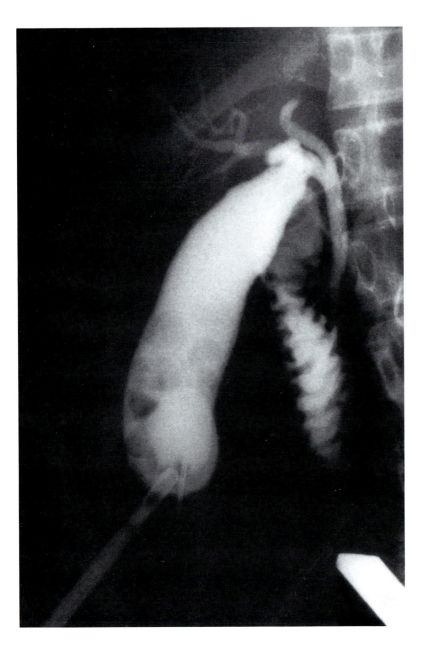

Figure 12-8
An example of abnormal cystic duct anatomy in which the cystic duct enters the right hepatic duct.

adhesions to the gallbladder of omentum, duodenum, or transverse colon mesentery, these may need to be lysed totally or partially to enable the surgeon to perform a cholangiogram. In many cases, the adhesions can be left until the cholangiogram has been completed.

If after the telescope has been introduced, the gallbladder is noted to be inflamed, that is, having the appearance of hydrops, a cholecystcholangiogram should not be performed. In this case, there is obstruction of the cystic duct and the biliary tree will not be visualized. The surgeon should proceed directly to cystic duct cholangiography.

There are other situations where a cholecystcholangiogram cannot be performed. These include conditions in which the bile is too thick to aspirate and when the anatomy of the liver is such that it cannot be brought down from under the chest wall into apposition with the abdominal wall to puncture it safely.

The situations in which an adequate study cannot be obtained occur in approximately 20 percent of the cases.

Cystic Duct Cholangiography

The other major method of cholangiography and the one that is most frequently employed is cystic duct cholangiography. This study is performed in a manner very similar to that used in open surgery.[2] The position of the abdominal wall trocars depends upon the specific system chosen by the surgeon for cholecystectomy.

The gallbladder is grasped and placed on stretch, putting tension on the cystic duct (see Fig. 12-9). Placement of a grasper near the infundibulum of the gallbladder will give maximum stretch on the duct. Placement of another trocar may be necessary to attain adequate tension on the duct (Fig. 12-10).

Once traction is adequately maintained then the dissection is begun. The cystic duct is isolated, beginning at the neck of the gallbladder. Once it is adequately exposed, a single clip is placed on the neck of the gallbladder. A microscissors is then used to make a small opening in the duct (see Fig. 12-11).

At this point, a cholangiography catheter device must be introduced into the abdominal cavity and then into the cystic duct. A number of methods can be employed to introduce the various cholangiography devices. If a catheter is used, it can be introduced through one of the trocars. If this is the method of choice, the catheter must be introduced through the most medial trocar in order to approach the duct in the proper direction (see Fig. 12-12). Alternatively, the catheter can be introduced percutaneously. The simplest technique appears to be direct percutaneous placement. There are a number of commercially available devices made specifically for laparoscopic cystic duct cholangiography. There are also a number of catheters, such as urologic catheters, that can be used. Some of the specialty catheters have securing mechanisms built into them and others do not.

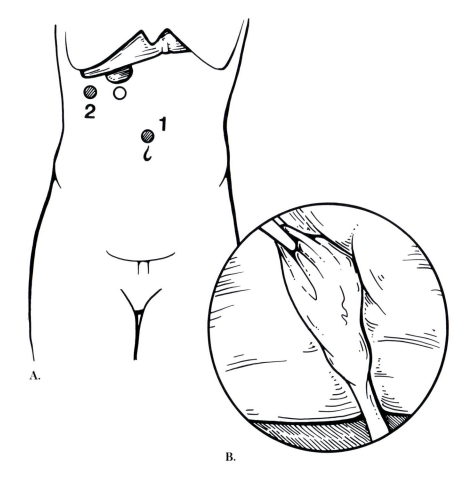

Figure 12-9
A. Two trocars are placed for telescope and gallbladder grasper.
B. Laparoscopic view of the gallbladder retracted, with the cystic duct on stretch.

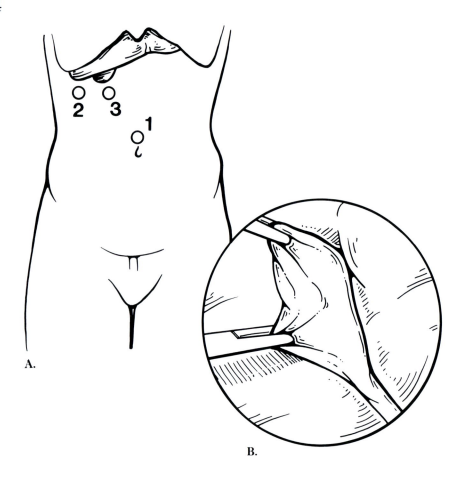

Figure 12-10
A. An additional (third) port placed for traction on the gallbladder.
B. Laparoscopic view of gallbladder traction, using two graspers.

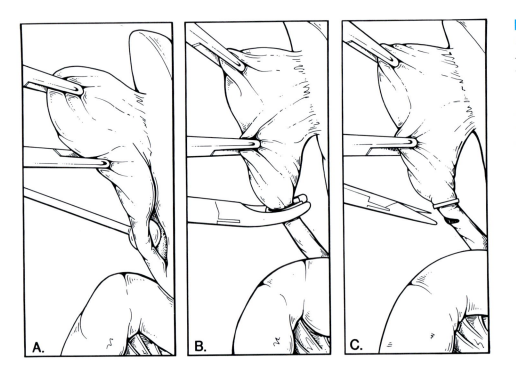

Figure 12-11
A. The cystic duct is dissected free of surrounding tissue. **B.** A clip is placed on the neck of the gallbladder. **C.** A small opening is made in the cystic duct.

Chapter 12 Laparoscopic Cholangiography

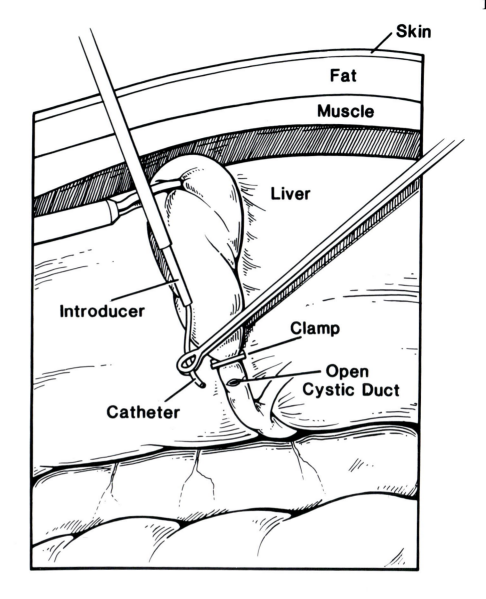

Figure 12-12
A cystic duct cholangiogram is performed by inserting a catheter into a small incision in the cystic duct. Many different commercially available catheters can be used.

Those that do not can be secured in place by passing them down a cholangiography clamp that is clamped down on the duct after the catheter has been introduced into the duct (see Fig. 12-13A and B). Alternatively, the catheter can be introduced into the duct, and then a single clip is applied. Saline should be injected while the clip is being placed to prevent inadvertent catheter occlusion with the clip (see Fig. 12-14A, B, and C).

Two films are taken. The first after the injection of 5 cc of 50% contrast and the second after the injection of an additional 5 cc. The quality of the studies are equal to those obtained with cholangiography performed during open cholecystectomy.

Cholangiography should be an integral part of laparoscopic cholecystectomy in a number of circumstances (see Table 12-1). Liberal use of cholangiography will help to minimize the complications associated with laparoscopic cholecystectomy, the most serious of which is common bile duct injury.

Cholangiograms can be performed after the dissection has begun in an effort to define anatomy that is somewhat confusing. It is better to

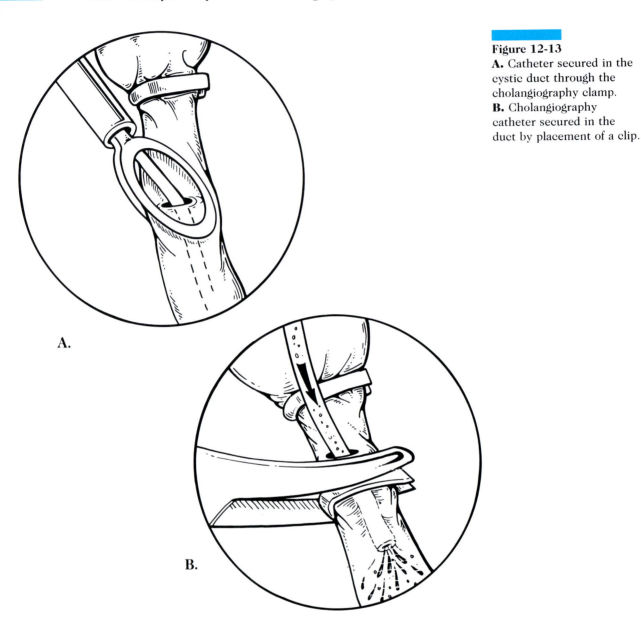

Figure 12-13
A. Catheter secured in the cystic duct through the cholangiography clamp.
B. Cholangiography catheter secured in the duct by placement of a clip.

TABLE 12-1 Indications for Intraoperative Cholangiography

Absolute Indications
- Suspected common bile duct stones
- Inexperienced surgeon performing procedure
- Confusing anatomy
- Dissection proceeding poorly
- A belief that cholangiography should be done in all cases

Relative Indications
- Extensive adhesions
- Acute cholecystitis
- Unusually scarred contracted gallbladder

perform a cholangiogram in a delayed fashion in order to "refigure" out the anatomy than it is to risk a serious complication.

Management of common bile duct stones identified via intraoperative cholangiography depends upon the surgeon's experience and available options. For surgeons just beginning to use laparoscopic techniques, a strong preoperative suspicion of common duct stones is best managed by preoperative endoscopic retrograde cholangiopancreatography (ERCP). Other more-experienced surgeons will be able to remove the stones using laparoscopic meth-

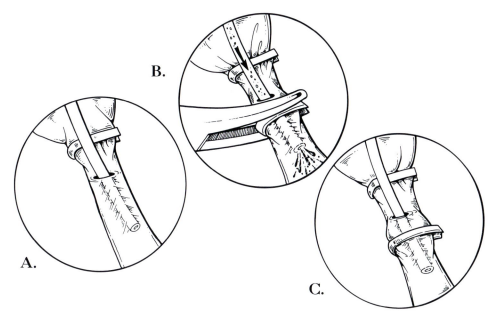

Figure 12-14
A. Cholangiography catheter introduced into the cystic duct. **B.** A clip is applied to secure the catheter into the duct while saline is injected through the catheter to assure catheter potency. **C.** Catheter secured in place for cholangiogram.

ods (see Chaps. 14 and 15). A surgeon who is not prepared to remove the common duct stones laparoscopically needs to choose between converting to an open common bile duct exploration or leaving the stones to be removed postoperatively with an ERCP.

Whatever rules the surgeon applies to the performance of cholangiography and whatever type of study is performed, the surgeon's decision should always be made with the best interest of the patient in mind and within the context of performing an efficient laparoscopic cholecystectomy without complications.

References

1. Phillips EH et al: The importance of intraoperative cholangiography during laparoscopic cholecystectomy. *Am Surg* 56(12):792–795, 1990.
2. Berci G, Sackier JM, Paz-Partlow M: Routine or selected intraoperative cholangiography during laparoscopic cholecystectomy? *Am J Surg* 161(3):355–360, 1991.
3. Blatner ME, Wittgen CM, Kaminski DL: Cystic duct cholangiography during laparoscopic cholecystectomy. *Arch Surg* 126(5):646–649, 1991.
4. Sackier JM et al: The role of cholangiography in laparoscopic cholecystectomy. *Arch Surg* 126(8):1021–1025, 1991.
5. Flowers JL et al: Laparoscopic cholangiography. Results and indications. *Ann Surg* 215(3):209–216, 1992.
6. Joyce WP et al: Identification of bile duct stones in patients undergoing laparoscopic cholecystectomy. *Br J Surg* 78(10):1174–1176, 1991.
7. Pietrafitta JJ et al: Cholecystcholangiography or cystic duct cholangiography. *J Laparoendosc Surg* 1(4):197–206, 1991.

Bibliography

Davidoff AM et al: Mechanisms of major bile duct injury during laparoscopic cholecystectomy. *Ann Surg* 215(3):196–202, 1992.

Handy JE et al: Intraoperative cholangiography: Use of portable fluoroscopy and transmitted images. *Radiology* 181(1):205–207, 1991.

13

Bleeding, Acute Cholecystitis, and Other Problems Encountered during Laparoscopic Cholecystectomy

John N. Graber

In most cases, laparoscopic cholecystectomy proceeds without difficulty. However, problems are encountered in many cases and a plan of action that prepares the surgeon to recognize and manage difficult situations is mandatory. Managing a freely bleeding cystic artery in an open incisional setting is not difficult for most surgeons. Tamponade the vessel, place the assistant and retractors appropriately, suction pooled blood, identify the source, grasp the vessel with a forceps and hold it in such a position so as to allow placement of a hemostat, use a clip, or cauterize it. It is a different scenario when you find yourself and the entire operating room staff watching the bleeding on the video screen. After trying to aspirate some of the pooled blood, you may find that the problem can get worse if you suction out the CO_2 and the pneumoperitoneum is lost along with the exposure. Having a contingency plan at hand to deal with such problems is helpful, and approaches to several of these difficult settings will be reviewed here. Above all, remember that when trouble arises during a laparoscopic procedure, you cannot let your "operative momentum" allow you to continue down a disastrous track. It should be apparent to everyone in the operating room that it is not a complication to convert to an open laparotomy, but, instead, it is good surgical judgment.

Management of Intraoperative Bleeding

Bleeding can be so difficult during laparoscopy that it is clearly better off avoided rather than dealt with as it occurs. Cauterizing tissue before it is cut cannot be overemphasized. Points where bleeding occurs most frequently during cholecystectomy are up and behind the cystic duct in the liver bed, along the inferiolateral gallbladder-liver margin, at the peritoneal reflection of the apex of the gallbladder fossa, and in the depth of the liver bed (Fig. 13-1). With

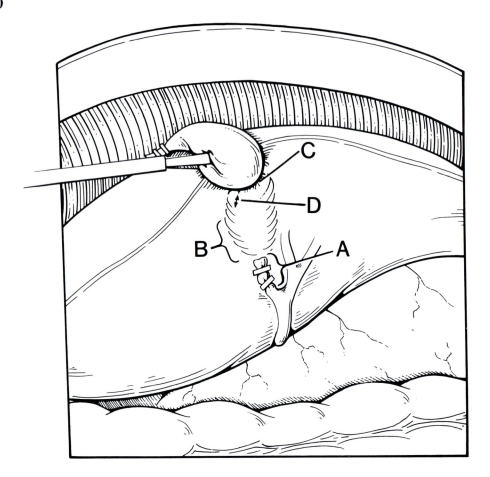

Figure 13-1
Typical sites of bleeding during cholecystectomy: **A.** In the liver bed up and behind the cystic duct at the neck of the gallbladder. **B.** Along the inferiolateral gallbladder margin. **C.** At the peritoneal reflection at the apex of the gallbladder. **D.** In the depth of the liver bed.

careful dissection and cauterization of vessels or by fulguration of tissue in these areas before they are cut, bleeding can be avoided.

Nonetheless, bleeding is part of surgery, and no matter how hard a surgeon tries to avoid it, some degree of hemorrhage is frequently encountered. The basic principles of obtaining hemostasis are not different with laparoscopy. It is just that it can be more difficult! When oozing or low volume bleeding is observed, the source must be found. This will require adequate exposure. Upward retraction on the gallbladder, reverse Trendelenburg positioning, or possibly downward traction on the colon or omentum will be needed. Then irrigation and suction of the pool of blood may be required before the vessel can be seen. Very judicious use of suction is necessary in order to avoid loss of the pneumoperitoneum. The high flow insufflators are absolutely necessary in this type of surgery to replace suctioned gas rapidly. Keep the suction pressure moderately low and make it count when you use it by suctioning with short duration directly on or in the target fluid.

An appropriate hemostatic method needs to be selected. Bipolar cautery is best if the bleeding is in the proximity of another organ such as the common bile duct or intestine. Unipolar cautery is excellent in the liver bed where a rim of necrosis around the vessel is generally not harmful. Laser can cut well with reasonably good hemostasis, but it is simply not as good as unipolar cautery once significant liver bed bleeding is encountered. This is true regardless if the laser is contact or free beam, Nd:YAG, argon, KTP, or Ho:YAG.

With excessive retraction on the gallbladder, the liver can be torn at the peritoneal reflection and cause worrisome bleeding. Accidental instrument punctures of the liver or other retraction injuries can also bleed, and many times, bleeding with these injuries is difficult to control with cautery because blood pools rapidly at the source. In this situation, apply pres-

Chapter 13 Bleeding, Acute Cholecystitis, and Other Problems

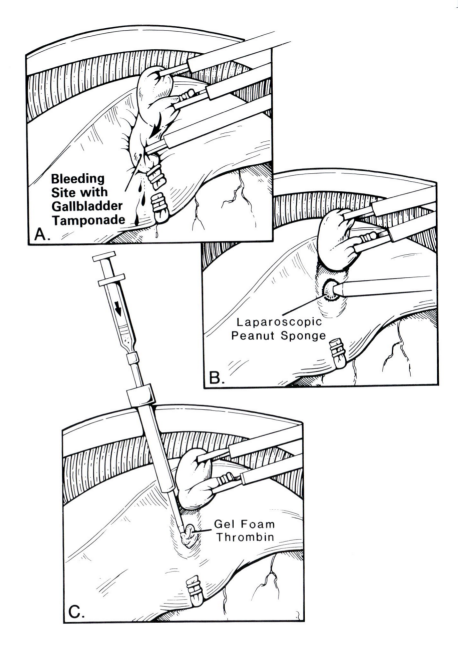

Figure 13-2
Various methods of controlling liver bed bleeding include: **A.** Tamponade the bleeding with the gallbladder, **B.** apply pressure with a laparoscopic Kittner peanut sponge, or **C.** inject Gelfoam powder and thrombin mixture into the site and reapply pressure.

sure to the source by pushing the graspers and gallbladder or a laparoscopic Kittner peanut sponge directly against the bleeding (Fig. 13-2). While controlling most of the bleeding in this manner, prepare a mixture of Gelfoam powder and thrombin that can be placed in a syringe and injected through an introducer passed through a 5-mm cannula directly onto the site of liver bleeding. Avitene pads can also be inserted into the peritoneal cavity through one of the larger cannulas and applied to the bleeding site. Then replace the pressure tamponade for several minutes.

Another tool that works well in this situation is the laparoscopic argon beam cautery. This device sprays a jet of argon gas directly into the target area, and an electrical cautery current passes through the gas into the tissue. The special advantage this offers in the setting of liver bed bleeding is that the gas stream blows away pooling blood so that the current is applied more directly to the bleeding target.

A freely cut cystic artery that is spraying blood around the peritoneal cavity presents a different set of problems (Fig. 13-3). A major obstacle is the spurting of blood directly into

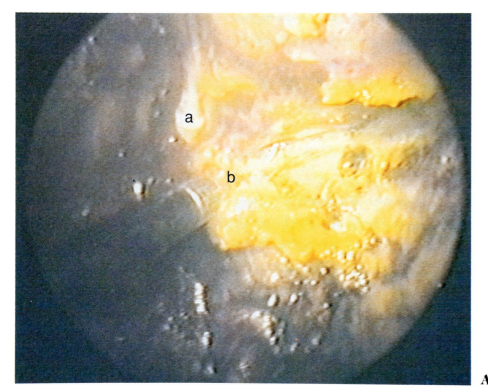

A.

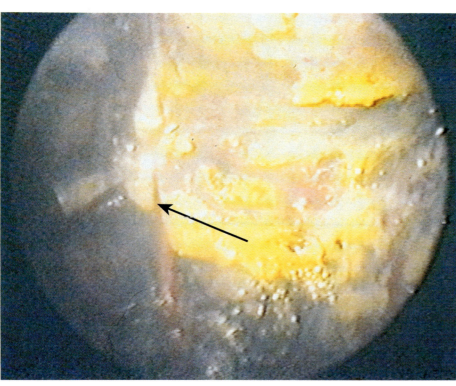

B.

Figure 13-3
Sudden severe bleeding from an unexpected branch of the cystic artery that sprayed into the telescope lens. **A.** Before the vessel was contacted (*a.* cystic artery branch, *b.* contact laser scalpel), **B.** the bleeding starts (notice the jet of blood [arrow]), and

Figure 13-3
C. the lens is hit, and **D.** then covered with blood. Total elapsed time is 0.25 s.

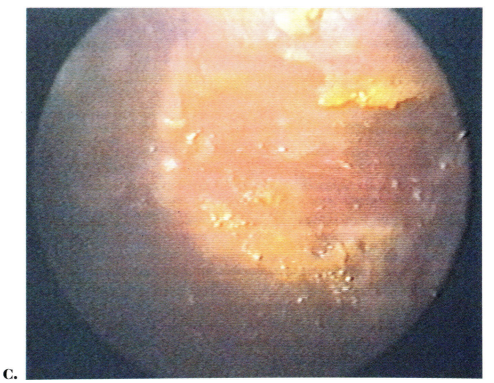

C.

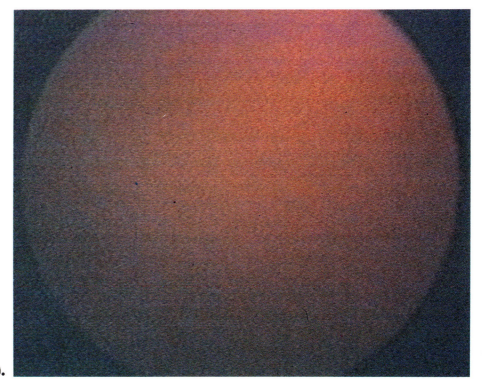

D.

the laparoscope's lens, completely "blinding" the surgeon—the classic weakness of the cyclops. A plan of action should be in place to manage this situation (Fig. 13-4). Once again, the gallbladder is a convenient object to use for at least partial tamponade of the bleeding. Immediately regain visualization by either rubbing the lens against intestine or the abdominal wall, or remove the laparoscope from the abdomen and wipe the lens with a sponge and antifogging solution. Once the visual field is restored, cautiously approach the bleeding site from the other side of the abdominal cavity. For this purpose a 45° viewing scope is helpful. Carefully move the scope to a site of visual advantage so that the lens doesn't become smeared again, and then with appropriate retraction and judicious use of suction, the vessel can be seen and controlled. If this fails with initial attempts, the problem of exposure gets worse quickly with the rising pool of blood that may not be readily suctioned. If you don't get it right away and you are unable to regain exposure of the vessel, tamponade the vessel with continued pressure and make an incision. All that is needed is a scalpel, suction, laparotomy pads, a Richardson retractor, and a clamp so there is no need to wait once you have made the decision. Remember, converting to an open laparotomy is not a complication, whereas a hypotensive myocardial infarction or stroke is.

Bleeding from the portal vein is a very different problem than any reviewed above. This serious complication would result from inadvertent puncture with an instrument or by aggressive dissection in the area behind the common bile duct.[1] It may be possible to tamponade the bleeding and apply a hemostatic pad, but little time should be spent on these efforts if there is any evidence of ongoing volume bleeding. Hepatic artery bleeding is also very worrisome and both of these situations would be best managed with immediate laparotomy and placement of the index finger into the foramen of Winslow and compression of the portal triad (Pringle maneuver) until the bleeding source can be found and repaired.

Trocar site bleeding can be massive (Fig. 13-5). Again, avoiding the problem is the best tactic, and this can usually be done by transilluminating the abdominal wall with the laparoscope to see vessels and then specifically missing them with the cannula puncture. Use the laparoscope to look at the puncture sites

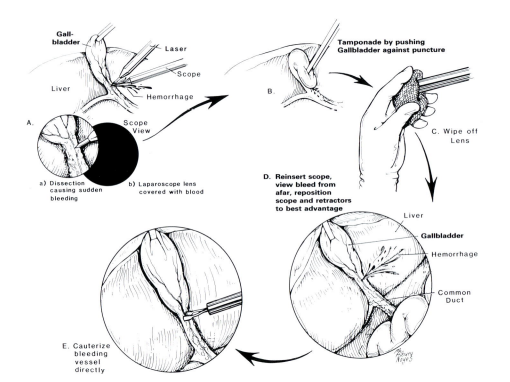

Figure 13-4
Protocol for managing a freely bleeding cystic artery: **A.** The vessel is cut (*a*) and blood spurts onto the lens (*b*). **B.** Immediate tamponade by shifting the gallbladder fundus into the area of bleeding. **C.** The telescope is removed and cleaned. **D.** After reinsertion, avoid the spurting blood but find a place to view the bleeding and reexpose it, suction carefully, and **E.** control the vessel with cautery or clip.

Figure 13-5
CT scan of patient who had a large bleed from a puncture site. Most of the hematoma was located in the right lower quadrant (arrow).

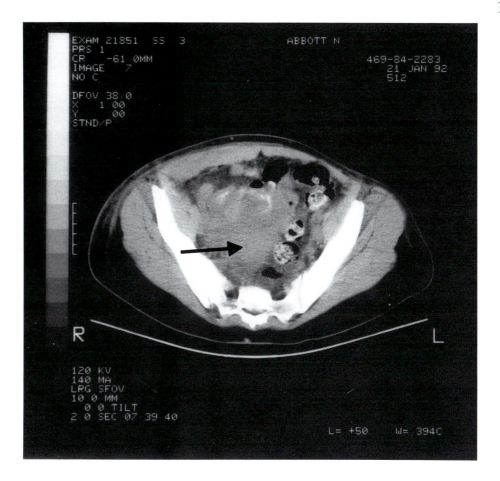

for any bleeding as the cannulas are being removed at the end of the procedure. If there is any, get as good a look into the defect as you can, and once again, a 45° scope is very helpful for this. Press with a finger from the outside to splay the tract open to view with the scope. If you can see the source of blood loss, bipolar cautery can be very useful from within the peritoneal cavity or from outside the abdominal wall. If the site cannot be identified, insert a Foley balloon through the puncture site into the peritoneal cavity, inflate the balloon, and withdraw it against the abdominal wall fascia for 5 to 10 min (Fig. 13-6). This will successfully tamponade small bleeding vessels in the muscle. If bleeding persists when the balloon is deflated, another method to control puncture site bleeding is to pass a straight Keith needle and a no. 00 nylon suture through the abdominal wall next to the site (Fig. 13-7). Then the needle can be grasped internally and directed back through the abdominal wall on the other side of the puncture.[2] This could be done again to create a figure eight stitch and knotted. This will almost certainly control the bleeding. Of course, the final option would be to extend the skin incision to allow external exploration of the tract and control the vessel.

Management of Acute Cholecystitis

Acute cholecystitis was once thought to be a contraindication to laparoscopic cholecystectomy.[3] Now management of this disorder can be treated safely using the video approach, but it is still a dramatically more difficult procedure than standard cholecystectomy.[4,5] A surgeon can never have absolute confidence that he or she can always accomplish gallbladder removal via the laparoscope in the setting of acute inflammation. One must be especially careful not

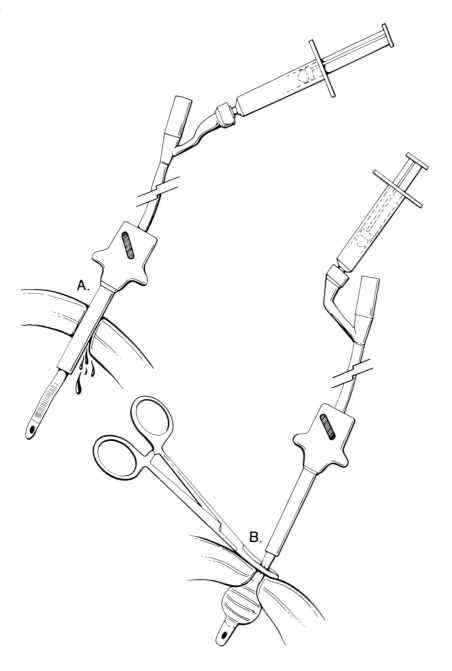

Figure 13-6
A Foley balloon is used to tamponade bleeding from a puncture site. **A.** The balloon is inserted through the cannula. **B.** After inflation, it is withdrawn against the abdominal wall and held in place with a clamp at the skin level for 5 min.

to let "operative momentum" carry him or her beyond what can be done safely and thus cause an injury.

There is a spectrum of presentation of acute cholecystitis that makes description of its management depend upon the specific degree of inflammation (Table 13-1) (Fig. 13-8). Often the most severe site of inflammation is in the body of the gallbladder, and the cystic duct will be moderately normal. This is an ideal situation

TABLE 13-1   Acute Cholecystitis

Spectrum of Presentation	
Mild inflammation	● Massive scarring
Pink and pliable	● Hemorrhagic and friable
Normal WBC* and afebrile	● Septic and hypotensive
Surgically anticipated	● Flabbergasted and bewildered

* WBC = white blood [cell] count.

Chapter 13 Bleeding, Acute Cholecystitis, and Other Problems

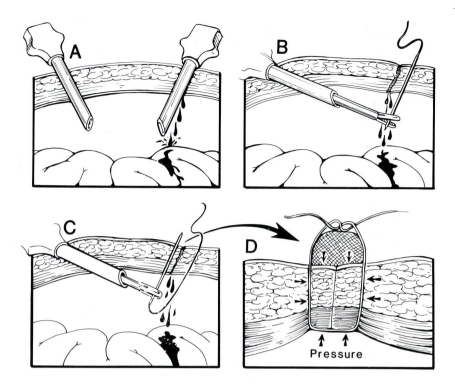

Figure 13-7
To control puncture site bleeding (**A**), a straight needle can be passed through the abdominal wall (**B**), grasped internally and passed back through the wall (**C**), to be tied around a bolster (**D**). The suture can be removed later.

because the major part of this surgery is cystic duct control. On the other hand, if a stone is lodged in the distal cystic duct, it can be inflamed and even necrotic. The variety of possible presentations makes the therapeutic approach largely dependent upon the situation.

The first and foremost consideration is obtaining adequate exposure. Dense hyperemic adhesions need to be taken down, using blunt traction and cautery. Larger than usual instrumentation may be helpful to grasp the gallbladder without tearing it. We have found a 10-mm claw tenaculum grasper to be most functional.

Secondly, decompression of the gallbladder by inserting a large needle into the lumen and aspirating the contents is very helpful by making it easier to grasp without tearing. The content may be a clear fluid (hydrops of the gallbladder), thick turbid bile, or frank pus. In any case, this material is best removed early rather than tearing the gallbladder and spilling it into the peritoneal cavity. Culture the aspirate.

Third, set out to identify the anatomy carefully. Stay close to the gallbladder wall to prevent injury to other structures. Encircle the cystic duct at the gallbladder; do not try to pick it up distal in a less inflamed more accessible area because the risk of inadvertently mistaking the common duct for the cystic duct is too great. Use a laparoscopic Kittner dissector. If this cannot be done without cutting structures of uncertain identity, change your angle of view and dissect at another site until the anatomy is clear. If you cannot figure out what the nature of the anatomy is, convert to an open procedure.

Once the cystic duct is identified, a cholangiogram should be done. A cholecystcholangiogram will not work because of the cystic duct obstruction associated with acute cholecystitis. A cystic duct cholangiogram is necessary. This study will not only confirm that there are no stones in the common duct but will also demonstrate that there is no ductal injury.

Next, the cystic duct is divided and the gallbladder is dissected from the liver bed. This may be dramatically more difficult than during elective cholecystectomy. If a plain between the gallbladder and the liver cannot be identified or is particularly bloody, consider removing the front wall of the gallbladder, leaving the back wall in the liver bed (see Chap. 11, Fig. 11-2). Remove all the stones and then ablate the residual mucosa with laser or cautery. In this set-

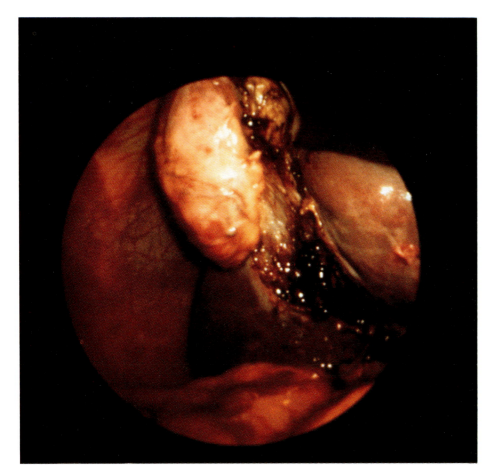

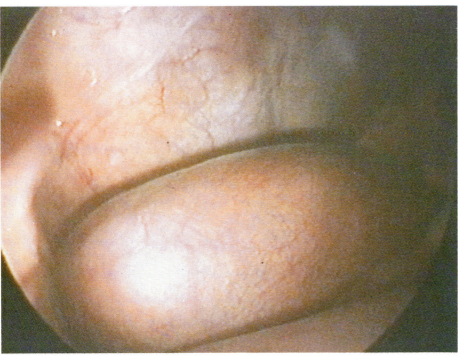

Figure 13-8
Acute cholecystitis: **A.** Gallbladder with severe acute adhesions and edema. **B.** Massively distended gallbladder found to have clear fluid within its lumen (hydrops of the gallbladder).

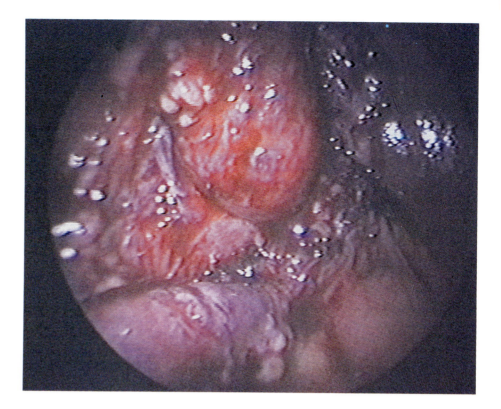

Figure 13-8
C. Gallbladder with hemorrhagic and gangrenous wall with frank pus within its lumen.

ting, we have found the laser (contact Nd:YAG) to work well to cut the friable gallbladder and then to ablate (free beam Nd:YAG) the posterior wall. Fulguration with electrocautery would work well, too.

Obtaining hemostasis and removing all debris, stones, and fluid is of considerable importance. Irrigate copiously at the close of the procedure with an antibiotic saline solution. Then a drain should be placed into the hepatorenal fossa (Fig. 13-9A and B).

Problems of Body Habitus

An obese patient presents several specific problems to the surgeon (Fig. 13-10). First, the Verres needle may not reach the peritoneal cavity and the instruments may not reach the gallbladder. Second, the thickness of the abdominal wall prevents easy manipulation of the instruments. Third, forceful redirection of the cannulas can cause injury to the peritoneal surface, the muscle fascia, and the skin. Fourth, the weight of the abdominal wall prevents the pneumoperitoneum from elevating it so that there is little room for anterior retraction of the gallbladder and consequently poor exposure of the cystic duct. Lastly, there may be extra fatty deposits next to the gallbladder, cystic duct, omentum, and transverse mesocolon, making dissection and exposure difficult. There are maneuvers that can improve on these matters, but very large patients will still be more of a challenge.

Use a special long Verres needle and direct it more perpendicular to the skin than usual. In these cases more than any other, pay attention to the two "pops" as the needle passes through the fascia and peritoneum. All of the typical checks usually made to confirm the intraperitoneal position of the needle are less definitive, and you may accept filling pressures 5 to 8 mmHg higher than usual.

In order to improve the ability to reach the gallbladder with the instruments, the cannulas need to be placed more superiorly in the abdominal wall. Be careful not to place the punctures too high so as to injure the costal margin because the ribs will be less easily palpable. The best position can usually be determined by placing the camera through the umbilical site as

Part Two Laparoscopic Abdominal Surgery

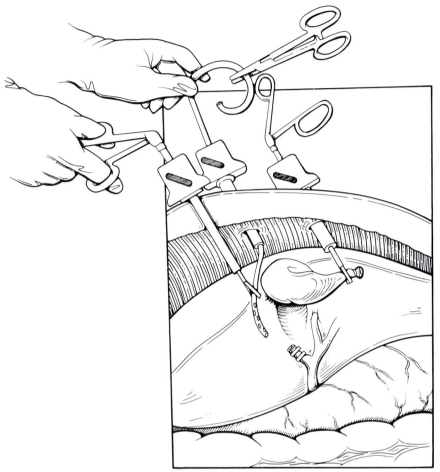

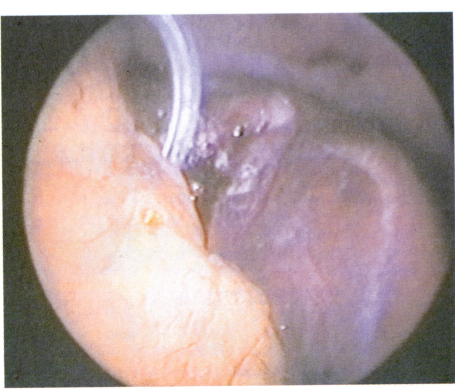

Figure 13-9
A and **B.** A drain placed into the hepatorenal fossa after cholecystectomy for acute cholecystitis.

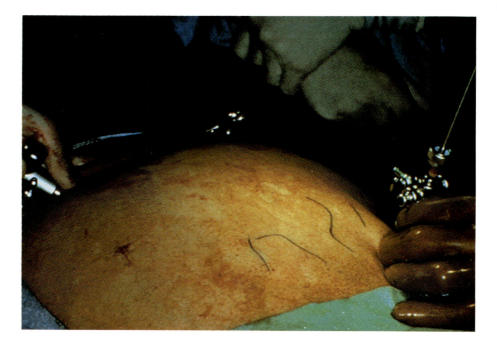

Figure 13-10
A 290-lb patient presents special problems.

usual. Then visualize the liver margin and push down on the upper abdominal wall to identify a site more directly in line with the gallbladder but below the costal margin. The rib margin is often more easily appreciated from the peritoneal side. More attention is necessary to be sure that the cannulas remain within the peritoneal cavity because they will tend to back out beyond the peritoneal surface. Patients who have an abdominal wall that is thicker than the length of the standard cannulas present one of the most frustrating problems to the surgeon, and until specific bariatric cannulas are made, these patients may be better served with an open incision.

The problem of redirecting a cannula that has been placed while aiming into the pelvis needs special mention (Fig. 13-11). The thicker

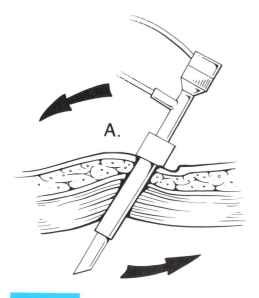
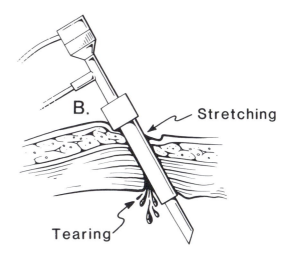

Figure 13-11
Redirection of the cannula after placement **(A)** in an obese patient can result in **(B)** tearing of the fascia and bleeding.

the abdominal wall, the more the skin, fascia, and peritoneum need to be stretched to redirect the cannula. This causes tearing and bleeding at these sites, which is very difficult to manage. The trocars need to be inserted while directing them into the upper abdomen, in line with their position of function. This can be done safely while observing the placement with the laparoscope, but placement of the initial cannula remains blind. For this reason, the use of a shielded disposable trocar is especially important. If the umbilical site turns out to be too low for adequate visualization, it can be abandoned, leaving the trocar unused and a new site made in the epigastrium.

The matter of poor exposure in obese patients is due in part to inadequate elevation of the abdominal wall. More room for dissection and exposure can be obtained by increasing the intraabdominal pressure to 20mmHg and tipping the patient into more reverse Trendelenburg than usual. These measures will combine to make for a greater resistance to venous return from the legs, which will increase the risk of deep venous thrombosis. Therefore, in these heavier patients, it is best to use lower extremity sequential pneumatic pressure support devices. Also, do not hesitate to place an extra cannula to improve retraction of the liver or the intestine if needed.

At times the falciform ligament can be quite large and obstruct the view of the cystic duct. If simple repositioning of the scope does not solve the problem, a straight Keith needle and a no. 00 nylon suture can be passed through the abdominal wall to enter the abdominal cavity next to the falciform ligament. Place this stitch high near the xiphoid. The needle can then be grasped internally, carefully redirected back through the abdominal wall on the other side of the ligament, and knotted in order to pull the falciform up and away from the operative field. The suture is cut at the end of the procedure.

Previous Abdominal Surgeries

Patients who have had previous abdominal surgeries will have adhesions that can interfere with placement of the Verres needle and the initial trocar. In order to avoid problems, the Verres needle can be placed in sites other than the midline. Insertion in the right or left lower quadrant, directing the needle into the pelvis

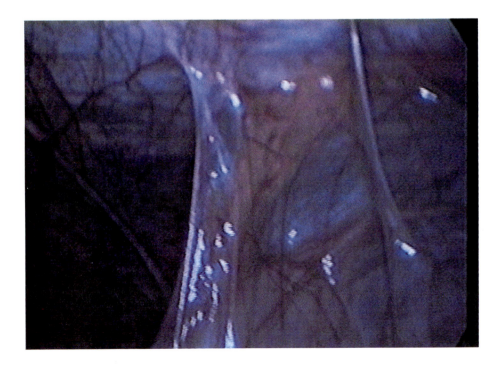

Figure 13-12
Severe intraabdominal adhesions from previous abdominal surgery.

or in the midline epigastrium, usually works well. Initial placement of a disposable 5-mm trocar with a retractable guard can be done safely lateral to the rectus sheath. Then, inserting a small laparoscope to visualize further trocar placement minimizes the potential for injury. An alternative is to use the Hasson cannula, which involves open incisional placement of the cannula without puncture insertion.[6] (This technique is described in Chap. 1.)

Adhesions can be taken down in order to access the right upper quadrant (Fig. 13-12). It is not likely to be of benefit to spend time taking down adhesions that do not interfere with the planned procedure. Cautious use of the hook cautery, cautery scissors, contact laser, or bipolar hook cautery all work well as do standard blunt and sharp dissection techniques. It is important to use traction and countertraction as much as possible. Always perform a postdissection inspection of the tissue to be certain that there is no intestinal injury or bleeding. Management of adhesions was further reviewed in Chap. 9.

Operating on the Pregnant Patient

Laparoscopic cholecystectomy during pregnancy is very controversial. Many authorities consider pregnancy a contraindication to the procedure. Others have accomplished laparoscopic cholecystectomy or appendectomy in pregnant patients multiple times without problems.[7–9] The primary complications to consider are potential injury to the fetus, loss of the pregnancy with fetal death, or initiation of labor and birth of a premature infant. The mechanism of these problems is through mechanical irritation of the uterus, toxic effect on the fetus by the anesthetic, or possibly by alterations in fetal or placental blood flow due to the pressure of the pneumoperitoneum or the anesthetic or by changing the acid base balance due to hypercarbia secondary to CO_2 absorption.

In general, surgery and anesthesia should be strongly discouraged during the first trimester of pregnancy because of the potential toxic effects on fetal development during this period. The third trimester offers different concerns of initiating premature labor or technical difficulties with negotiating around the sizable uterus. Consequently, if laparoscopic or incisional cholecystectomy is considered in a pregnant patient, preferentially, it should be accomplished during the second trimester.

The specific technical problems encountered during the procedure relate to fundal height causing uterine interference with obtaining the pneumoperitoneum and placement of trocars, uterine contact with instruments or cannulas during the operation, and difficulties in gallbladder and bile duct exposure. At 20 weeks of gestation, the fundus of the uterus is typically located at the level of the umbilicus. Placement of a Verres needle may be overly dangerous and an open laparoscopic technique employing a Hasson cannula is always warranted. In the setting of the uterus being palpable well above the umbilicus (i.e., the third trimester), the Hasson cannula can be placed in the midline between the umbilicus and the xiphoid process. Even in such situations, after the pneumoperitoneum has been satisfactorily administered, upper abdominal exposure can be surprisingly good.

Sequential pneumatic support devices need to be placed on the lower extremities before the anesthetic is administered. Then the patient needs to be placed in steep reverse Trendelenburg position. Fetal monitoring can be obtained during the surgery; however, little can be done in most settings to interrupt fetal distress (e.g., deliver the baby). Continuous endtidal CO_2 measurement is mandatory to minimize a potential disruption of fetal physiology by the pneumoperitoneum.

Routine cholangiography should be avoided in the pregnant patient. If a cholangiogram is specifically indicated, the uterus should be protected with a lead apron covered with a sterile sheet. A strategically located metal Mayo stand may work satisfactorily.

Postoperative fetal monitoring is helpful to determine if the uterus is contracting. Administration of terbutaline sulfate may be warranted to control early contractions. If the fetus is stable and there are no contractions, the patient can usually go home the day after the surgery.

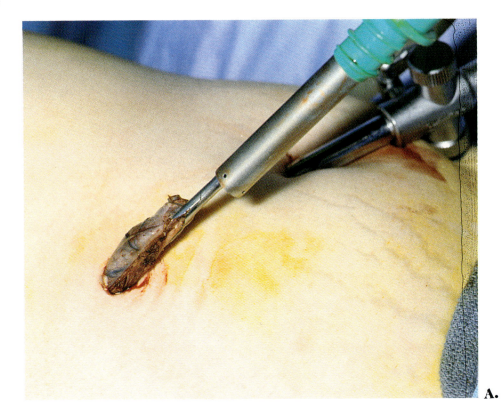

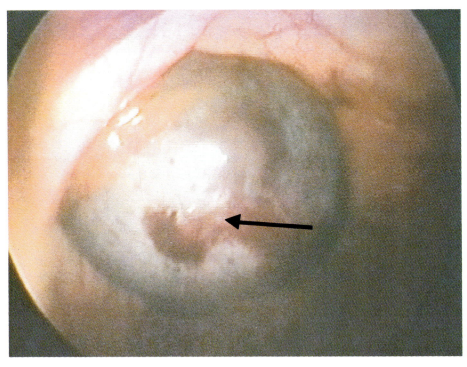

Figure 13-13
In order to get a gallbladder full of stones through the abdominal wall, it can be (**A**) partially pulled through a puncture site. **B.** The stones will ball up in the fundus that will remain intraperitoneal (arrow).

A.

B.

Figure 13-13
C and **D.** The stones can then be removed through the neck of the gallbladder with a ring forceps before it will squeeze through the puncture site

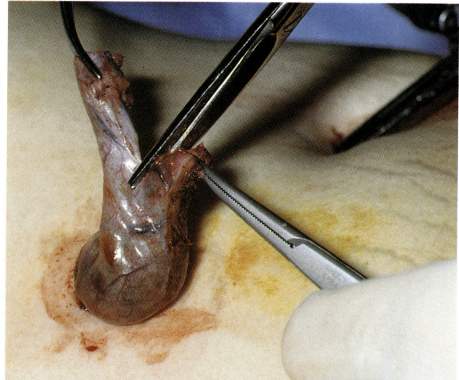

C.

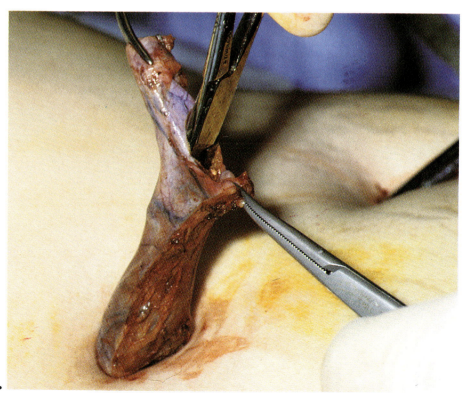

D.

Part Two Laparoscopic Abdominal Surgery

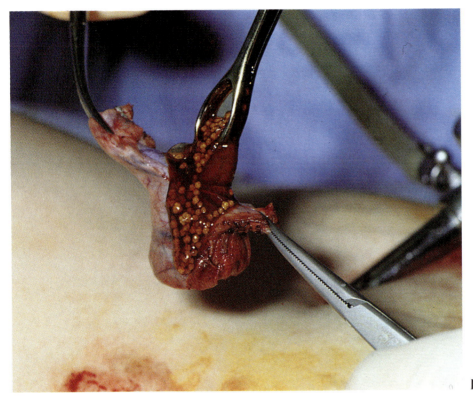

E.

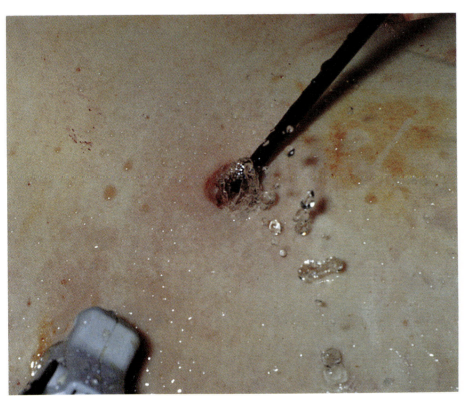

F.

Figure 13-13
(E) without enlarging the incision. **F.** The tract is irrigated with saline while the escaping CO_2 gas blows all debris and irrigant out onto the abdominal wall. A cannula can then be replaced.

Removal of Tissue

As the laparoscopic techniques progress, larger organs are approached and one of the more perplexing problems is removing the tissue once the organ has been dissected from its attachments. Often the gallbladder is full of stones or too thick to remove through the cannula intact. There are at least six basic ways to handle this: morcellation of the gallbladder and fracture of stones, open the gallbladder and remove the stones individually and then pull out the gallbladder, pull the neck of the gallbladder through a puncture site and remove stones individually, place the gallbladder and stones into a bag or extraction device and pull them out through a puncture site, enlarge the fascia and skin incision at a puncture site and pull out the gallbladder intact, and, lastly, leave the gallbladder and or stones within the peritoneal cavity.

All of these techniques have their potential advantages and to one degree or another can be used depending upon the situation. Morcellation prevents contamination and stretching of the puncture sites but has the propensity to leave debris within the abdominal cavity. The same is true of opening the gallbladder to remove stones.

Pulling the neck of the gallbladder through the abdominal wall while the stones bunch up in the fundus of the gallbladder within the peritoneal cavity seems to be the best routine solution (Fig. 13-13A to F). Once the neck of the

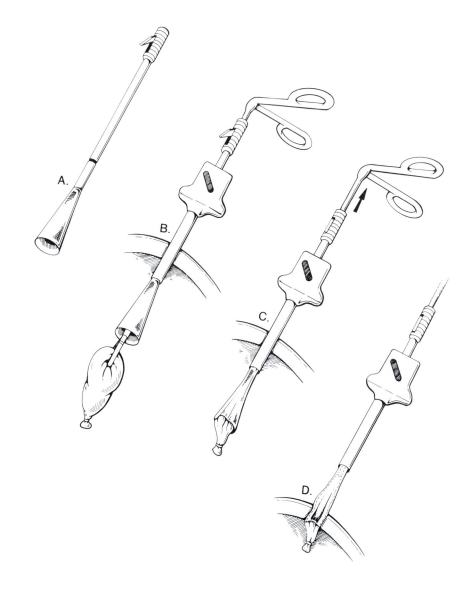

Figure 13-14
A tissue and organ extractor (**A**) works by (**B, C**) drawing tissue into a metal shroud or fabric sheath with a grasper that can be passed through the handle. The device can be withdrawn through the cannula or, if necessary, directly through the abdominal wall (**D**) by compressing and elongating the tissue as it squeezes through a channel too small for it to otherwise pass. The device can also be made with a plastic bag attached to collect fluid and debris compressed out of the gallbladder.

gallbladder is grasped outside the abdominal wall, the stones can be grasped by inserting a ring forceps or a stone forceps through the neck of the gallbladder to grasp the stones still stuck in the fundus. After enough of the stones have been removed, the gallbladder will squeeze through the puncture site. There is some contamination of the tract, and it should be irrigated immediately with antibiotic saline solution (Fig. 13-14). The escaping CO_2 gas from the pneumoperitoneum will blow the irrigant and the debris out of the tract.

The use of new devices such as the Endobag (see Chap. 1, Fig. 1-20) or the "tissue and organ extractor" (Fig. 13-14) is helpful in certain cases to remove particularly large or contaminated tissue.

Discussion

There are an enormous number of potential problems that can be encountered in these new approaches to old procedures. As each frustration is identified, a solution is found. Problem-solving abilities need to be developed along with the other new skills. Having a contingency plan for the many difficulties that may arise is the most important step to confident and proper management.

References

1. Deyo GA: Complications of laparoscopic cholecystectomy. *Surg Laparosc Endosc* 2(1):41–48, 1992.

2. Ko ST, Airan MC: Therapeutic laparoscopic suturing techniques. *Surg Endosc* 6:41–46, 1992.

3. Sackier JM, Berci G: Diagnostic and interventional laparoscopy for the general surgeon. *Contemp Surg* 37(4):15–26, 1990.

4. Cooperman AM: Laparoscopic cholecystectomy for severe acute embedded, and gangrenous cholecystitis. *J Laparoendosc Surg* 1(1):37–40, 1990.

5. Flowers JL et al: The Baltimore experience with laparoscopic management of acute cholecystitis. *Am J Surg* 161:388–392, 1991.

6. Fitzgibbons FJ, Salerno GM, Filipi CJ: Open laparoscopy, in Zucker KA: *Surgical Laparoscopy.* St. Louis, Quality Medical Publishing, 1991.

7. Battista JC, Pequet AJ: Personal communication. Milwaukee, May 1992.

8. Schriber JH: Laparoscopic appendectomy in pregnancy. *Surg Endosc* 4:100–102, 1990.

9. Soper NJ, Hunter JG, Petrie RH: Laparoscopic cholecystectomy during pregnancy. *Surg Endosc* 6:115–117, 1992.

14

Laparoscopic Common Bile Duct Exploration

Stephen J. Shapiro
Leo Gordon
Leon Daykhovsky

> Horrible and stupendous calculi, coagulated in the gallbladder. Their shape, color, number, and wonderful effects producing vomiting, nausea, heaviness, low spirits, heavings of the stomach and hypochondria, atrophy, tabes, obstruction of the viscera, inflammation, incurable jaundice, sleeplessness, lassitude, sadness and melancholic affections, inclination to anger, difficulty, and heat of urine, lepra of the skin, fever, sudden death by a hidden and generally unknown seminary and foment of diseases and symptoms of a mysterious and perplexing character.
>
> Schenk, 1609.

As our knowledge of biliary tract disease increased, earlier intervention became the rule. The remarkably accurate description above of the effects of common duct pathology serves as a reminder of the complications of delayed treatment. Although nearly 400 years have passed since this description, the issue remains just as prominent in today's surgical world. The laparoscopic revolution now centers about the issue of common duct stones and how best to deal with them. Our goal in this chapter will be to describe and detail the technique of laparoscopic common bile duct exploration. The "mysterious and perplexing character" of this particular problem in laparoscopic surgery today will be explained.

Since Courvoisier performed the first successful choledochotomy on January 21, 1890, common bile duct exploration has evolved to become a standard part of the surgical approach to biliary tract disease. Surgery of the gallbladder and common duct became a frequent event in the surgical practice of the 1940s through the 1980s. Cholecystectomy and bile duct exploration were streamlined by the use of intraoperative cholangiography and flexible choledochoscopy. The sudden appearance of laparoscopic cholecystectomy in 1989 and 1990 has dramatically changed the traditional approach to biliary tract disease.[1,2]

Laparoscopic cholecystectomy has presented a variety of new challenges to the surgical endoscopist. Common bile duct stones that were identified early in the experience of laparoscopic cholecystectomy were generally treated by one of three ways:

1. The cholecystectomy was completed, allowing for spontaneous passage of the stone(s).
2. The patient was referred for endoscopic sphincterotomy following the laparoscopic cholecystectomy, or
3. The laparoscopic case was converted to an open case for choledochotomy and stone extraction.

All of these options have created problems.

To convert to an open laparotomy and a standard common bile duct exploration defeats the original intent of the less invasive laparoscopic approach. Allowing for the stones to pass spontaneously creates the risk that they will become obstructed and the patient will develop cholangitis or biliary pancreatitis.[1] At that time, the patient would need emergency decompression of the common bile duct. The final option being a referral for an ERCP is worrisome on several accounts.

Endoscopic sphincterotomy carries significant morbidity and potential mortality.[3,4] In the most expert hands, the mortality of this procedure is approximately 1 percent, and the morbidity is between 8 and 12 percent. Some investigators have been concerned about the destruction of the ampullary sphincter mechanism and the result in chronic bacto-bilia. This may be especially important in the younger patient. The success of this procedure is approximately 85 percent.[5] Therefore, a significant number of patients would be technical failures and would certainly require an additional laparotomy. Early in the history of laparoscopic cholecystectomy, the alternative of postoperative ERCP was attractive because it afforded a nonsurgical way out. More recently, we have embarked on the laparoscopic common duct exploration.

The position of laparoscopic common duct exploration is in evolution. The surgeon should not give up the domain of the common bile duct.

In general, common bile duct exploration is indicated when stones are identified in the common bile duct on a cholangiogram. The intraoperative cholangiogram is a road map for avoiding ductal injuries. It is a guide to common duct pathology and has a central role in the performance of laparoscopic cholecystectomy. Once stones are identified in the common duct, there are basically two laparoscopic techniques available to remove them. They are an exploration performed through the cystic duct or direct access to the common duct by use of a choledochotomy.

Common Bile Duct Exploration through the Cystic Duct

The intraoperative cholangiogram is an essential part of laparoscopic cholecystectomy. Care-

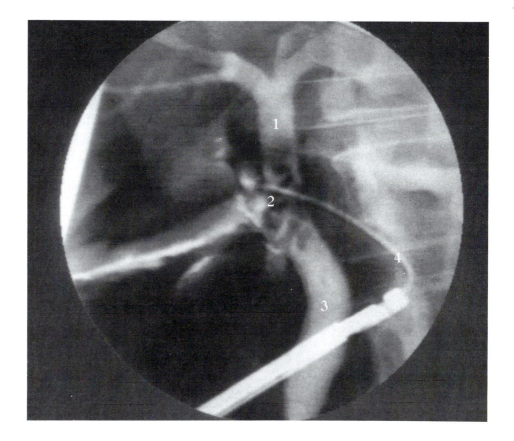

Figure 14-1
Cystic duct cholangiogram performed during routine laparoscopic cholecystectomy showing multiple common duct stones. 1 = Common hepatic duct. 2 = Multiple common duct stones. 3 = Common bile duct. 4 = Cholangiocatheter in cystic duct.

ful and thoughtful assessment of this study is the initial step in the process of common bile duct exploration through the cystic duct. After the cholangiogram has been obtained, there are several very important points to observe (Fig. 14-1). First, the length of the cystic duct should be measured from the cystotomy to the common bile duct. Secondly, the diameter of the largest common bile duct stones should be noted. Thirdly, identification of abnormal or anomalous cystic duct insertions is imperative so as to avoid injury during exploration.

The appropriate balloon catheter is chosen with specific reference to the cystic duct anatomy noted on the cholangiogram. A 0.035 in. hydrophilic coated guide wire is lubricated with saline (Terumo wire, Microvasive Boston Scientific Group). The white port of the no. 5 French shaft balloon dilating catheter is also lubricated with saline. The guide wire is then preloaded through this port.

The preloaded balloon catheter is then placed through a 3-mm reducer and is inserted through the midclavicular trocar. The wire and catheter are advanced to the ductotomy. The guide wire is advanced under fluoroscopic and visual control into the common bile duct (Fig. 14-2A and B).

The balloon dilation catheter (Fig. 14-3) is then advanced over the wire through the cystic duct toward the common bile duct. It is positioned so that the proximal radio-opaque marker is outside the incision in the cystic duct.

The balloon is then inflated, using saline and a 10 cc syringe attached to a pressure gauge. The syringe is used to generate the recommended 6 to 12 atm of pressure. The dilation is performed under direct vision (Fig. 14-4A and B). Fluoroscopic confirmation of the balloon position can be obtained if the operating room is so equipped. The balloon is kept inflated for 3 to 5 min. It is not unusual to see the balloon directly through the wall of the cystic duct during this maneuver.

The dilation of the cystic duct as described requires significant additional training for the general surgeon. Although there has been concern over cystic duct necrosis, it has not been

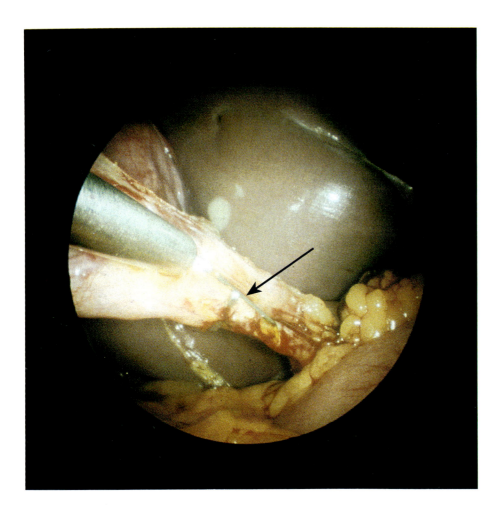

Figure 14-2
A. The guide wire (arrow) is preloaded on the balloon dilation catheter and advanced into the common duct through a cystic duct incision.

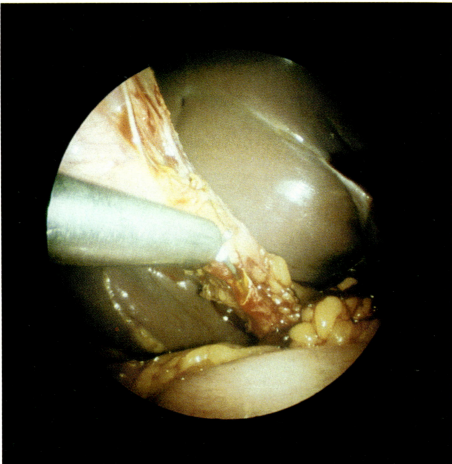

Figure 14-2
B. The metal introducer is placed near the cystic ductotomy to prevent buckling of the guide wire as it is passed.

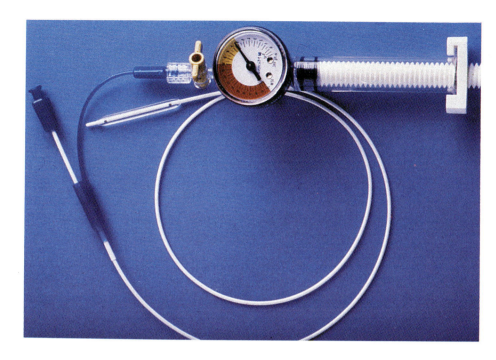

Figure 14-3
A balloon dilation catheter with a central lumen for a guide wire and another lumen for balloon inflation connected to a special syringe inflator with a dial readout to measure inflation pressure and a screwing mechanism for accurate adjustment (Microvasive, Inc.).

reported. Temporary cystic duct stents are currently being developed that may make this approach technically easier.

The balloon is then deflated and withdrawn over the wire. The cystic duct will now accommodate passage of a choledochoscope. We employ a no. 9 French disposable deflectable choledochoscope (Fig. 14-5A and B). The scopes have a relatively high resolution image with zero to infinity focus. There is a 1.1 mm working channel that will allow passage of other instrumentation or laser fibers. The choledochoscope is bidirectional, with 90° and 30° deflection capacity. The 90° deflection capacity offers steerability over the catheter. At present, most of these choledochoscopes have a relatively rigid tip for the lens mechanism, and the deflection segment is located 1.5 or 2.5 cm from the tip. In time, the deflection point will be closer to the tip, allowing for easier manipulation in ducts that are less than 1 cm in diameter.

The choledochoscope image bundle has 6000 fibers and consequently provides a high resolution image from within the duct. The images obtained from the choledochoscope are then relayed through a CCD camera to a video monitor. Illumination of the choledochoscope is achieved through the use of a separate 300 W xenon light source.

Critical to the use of this choledochoscope is a Touhy-Borst adapter attached to the working channel. This permits passage of irrigation fluid or wires down the working channel of the choledochoscope.

The choledochoscope can be passed over the guide wire that had been previously placed in the cystic duct. The guide wire allows the safe passage of the choledochoscope past the valves of Heister. Irrigation provides a clear image and slightly dilates the duct as the choledochoscope is passed. The scope can be advanced over the wire to the more distal common bile duct (Fig. 14-6).

Transcystic choledochoscopy requires vigilant attention to both the intraabdominal laparoscopic image as well as to the image generated from the choledochoscope. The assistant surgeon must observe the passage of the choledochoscope to avoid tearing or evulsion of the duct. The choledochoscope may coil or abut adjacent structures if it is not observed. Once the common bile duct stone (or stones) has (or have) been visualized (Fig. 14-7), the wire is withdrawn and the stone manipulation and extraction begins.

If the stone in the common bile duct is free-floating and not impacted in the ampulla, the 4-wire Segura stone basket is advanced through the Touhy-Borst connector and positioned just beyond the stone (Fig. 14-8A, B, and C). Irrigation continues to permit adequate visualization. Under direct vision, the basket is opened by moving the slide on the Segura basket handle forward. Opening the basket is observed directly. The basket is withdrawn gently toward the stone. If the stone is not trapped in the basket at this point, several maneuvers can be performed to grasp the stone. Initially, the wire may be twisted. The choledochoscope may be used to position the basket by using its deflection capabilities. Finally, both maneuvers may be performed simultaneously. These maneuvers must be performed with attention to both the abdominal and common bile duct monitors.

Once the stone is entrapped in the basket, the basket is gently closed. Gentle retraction is used to abut the stone to the tip of the choledochoscope. Once this is done, the choledochoscope is removed and the stone is placed into Hartmann's pouch for later retrieval (Fig. 14-9A and B).

If the stone is too large to be extracted, there are several strategies that can be employed. The first option is to repeat the dilation of the cystic duct, using a slightly larger balloon. Care must be taken to do this under direct vision to prevent duct disruption. The second option is to use the stone basket as a crushing device to morselate the stone. In our experience, pigmented stones are easier to crush than pure cholesterol stones. A third option is to use a tunable pulsed dye laser that can safely fragment a large common bile duct stone (Fig. 14-10). It is also helpful to fragment stones that are impacted in the ampulla.

Experimental work done at the Laser Research Laboratory at the Cedars-Sinai Medical Center in Los Angeles has shown that this laser

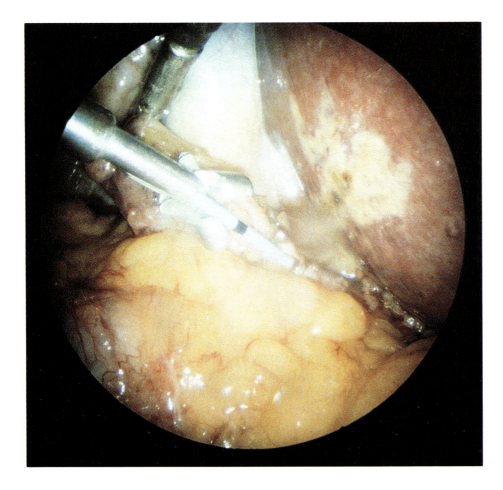

Figure 14-4
A. The balloon is guided into the cystic duct while deflated. One-third of the balloon is left outside of the duct for correct positioning.

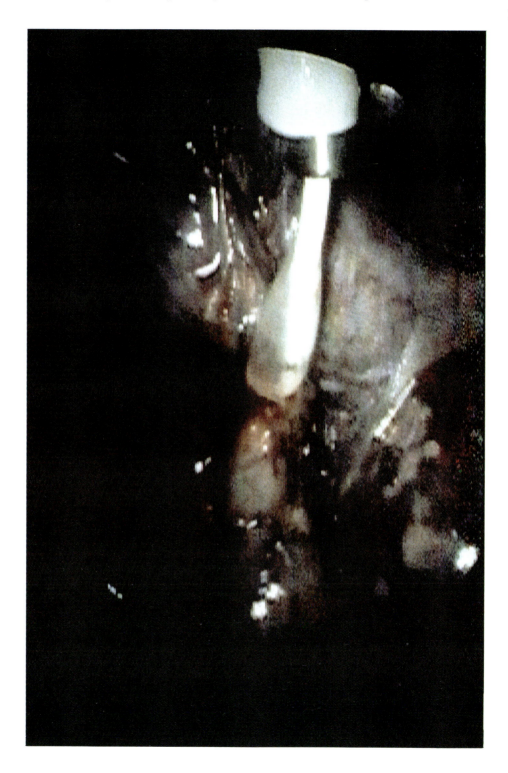

Figure 14-4
B. The balloon is then inflated to the recommended pressure for up to 3 min under direct laparoscopic visual control.

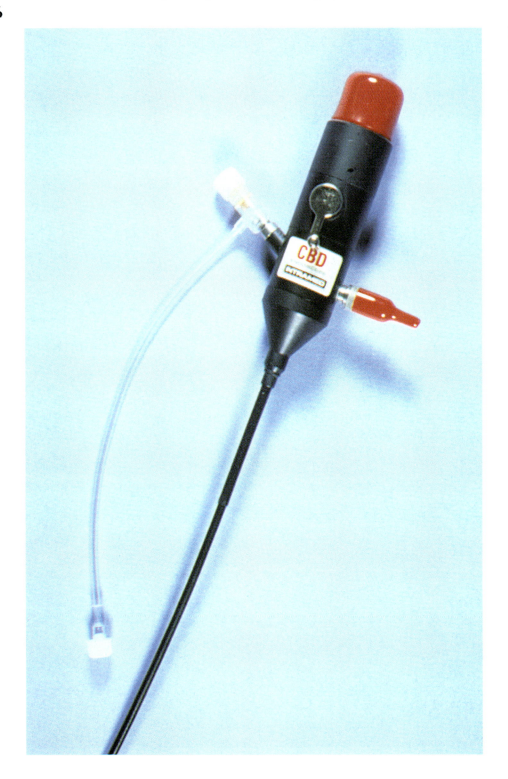

**Figure 14-5
A.** The disposable laparoscopic choledochoscope is no. 9 French in diameter, has a 1 mm working/irrigation channel, and (*continued on page 177*)

Figure 14-5 (B) has 90° deflection capabilities.

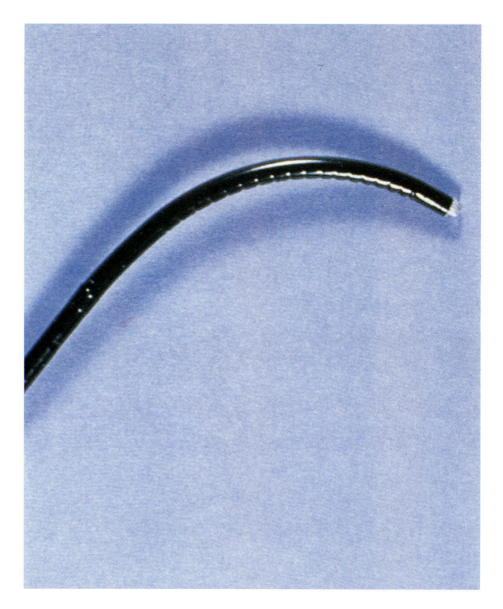

can effectively fragment the stone without the risk of common duct injury even if there is a direct contact with the laser tip to the common duct wall.[6] This device can be used even in the setting of a small cystic duct that will allow entry of only a 1.5-mm choledochoscope. The fragments can then be washed through the ampulla into the duodenum. The laser affords great flexibility in dealing with the anatomic variations in differing stone sizes in the biliary tree.

Use of this device requires that the laser fiber actually touches the stone when it is fired. The pulsing nature of the laser causes plasma formation on the surface of the stone that causes an acoustic shock wave that causes fragmentation of the stone. This works best with calcified stones, quite well with cholesterol stones, and less effectively with pigmented stones.

A final option for the irretrievable stone is to dilate the ampulla with the balloon in an attempt to dislodge the stone through the ampulla. There is little experience with this method. Because of the putative risk of duct disruption and pancreatitis, further experience is required prior to clinical use.

If stones are fragmented in the duct, irrigation is used to wash them through the ampulla. For adequate lavage, the basket should be with-

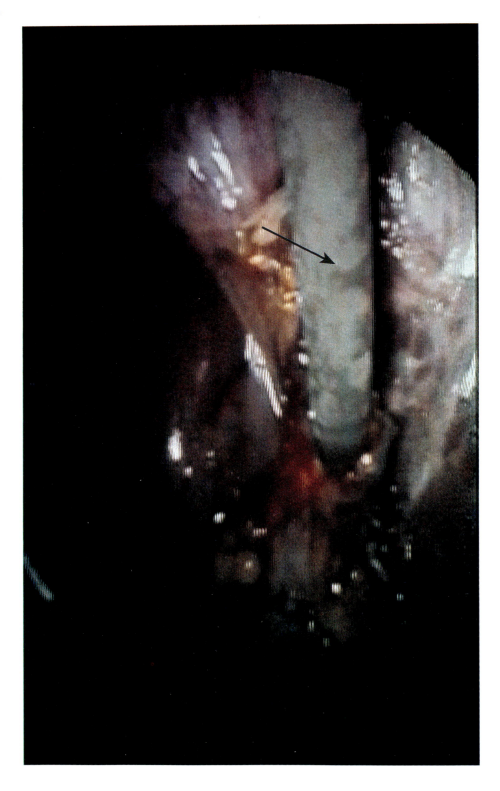

Figure 14-6
The choledochoscope (arrow) can be advanced over the guide wire into the cystic duct and common duct.

drawn and the choledochoscope is positioned proximal to the fragments. This allows high flow rates of the irrigant.

Just as the impacted stone is troublesome in open bile duct exploration, so also does it present a challenge to the biliary laparoendoscopist. As with an open case, a biliary Fogarty catheter may be passed through the choledochoscope beyond the stone and inflated. The soft tip of the Fogarty provides a margin of

Chapter 14 Laparoscopic Common Bile Duct Exploration

Figure 14-7
Several stones impacted in the ampulla are visualized with the choledochoscope in the common bile duct.

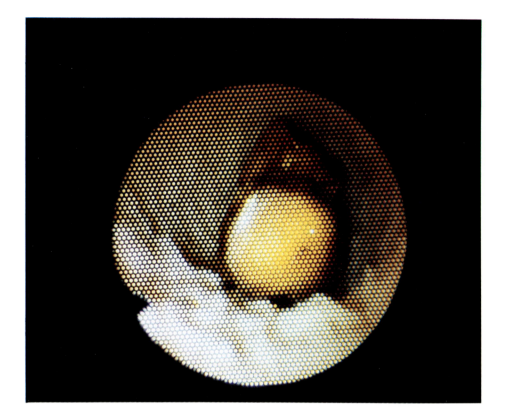

safety that the stone basket does not have. If the Fogarty catheter cannot dislodge the stone, the pulsed tunable dye laser may be used to fragment it as mentioned earlier.

When the stones have been removed or the fragments flushed through the ampulla, a completion cholangiogram is necessary.

Completion cholangiography is an essential

Figure 14-8
A. The Segura baskets come in several sizes and basket conformations. The basket is extruded by pushing the thumb slide on the handle (Microvasive, Inc.).

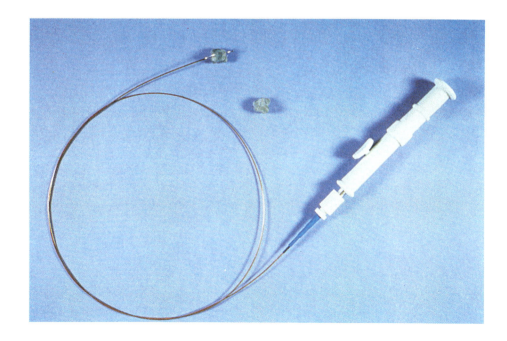

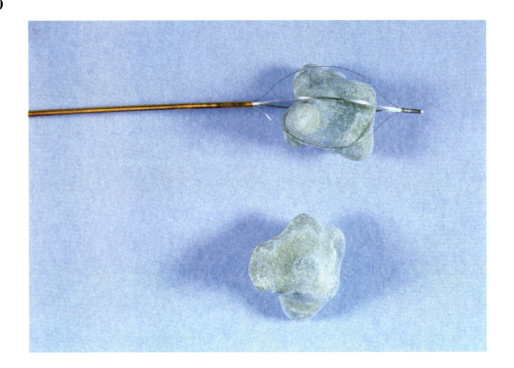

Figure 14-8
B. A four-wire basket drawn up around a stone.

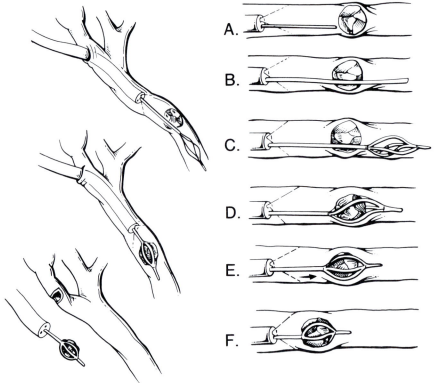

Figure 14-8
C. The technique involves passing the device around the stone (*a,b*), extruding the basket (*c*), slowly withdrawing the basket past the stone (*d*), drawing up the basket around the stone (*e,f*), and pulling the scope and basket/stone slowly out of the duct while observing the process on the choledochoscopic and laparoscopic monitors.

part of transcystic duct common bile duct exploration (Fig. 14-11). In addition to proving the adequacy of stone extraction, it also demonstrates integrity of the bile duct. This study can be done in the same fashion as cystic duct cholangiography prior to common bile duct exploration.

Because the cystic duct has been dilated and repeatedly cannulated, an adequate cystic duct closure is essential. The PDS Endoloop is rec-

Figure 14-9
A. The common duct stone is trapped in the basket and is withdrawn from the duct while it is observed through the choledochoscope.

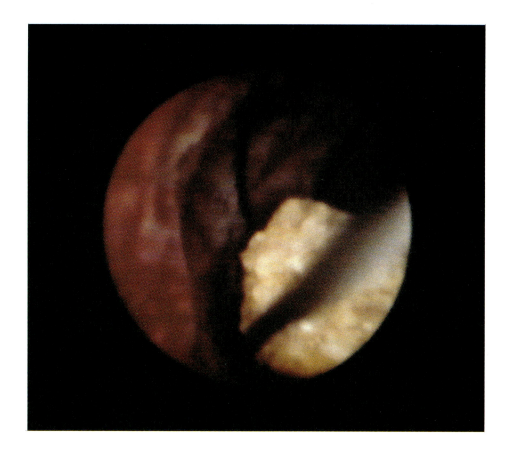

Figure 14-9
B. Once outside of the duct, the stone can be temporarily placed into Hartmann's pouch and the scope reinserted into the duct.

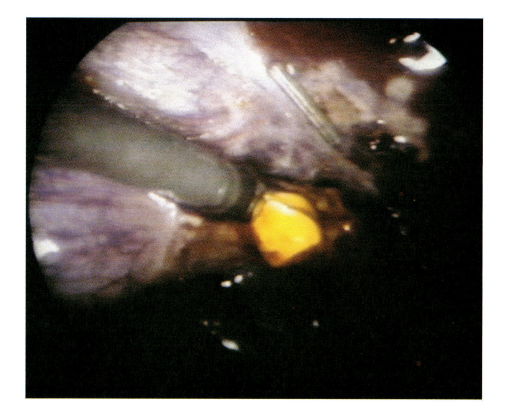

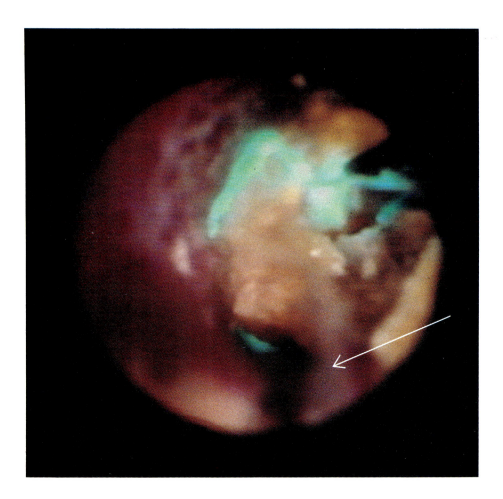

Figure 14-10
A pulsed dye laser can be used to fragment the stones that may allow the pieces to be removed with a basket, or the fragments may be flushed through the ampulla into the duodenum (arrow marks the laser fiber).

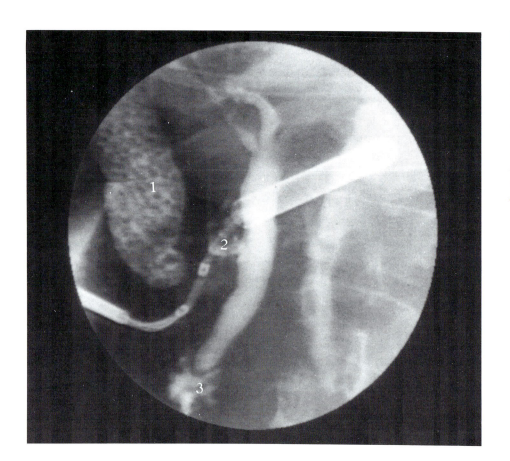

Figure 14-11
A completion cholangiogram showing no residual stones and free flow of contrast into the duodenum.
1 = Gallbladder filled with stones. 2 = Cystic duct with catheter. 3 = Free flow of bile into duodenum.

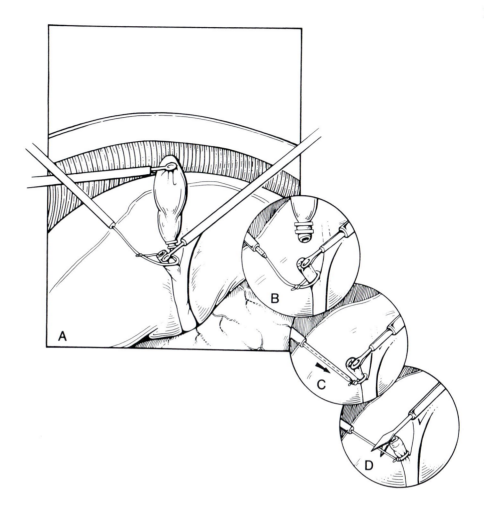

Figure 14-12
Placement of a loop knot on the cystic duct is recommended. The technique involves **(A,B)** placing the loop around the cystic duct, **(C)** cinching down the knot with the knot pusher, and **(D)** cutting the suture.

ommended (Fig. 14-12). After cystic duct ligation, the standard laparoscopic cholecystectomy is completed.

In our experience, 87 percent of the common duct stones encountered were in the common bile duct. The remaining calculi were distributed in the common hepatic, right, and left intrahepatic ducts. These calculi present a difficult problem for transcystic duct method. The cystic duct does not necessarily enter the common duct at right angles. Berci, reporting on more than 4000 intraoperative cholangiograms, states that only 17 percent of the cystic ducts enter the common bile duct from the lateral side.[3] Anterior, posterior, and medial insertions occurred in the other instances. In 7 percent of the cases, the cystic duct presented with parallel drainage entering just proximal to the ampulla.[7] From this assessment, it can be seen that the endoscopic approach to the upper ducts may be anatomically difficult in 17 percent of the cases. For these specific instances, we have developed a method of direct common bile duct exploration performed through the laparoscope.

Direct Laparoscopic Common Bile Duct Exploration

In order to access the common bile duct through a direct choledochotomy, the anterior wall of the common bile duct must be identified. Overlying connective tissue is dissected using atraumatic grasping forceps and bipolar cautery. Small vessels are carefully coagulated. Care must be taken with electrified instruments when dissecting the common duct. The operating surgeon as well as the assistant must be vigilant in their observation of uninsulated portions of dissecting instruments.

A choledochotomy is made, using a needle tip electrocautery (Fig. 14-13*A*, *B*, and *C*). Once

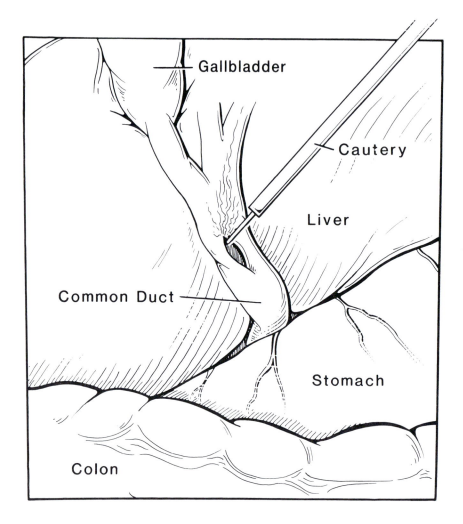

Figure 14-13
A. The choledochotomy for direct access to the common bile duct is made with the needle cautery on the anterior surface of the duct.

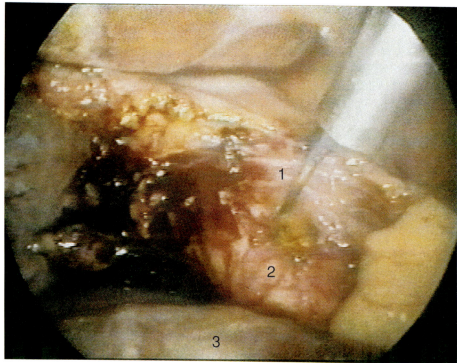

Figure 14-13
B. 1 = Needle cautery.
2 = Common bile duct.
3 = Duodenum.

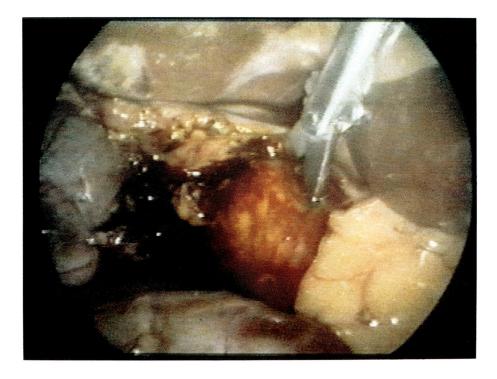

Figure 14-13
C. The incision is then enlarged to about 6 or 7 mm with laparoscopic scissors.

the duct is entered, bile will be seen and the electrocautery is exchanged for a straight or laparoscopic Potts scissors. An additional trocar placed in the left upper quadrant will frequently facilitate the procedure. This will allow additional retraction or manipulation of the choledochoscope and eventual T-tube placement. The no. 9 French choledochoscope is then placed through the subxiphoid trocar. It can be directed either distally into the ampulla or proximally into the common hepatic duct. The stone extraction then proceeds as has been described with the transcystic duct approach. When using a direct choledochotomy, it is necessary to use a T-tube to decompress the biliary tree after exploration has been completed.

A 12–14 French T-tube is placed through the subxiphoid trocar into the abdominal cavity (Fig. 14-14A and B). Using atraumatic graspers, the surgeon inserts the T-tube into the common bile duct. This frequently requires coordinated teamwork between the surgeon and the assistant surgeon. Occasionally a second assistant is required. The common duct is then closed with interrupted sutures of 4–0 Vicryl. Endoscopic suturing and knot placement requires practice and direct familiarity with both intra- and extracorporeal techniques of tying. We employ a "ski" needle passing transversely through the duct edges and using intracorporeal knot-tying technique.

The duct should be closed securely around the T-tube to avoid leakage. Once the T-tube is secure, the cystic duct is ligated and the gallbladder is removed in the usual laparoscopic fashion. A drain is placed in the pouch of Morrison. Completion T-tube cholangiography is then performed.

The transcystic duct method is our preferred approach to laparoscopic common bile duct exploration because the patients have the same postoperative course as routine laparoscopic cholecystectomy. The direct approach to the common duct may be more familiar to surgeons; however, it does not appear to offer significant advantages to the patient. In our experience, this approach lengthens hospital stay, obviating one of the main advantages of laparoscopic cholecystectomy.

It is not a treatment failure or a surgical failure if an open laparotomy and choledochotomy is performed for bile duct stones. The morbidity and mortality of this procedure is extremely low and has long been proven to be efficacious and well-tolerated.[8] The decision to convert a laparoscopic cholecystectomy to an open laparotomy in order to treat common bile duct stones that have been discovered on cholan-

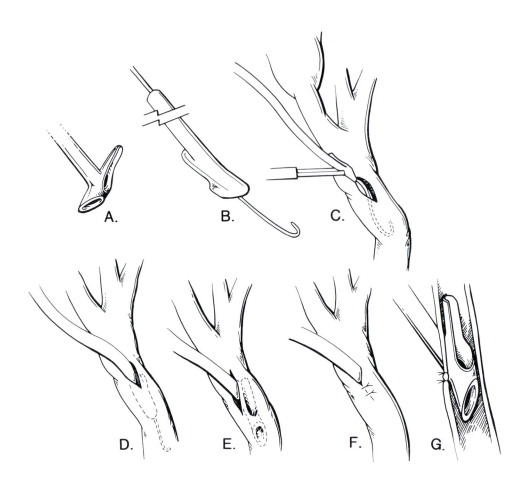

Figure 14-14
A. The T-tube is cut (*a*) and then inserted over a guide wire into the choledochocotomy (*b,c,d,e*). Laparoscopic suture placement is used to close the incision around the tube (*f,g*).

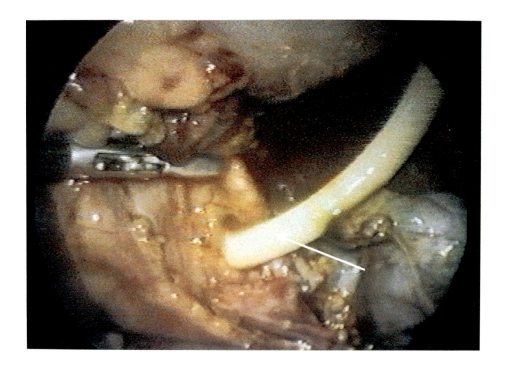

Figure 14-14
B. The T-tube (arrow) is observed closely to avoid inadvertently dislodging it when removing instruments and ports.

giogram is an exercise in surgical judgment. It is a judgment based on the anatomic findings and the experience of the surgeon.

We are early in the evolution of the transcystic duct approach to common bile duct stones.[9] At the Cedars-Sinai Medical Center, approximately 105 laparoscopic common bile duct explorations have been done. Ninety-five percent of these have been accomplished using the cystic duct approach. This technique involves a new set of manual and cognitive skills. The use of wires, baskets, and balloons, as well as the skillful use of intraoperative fluoroscopy, are essential to the success of the procedure. Furthermore, skillful choledochoscopy and transcholedochal instrumentation are needed. Transcystic bile duct exploration needs a primary surgeon and two assistant surgeons trained as a team. It must be clear that all members of that team have a commitment to refining their laparoscopic skills.

These new and exciting procedures represent an early experience. Our experience at Cedars-Sinai Medical Center has lead us to recommend it to the endoscopist who is willing to undergo the requisite didactic and laboratory education. Each surgeon must seek additional training to become familiar with the tools as well as the nuances of the procedure. Proper training and experience will make laparoscopic common bile duct exploration a safe and valuable tool.

References

1. Meador John H et al: Laparoscopic cholecystectomy. *South Med J* 84(2):186–189, 1991.
2. Sackier J et al: The role of cholangiography in laparoscopic cholecystectomy. *Arch Surg* 126:1021–1026, 1991.
3. Hart R, Classen M: Complications of diagnostic gastrointestinal endoscopy. *Endoscopy* 22:229–233, 1990.
4. Scheeres DE: Endoscopic retrograde cholangiopancreatography in a general surgery practice. *Am Surg* 56(3):185–191, 1990.
5. Heinerman MP et al: Selective ERCP and preoperative stone removal in bile duct surgery. *Ann Surg* 209(3):267–272, 1989.
6. Berci G et al: Common bile duct laser lithotripsy. *Gastrointest Endosc* 36:137–139, 1990.
7. Hamlin JA: Biliary ductal anomalies, in Berci G, Hamlin JA: *Operative Biliary Radiology*. Baltimore: Williams & Wilkins, 1981, vol 8, p 109.
8. Morgenstern L, Wong L, Berci G: 1200 open cholecystectomies before the laparoscopic era: A standard for comparison. *Arch Surg* 127:400–403, 1992.
9. Shapiro S, Gordon L, Daykhovsky L: Laparoscopic exploration of the common bile duct: Experience in 16 selected patients. *J Laparoendosc Surg* 1(6):333–341, 1991.

15

Sheath Access via the Cystic Duct for Common Bile Duct Choledochoscopy

John N. Graber

Unless the common bile duct can be accessed in a routine fashion during laparoscopic surgery, management of common bile duct stones will no longer remain in the domain of the general surgeon.[1-3] We have developed a guide wire and catheter-based system to explore the common duct via the cystic duct that can be done routinely, without excessive risk, and is within the technical abilities of most laparoscopic abdominal surgeons. The alternative of referring these cases to gastroenterologists or radiologists to manage following cholecystectomy lowers the overall quality of patient care.

There are four plausible ways to enter the common bile duct during a laparoscopic procedure: transhepatic, via the cystic duct, direct choledochotomy, and transduodenal through the ampulla. Of these, we have found the cystic duct access to be superior for choledochoscopic assessment of stones in the common duct.[4,5]

Transcystic Duct Common Bile Duct Access

In short, cystic duct access involves passage of a guide wire through the cystic duct and into the common bile duct. Then a balloon dilation catheter is used to dilate the cystic duct before passing a sheath with a pneumostatic valve into the cystic and common duct. Once this sheath is in place, a choledochoscope can easily be passed into the common duct and the stones can then be dealt with in many ways.[6] The use of a sheath is important for specific reasons.

First, a sheath offers precise control for the manipulation of the choledochoscope. If the choledochoscope is inserted through an abdominal wall cannula and into the cystic duct directly, there are several problems encountered. For one, the valves of Heister are quite difficult

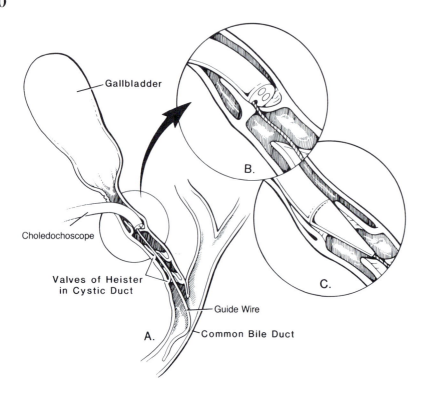

Figure 15-1
A. Passage of a choledochoscope is made difficult by the valves of Heister.
B. This can be true even when it is passed over a guide wire.
C. Passage of the sheath with the internal dilator avoids this problem.

to navigate even if a guide wire is inserted first and the scope passage is attempted over the wire (Fig. 15-1). The present-day scopes are eccentric with regard to the wire channel, and this leads to the scope getting hung up on the valves. The sheath also prevents looping and buckling of the choledochoscope within the abdominal cavity. Without a surrounding support such as a sheath, the flexible nature of the choledochoscopes causes them to kink, buckle, and loop inside the abdominal cavity when they are passed through the cannula and meet minor resistance in the duct (Fig. 15-2A and B). Once there is any loop or slack in the scope, you lose control over the tip. This problem is eliminated because the sheath offers complete support to the body of the scope. These factors result in complete control over the scope so that it can be rotated, pushed, pulled, or deflected without problems.

A second advantage is that the sheath can be used as another source for irrigation. This is especially valuable when the instrument/irrigation channel of the choledochoscope is occupied with a "large" instrument preventing adequate irrigating flow around it. Also, the sheath protects the posterior wall of the duct by directing instruments and the scope into the common duct lumen.

Lastly, a completion cholangiogram can be accomplished easily through the sheath after removing the scope.

In order to make the transition into common bile duct exploration during routine laparoscopic cholecystectomy, a plan and instrumentation must be at hand. A system that allows flow from one step to the next depending upon the situation makes routine duct exploration much more efficient and less time consuming.

The decision to explore the common bile duct is usually made by identification of stones in the duct on a cholangiogram (Fig. 15-3). The technique of the cholangiogram affects the routine of how the common duct is to be accessed. If a cholecystocholangiogram is done, that is, direct injection of dye into the gallbladder, then the cystic duct would need to be exposed and accessed. If a cystic duct cholangiogram is done, a system should be used that allows direct continuation to common duct access after stones are identified.

In the case of a cystic duct cholangiogram, the catheter should be inserted from a site that is convenient for common duct exploration if

Figure 15-2
A. Without internal support the choledochoscope can buckle and loop within the abdominal cavity.

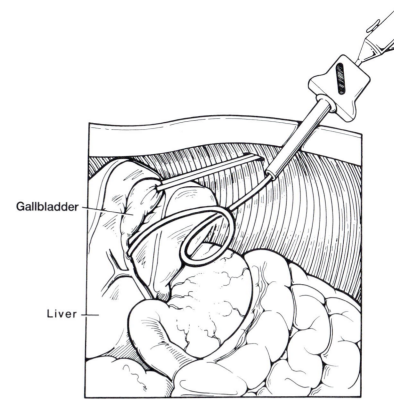

Figure 15-2
B. A sheath prevents looping, which increases fingertip control over the scope.

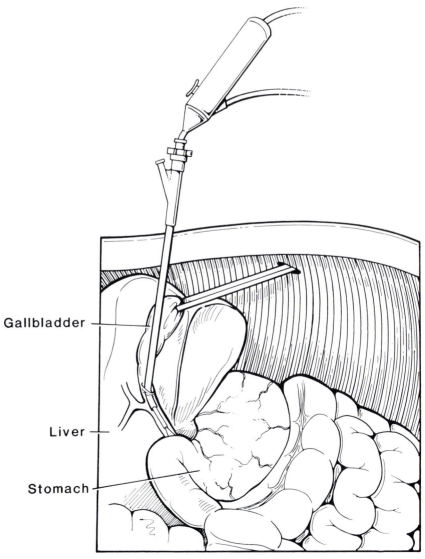

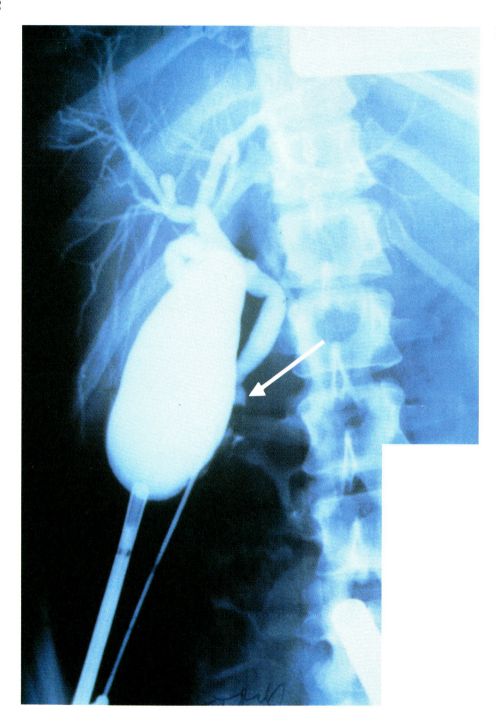

Figure 15-3
A cholecystocholangiogram showing a stone lodged in the ampulla, causing ductal obstruction (arrow).

needed. After the cholangiogram is done, the same catheter should allow passage of a guide wire to facilitate insertion of the sheath. We have found that rather than inserting the catheter for the cholangiogram through a cannula, inserting it percutaneously at a strategically advantageous point on the abdominal wall works best. This site on the abdominal wall should be the ideal spot to carry out common bile duct access if it is warranted. It can be identified after the cystic duct is exposed and retracted by lifting the gallbladder anteriorly and then noting the trajectory of the cystic duct to the abdominal wall (Fig. 15-4). This is the point from which the common duct exploration devices should be inserted so as to avoid difficult

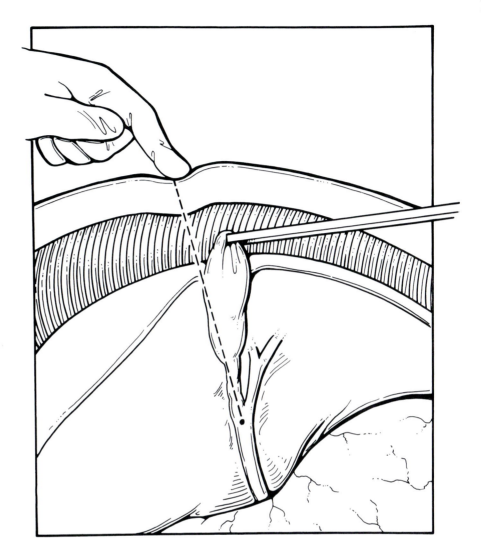

Figure 15-4
A strategic site on the anterior abdominal wall is found by pressing a finger on the skin to locate the spot directly in line with the retracted cystic duct.

angles of entry into the cystic duct. Consequently, this is also the point through which the percutaneous cholangiocatheter needs to be passed. This specific device is available as a thin metal needle with a blunt obturator such as in the Verres needle. It can be passed directly through the skin and directed into the cystic duct. The obturator can then be removed and a guide wire passed if stones are seen on the cholangiogram. Then the sheath can be inserted.

If a cholecystocholangiogram has been done revealing common duct stones, then it is followed by routine exposure and 360° control of the cystic duct. In the same manner as noted previously, the advantageous point on the abdominal wall is identified. At this site an Amplatz needle or another needle that will accept a 0.035 in. or 0.038 in. guide wire is passed through the abdominal wall in appropriate alignment with the cystic duct. Once the needle is placed, the guide wire is passed into the abdominal cavity and the needle removed.

With either method of cholangiography, the same guide wire and access sheath is used to access the common duct. The specific guide wire that works best for negotiating the cystic duct is a 30° angled tip hydrophilic coated device. The sheath and introducer are similar to vascular access devices with a hemostatic valve (Fig. 15-5). In this case the valve system is pneumostatic. The size of the sheath depends upon the size of the choledochoscope to be used. Most of these scopes are 9F and consequently a 10F sheath 20 cm in length works very well. We have used a scope that is 7F yet still has a 1

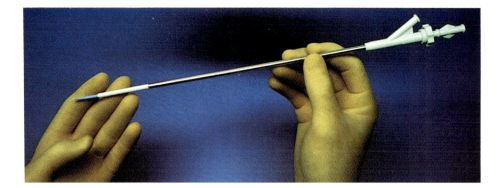

Figure 15-5
The guide wire is 0.038 in. diameter and hydrophilic coated. The sheath has a pneumostatic valve with an internal dilator, a stiff shaft with a flexible distal segment, and an irrigation port (Clarus Medical).

mm interventional channel (Fig. 15-6A and B). Another advantage of this scope is that it has fiberoptic connections for the light source and the camera to the main body of the scope, making it more manageable during use. For this scope an 8F sheath is used.

The sheath and dilating introducer can now be inserted over the guide wire into the abdomen. It is helpful to use a no. 11 blade scalpel to create a small tract for the sheath. In the setting of the cystic duct cholangiogram, the guide wire is already in the cystic and common ducts; but if a cholecystocholangiogram has been done, the guide wire must be advanced. The sheath and introducer are then used to direct the guide wire toward the cystic duct. A clip or two should be placed at the base of the gallbladder, and a small transverse incision is then made in the cystic duct, leaving enough proximal cystic duct to hold several clips at the end of the procedure. With the guide wire extending only 1 or 2 cm from the tip of the sheath's introducer, the guide wire is directed into the cystic duct; and by twisting or twirling it with the surgeon's fingers, it is passed into the common duct (Fig. 15-7A and B). The guide wire should not be forced because it should slide easily. Forcing it may cause perforation of the posterior wall of the common duct. The angled tip and the twirling action should keep it within the lumen and through the often difficult valves of Heister. Although fluoroscopic visualization can be helpful, we have not used it routinely. From this point on, the system is the same regardless of the method of cholangiography.

Next the cystic duct must be dilated to accommodate the sheath, the exploration devices, and the size of stone or fragments to be removed. The introducer is removed from the sheath with care taken not to withdraw the guide wire from the duct. A balloon dilation catheter similar to those used in balloon angioplasty or ureteroplasty is chosen (Fig. 15-8). A balloon catheter with a 30-cm shaft is needed but remains to be developed. A 4-mm diameter balloon would be sufficient to allow passage of a no. 10 French sheath, but the stone material may be somewhat larger and a 6-mm balloon may be necessary. The balloon size can be determined by measuring the size of the largest common duct stone seen on the cholangiogram. In most cases, the larger the common duct stone, the larger the cystic duct so that you can usually safely dilate the duct to the size of the stone as measured on the cholangiogram. Dilations of greater than 1 cm have been described. A balloon length of 2 to 4 cm is adequate to dilate the length of the cystic duct, and this should be determined by estimating the duct length on the cholangiogram.

The balloon is passed over the wire through the pneumostatic valve and sheath to the cystic duct (Fig. 15-9A and B). When deflated, the balloon can usually be passed through the duct easily while maintaining upward retraction on the gallbladder. It is necessary to keep the sheath near the entrance into the duct in order to prevent buckling and looping of the balloon catheter in the abdominal cavity as it is passed into the cystic duct. The balloon is positioned so that three-quarters of it is within the cystic duct and one-quarter out (Fig. 15-9C). Then it is inflated to the recommended pressure, usually around 6 atm. Most investigators suggest

Figure 15-6
A. The choledochoscope has a 7F shaft with a 1-mm working channel and steerable tip.

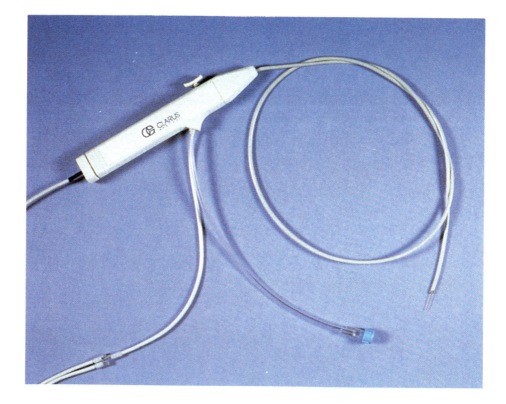

Figure 15-6
B. The camera and light source connections are separated from the body of the scope by fiberoptic leads that make the scope more manageable during use (Clarus Medical).

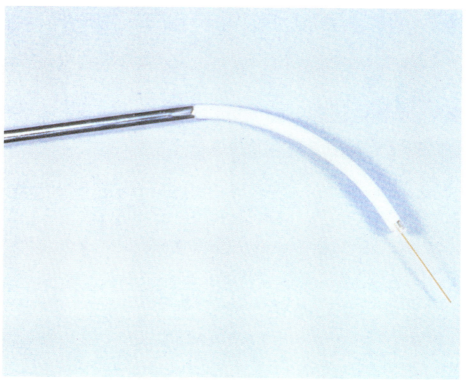

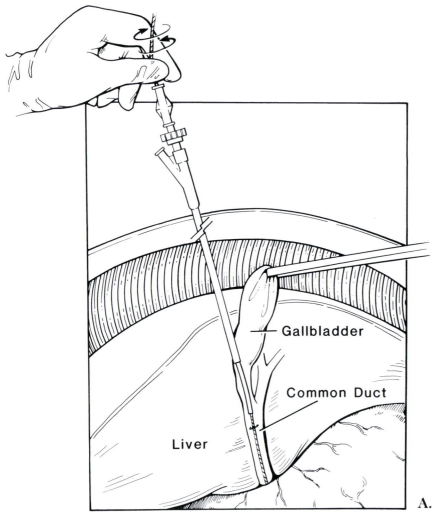

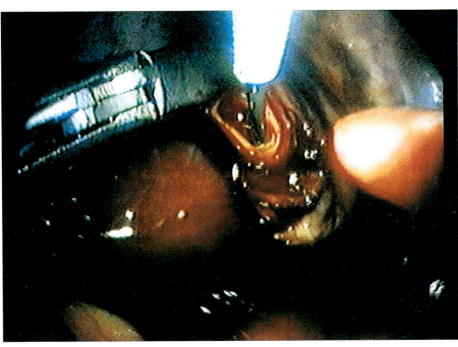

Figure 15-7
A and **B.** With a twirling motion of the fingers, the guide wire should pass easily into the common duct.

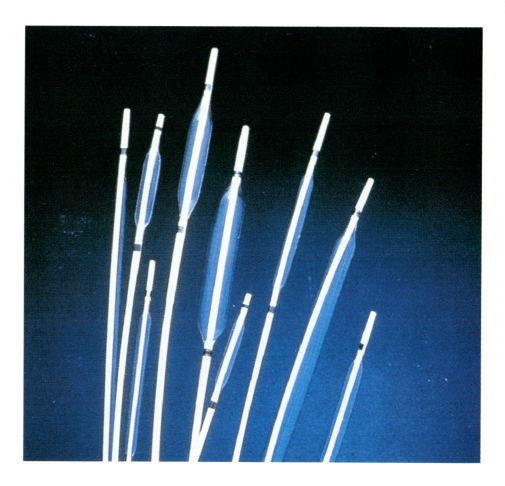

Figure 15-8
Balloon dilation catheters are available in any size; hand-held disposable insufflators are used (Microvasive).

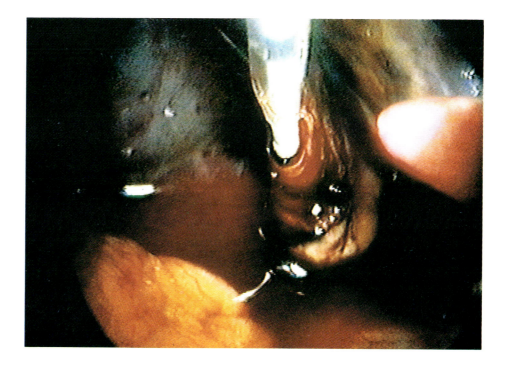

Figure 15-9
A. The dilation balloon is passed over the guide wire into the cystic duct (*continued on page 198*)

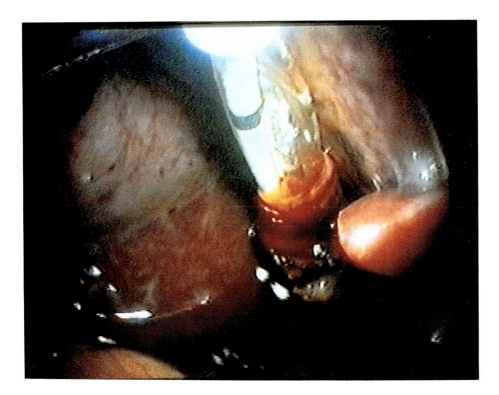

**Figure 15-9
B.** and inflated to 7 atm of pressure.

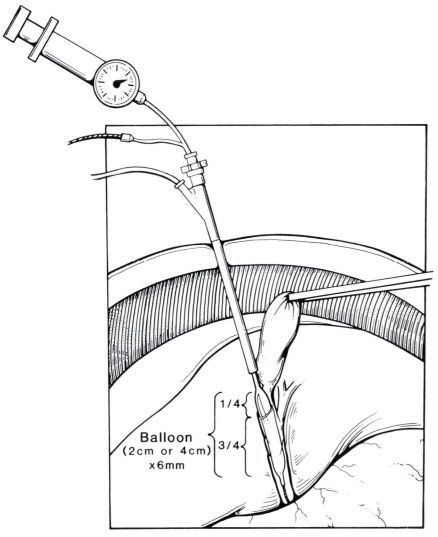

**Figure 15-9
C.** Leave one-quarter of the balloon visible outside of the duct.

Figure 15-10
A. With the sheath in place, the scope **(B)** can be passed with little resistance and with improved control.

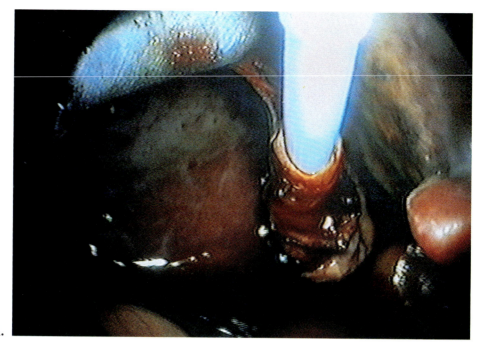

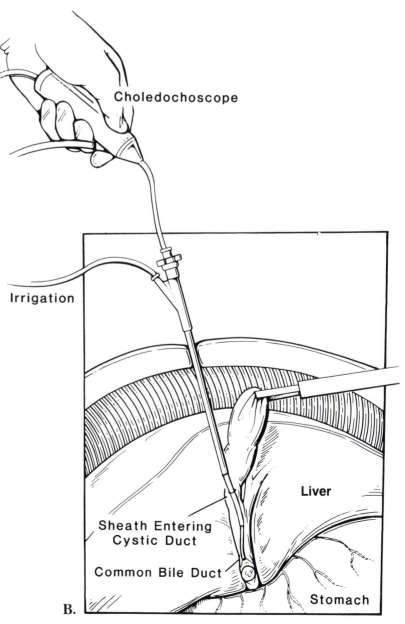

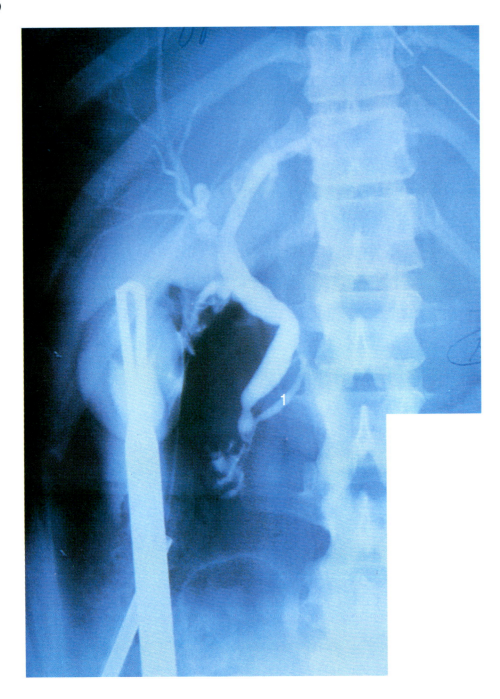

Figure 15-11
Completion cystic duct cholangiogram showing the common bile duct, pancreatic duct, and free flow of dye into the duodenum.
1 = Pancreatic duct.

leaving the balloon inflated for 3 min, but it is not clear that more than 15 or 30 s is necessary. The balloon is then deflated and removed again with care taken not to withdraw the guide wire. If the guide wire is dislodged, simply reinsert the dilating introducer over the wire and through the sheath and then replace the guide wire into the cystic and common duct as before. Now the sheath system can be advanced through the dilated cystic duct into the common duct (Fig. 15-10A and B). Again, this passage should not be forced.

Once the sheath is appropriately placed, the guide wire and introducer can be removed. Low pressure irrigation can be accomplished through the side port of the sheath from a gravity controlled bag of normal saline and a three-way stopcock. Passage of a choledochoscope and other devices is now greatly facilitated (Chap. 14). Once the stones have been treated, a completion cholangiogram should be done (Fig. 15-11). The cystic duct can then be clipped or ligated.

Discussion

Analysis of this system to access the common bile duct during a laparoscopic procedure shows some positive and some negative features. On the positive side is the relative ease with which the access is accomplished in the majority of cases. Use of the sheath allows for better manipulative control of the choledochoscope without having to deal with the scope buckling and looping within the abdominal cavity. The sheath and valve also offer minimal resistance to the scope and afford better tactile sensation. The side port irrigation is also helpful because the irrigation channels in the scopes are generally too small to attain adequate flow. Also the sheath offers some protection to the posterior wall of the common duct by directing devices down the common duct lumen.

On the negative side, this system offers no way to access the common hepatic duct. Fortunately, 90 percent of common duct stones are found in the distal common bile duct obviating the need to explore the common hepatic duct. If stones are seen in the common hepatic duct on the cholangiogram, this access system should not be used and other alternatives should be employed. The presence of the sheath within the duct acts as a formidable barrier preventing stones in the common duct from being unintentionally flushed up into the common hepatic.

Another concern is that if a stone is snared with a basket, it will usually be too large to be pulled out through the sheath. In this case, the stone, scope, and sheath will have to be pulled out in unison through the cystic duct. After the stone is dropped into the pouch of Douglas, the sheath would need to be reinserted for each stone. An alternative that has a great deal of promise is to use a device such as a pulsed laser or an electrohydrolic lithotripper to fracture the stone into smaller pieces that will pass through the ampulla.

As each problem is identified, it is solved in turn. Over time, these and other techniques and the instrumentation will become more refined, and surgeons will again find common bile duct exploration a routine part of surgery.

References

1. Arregui ME et al: Laparoscopic cholecystectomy combined with endoscopic sphincterotomy and stone extraction or laparoscopic choledochoscopy and electrohydraulic choledocholithiasis. *Surg Endosc* 6:10–15, 1992.

2. Shapiro SJ et al: Laparoscopic exploration of the common bile duct: Experience with 16 selected patients. *J Laparoendosc Surg* 1(6):333–341, 1991.

3. Carrol BJ et al: Laparoscopic choledochoscopy: An effective approach to the common duct. *J Laparoendosc Surg* 2(1):15–21, 1992.

4. Hunter JG: Laparoscopic transcystic common bile duct exploration. *Am J Surg* 163:53–58, 1992.

5. Reid DA: Choledochoscopy of the cystic duct as a new approach to the biliary tree. *Surg Gynecol Obstet* 169(1):68–70, 1989.

6. Graber JN: Laparoscopic common bile duct access. *Surg Alert* 8(7):30–32, 1992.

16

Cholelithiasis: The Alternatives to Surgery

Robert Mackie

Introduction

The competition for medical removal or destruction of gallbladder stones has intensified in the past few years. Is there a revolution in the management of cholelithiasis with the many new nonsurgical approaches, or are we merely embarking on several new errors in management rather than a new era? Will the new minimally invasive procedure of laporoscopic cholecystectomy obviate the need for nonsurgical approaches? The answers to these questions are probably at least 10 years away, but the idea of nonsurgical management is really not new.[1] While major advances have been made in both our understanding of the development of cholesterol predominant stones and what might be done to rid the gallbladder of them, certainly the ultimate means of prevention or control for stones already present while leaving the gallbladder intact does not exist at this time.

Asymptomatic Stones

Sir William Osler once observed that "most gallstones caused no symptoms." William Mayo refuted this claim early in this century, however, and for decades surgeons were taught that most if not all gallbladders containing stones should be removed.[2]

If there is a new era in gallstone management, the first stage was probably the realization that many patients live and die with their gallstones having never caused pain or medical problem. Autopsy surveys showed that more than 90 percent of autopsied patients with gallstone disease died from unrelated causes, and cholelithiasis was a factor in only 3 to 7 percent of deaths.[3,4] It is probably not true that the longer patients live with gallstones, the more likely they are to experience pain or complications. In fact, just the opposite may be the case. Gracie and Ransohoff followed 123 asymptomatic patients (mostly men) for up to 15 years with only 18 percent developing symptoms.[5] In addition, the probability of developing symptoms fell steadily with time. That is, the longer patients were asymptomatic, the less likely they were to develop symptoms. This study has been criticized for its small size, and for the fact that only 13 of the 123 patients were women. Some further supporting data do exist, however. A study from the Health Insurance Plan of Greater New York showed that only approximately 10 percent of asymptomatic patients with gallstones developed symptoms over a limited follow-up period (median 46.3 months), and only 7 percent of these patients required cholecystectomy.[6]

The fact that 80 percent of cancerous gallbladders contain stones is sometimes raised as a reason for prophylactic cholecystectomy in patients with asymptomatic stones. While the presence of gallstones probably predisposes to the development of gallbladder adenocarcinoma, this is a relatively rare occurrence.[7,8] In addition, gallbladder adenocarcinoma occurs late (mean age 69), so that the increase in life span brought about by prophylactic cholecystectomy would be offset by greatly increased cost and some increased morbidity and mortality in young people. Further statistical analysis of the risks and benefits of removal of asymptomatic stones would seem to agree with these conclusions.[9] The majority of clinicians agree currently, then, that patients with asymptomatic stones should usually be observed expectantly. A well-controlled study to prove this to be the correct conclusion from the existing noncontrolled data can probably never be done.[10]

Groups at increased risk for complications have been proposed for a more aggressive approach even in the asymptomatic stage. These include patients with porcelain gallbladders (association with gallbladder carcinoma), young American Indian females (increased long-term risk of complication), and diabetics, although a recent report discounts an increased risk in this last group.[11] Finally, asymptomatic patients with stones in the common duct may be another group at considerably more risk for future complications. While little prospective data is available on the natural history of choledocholithiasis, Bateson's postmortem studies found that the presence of ductal stones contributed to the patient's death in about half of the cases.[12,13]

If asymptomatic stones are to be left alone, it becomes important to try to refine our ability to distinguish true symptoms of biliary cholic. It may be helpful to consider four subgroups of patients: First, truly asymptomatic patients. Presumably, their stones have been found incidentally during the course of other diagnostic studies (fetal ultrasound, abdominal flat plate, etc.); second, patients with nonspecific symptoms, such as dyspepsia, atypical intermittent abdominal pain, fatty food intolerance, and bloating; third, patients with mild, intermittent, but credible symptoms of biliary pain; and fourth, patients with unequivocal symptoms due to inflammation and cystic or common duct obstruction.[14] Accurate results as to the efficacy of either medical or surgical management of patients in subgroup 2 will be threatened by the inclusion of many patients who probably do not have symptomatic stones. Many of such patients will have the same or similar symptoms when interviewed 6 to 12 months after conclusion of treatment.

The natural history of patients with symptomatic stones as opposed to asymptomatic stones continues to favor early intervention. Wenckert and Robertson's 11-year review of 781 mildly to moderately symptomatic patients showed that severe symptoms developed in 35 percent, and serious complications developed in 18 percent. Mortality in patients over the age of 60 who did not have biliary tract surgery was more than 15 percent, significantly higher than the rate for those who elected surgery.[15] McSherry's study also concluded that almost half of the symptomatic patients developed worsening of symptoms during conservative follow-up, and surgery was eventually performed in 44 percent.[6] Patients selected for nonsurgical therapy of symptomatic biliary stones probably should be in the early course of their disease and experience mild to moderate symptoms without evidence for complicated disease.

The advent of nonsurgical management of gallstones, including bile acid therapy, lithotripsy, contact dissolution, etc., has changed the radiographic determination of cholelithiasis. What was once a question of binary proportions—are there stones, yes or no?—has now become a complex one of determining gallbladder functional status, as well as determining size, number, and radiographic density.[7] Nonsurgical trials have required a functioning gallbladder. Thus, most trials have included an oral cholecystogram (OCG) for primary evaluation of function. Size and number have been determined by best estimate on OCG and/or sonographic imaging. For treatment modalities that work only on cholesterol predominant stones, the need for determination of stone density beyond that provided by plane radiographic view of the right upper quadrant (i.e., to rule in or out calcium predominant stones) has yet to be determined. Density as determined by computed tomography (CT) evaluation would be an expensive but accurate method of determining density because a number of studies have shown correlations between cholesterol and calcium content and CT attenuation coefficients.[16–18] However, there has been great variation in results, probably owing to the complex nature of gallstone composition, and some investigators have questioned whether CT might be too sensitive to provide relevant clinical information for nonsurgical therapy.

Oral Dissolution

Certain naturally occurring bile acids have the ability to desaturate bile and pull cholesterol back out of gallstones, theoretically allowing dissolution of stones within the gallbladder. Therapy relies on the fact that the majority (70 to 85 percent) of gallstones in the Western world are cholesterol predominant. Two such bile acids have received extensive study and are currently on the market for gallstone dissolution: chenodeoxycholic acid (CDCA), and ursodeoxycholic acid (UDCA). These two bile acids are structurally very similar, differing only in the orientation of the hydroxyl group at the 7 carbon position (Fig. 16-1).

Danzinger et al., in 1972, noted that the primary bile acid CDCA reduced the cholesterol saturation of bile and effected cholesterol stone dissolution.[19] CDCA was the first studied and marketed in this country (1983). CDCA acts primarily by decreasing biliary secretion of cholesterol and secondarily through expansion of the bile acid pool. It has been used infrequently because it was effective in only a limited number of patients in the National Cooperative Gallstone Study, is relatively expensive, occasionally hepatotoxic, causes diarrhea frequently, and increases serum concentrations of low-density lipoproteins (LDL) cholesterol.[20] The National Cooperative Study was a 2-year trial using 2 regimens: 350 mg and 750 mg per day that were also compared with placebo. The patients receiving 750 mg daily had a 14 percent rate of complete dissolution and a 41 percent rate of partial dissolution when all patients with greater than 50 percent stone dissolution were included. Patients with less than ideal body weight had a 36 percent complete dissolution rate and a 76 percent partial or complete dissolution rate. This "thin" group may have been nearer the current recommended optimal dosage for CDCA of 12 to 15 mg/kg/day. At this dosage with highly selective criteria, complete

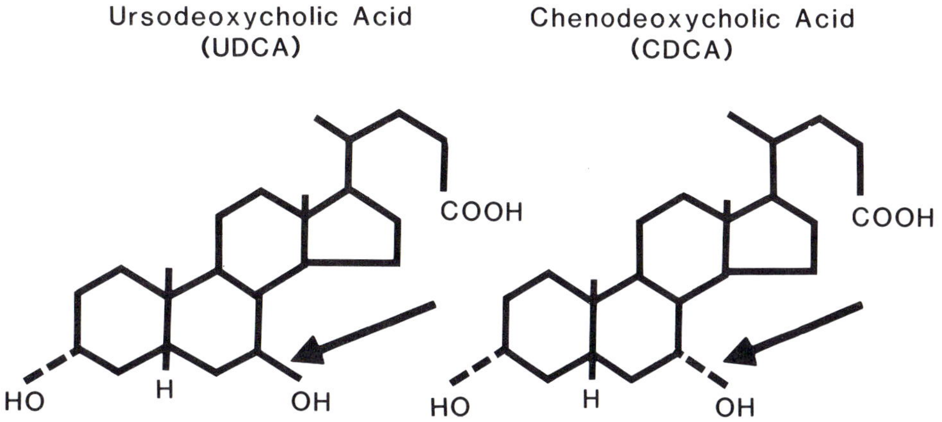

Figure 16-1
These two bile acids are structurally very similar, differing only in the orientation of the hydroxyl group at the 7 carbon position (arrows).

dissolution success rates of greater than 70 percent have been obtained.[21]

Because of much improved side-effect profile, UDCA has largely replaced CDCA for dissolution except when both are used in combination therapy. Urso (meaning *bear*) is the primary bile acid in polar bears, as well as Chinese black bears, and has been used for years in Japan for a variety of hepatic and intestinal diseases. It is normally found in human bile in small quantities, produced from CDCA by intestinal bacteria.

The structural change from CDCA to UDCA is again minor, the 7 carbon hydroxyl being axial (alpha) in the former, equatorial (beta) in the latter. This shift, however, pushes the charged hydroxyl group onto the lipophilic side of the molecule. This change makes UDCA a "poor" classic bile acid. That is, it is relatively poor at forming classic micelles to carry cholesterol in solution. However, toxicity of all bile acids may well be related to their ability to interact with biologic membranes. High concentrations of UDCA probably has less effects on hepatic cell membranes and may well be to some extent protective against the toxic effects of other bile acids. This theory is further supported by studies using combined CDCA + UDCA, showing that the combination is largely free of side effects,[22] while liver test abnormalities occur in patients who receive CDCA alone at the same low doses.[20] Finally, multiple studies are underway using UDCA in cholestatic liver diseases specifically for its possible protective effect.

UDCA seems to compensate for its inability to act a highly effective micelle former by enhancing a second mechanism for pulling cholesterol out of gallstones into solution. Phospholipids alone (e.g., lecithin) have the ability to hold cholesterol in solution in the form of large lipid vesicles. UDCA rich bile enhances the formation of these large unilamellar vesicles from the surface of stones. The ability of UDCA to promote this mesophase may explain why some studies show successful dissolution despite failure of patients' bile to desaturate.[23,24]

UDCA, when given in doses of 10 to 12 mg/kg/day, has been successful in dissolving 30 to 70 percent of stones in various studies. Salen et al. reported successful clearance of gallstones in 40 to 50 percent of treated patients in 2 to 3 years of treatment with CDCA.[25] Selection of patients is probably very important in dictating success rates. To obtain higher success rates, several favorable predictors are necessary. Patency of the cystic duct and/or a functioning gallbladder should be confirmed. Calcium containing stones should not be treated. A flat plate of the right upper quadrant (RUQ) will screen grossly for calcium content. Small stones (less than 5 to 7 mm) probably need no further screening. OCG can also be of predictive value in screening for cholesterol predominant stones.[26] Larger stones are more reliably screened by a limited CT scan of the gallbladder to assess stone density.[16–18] Stones above 1.5 cm in diameter are less likely to be dissolved successfully even without calcification. Gallbladders with a large stone load (i.e., greater than 50 percent of the volume filled) also have a poor prognosis for complete dissolution. The ideal gallbladder for dissolution is a well-functioning one with small floating stones (Fig. 16-2).

Therapy should be begun at 10 to 12 mg/kg/day in divided doses, and the ultrasound monitored every 6 months. If there has been no progress made in either size and/or number of stones in 6 months, therapy should probably be abandoned because complete dissolution with continued therapy is unlikely. Failure may indicate poor medication compliance, cystic duct obstruction, or stones of high calcium content.[27] If progress is being made, therapy is continued for 6 months to 2 years until the ultrasound is negative for stones or fragments. Because small fragments missed on ultrasound may act as a nidus for early recurrence, we recommend continued therapy for an additional 3 months with a repeat ultrasound at that time. If this is also negative, treatment is stopped and ultrasounds are repeated every year for 5 years.

Gallstone Lithotripsy

Extracorporeal shock wave lithotripsy (ESWL) rode a roller-coaster ride of enthusiasm and in-

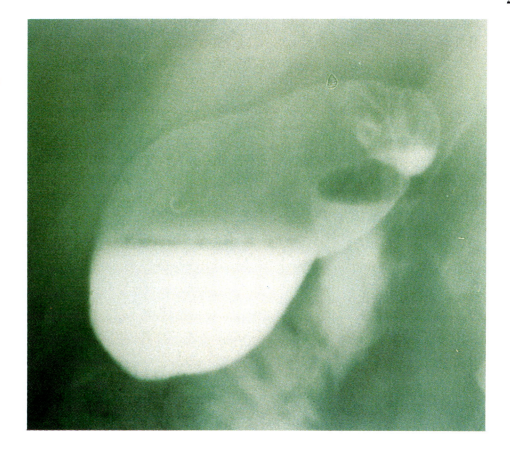

Figure 16-2
A cholangiogram that shows the heavier contrast material layered beneath multiple small floating stones. This is the best combination for successful stone dissolution therapy.

terest in the United States over the past several years. A number of manufacturers from several other countries developed lithotripters and initiated clinical trials in the United States. ESWL revolutionized the treatment of kidney stones and showed an impressive growth curve from its introduction into the United States with Food and Drug Administration (FDA) trials in the early 1980s.[28] Because the kidney program was so successful and because it was estimated that there are six gallstone patients in this country for every kidney stone patient, it was perhaps inevitable that this technology would soon be applied to the biliary tract. Unfortunately, engineering advances and enthusiasm for application of the new technology outpaced the ability of medical investigators to determine which parameters will be important clinically and which patients will truly benefit by treatment with lithotripsy. Whether it will survive as a viable option for the treatment of mildly to moderately symptomatic gallstones has been severely questioned.[29]

The use of shock waves was initiated in mining engineering in the Commonwealth of Independent States (CIS) (former Soviet Union). The tissue effects of shock waves were first realized from reports of blast injury to miners. The clinical use of shock waves to crush renal stones was first proposed in CIS in the 1950s. The basic principles of modern extracorporeal shock wave lithotripsy evolved further from Dornier's (German manufacturer) investigations into causes of the pitting often seen on spacecraft and supersonic aircraft after high speed flight. Studies revealed that when the craft collided with tiny water droplets at supersonic speeds, shock waves were generated. These shock waves are capable of producing pitting in titanium. Further investigations demonstrated that a destructive effect occurred when the shock waves traversed the interface of materials with different acoustical properties, such as a fluid and a brittle solid.

All lithotripters create, by various means, a high intensity pressure wave of short duration in water or similar fluid medium, then apply a convergence mechanism to direct the wave to a small area (envelope) in which stones are to be fragmented (Fig. 16-3). Such shock waves are characterized by a large positive front lasting in the microsecond range followed by a smaller negative front of longer duration.[30] An externally generated shock wave enters the body and propagates without interference as long as water-dense material is seen, as in body soft tissues. When the shock wave meets an acoustic interface, as in the surface of a gallstone, a significant portion of its energy is converted to destructive tensile forces.

To assure that the shock waves passed only through water-dense material until they entered the patient, the first lithotripters coupled the patient to the machine by immersion into the water bath in which the shock waves were generated.[31] The first large series of gallstone lithotripsy from Europe used an immersion machine modified for gallstones.[32] The immersion arrangement has obvious problems in patient handling, emergency access, anesthetic delivery, etc. Therefore, all manufacturers were designing the second generation of machines while gallstone trials were being proposed for the United States. These machines all allow the patient to remain out of the water bath by various means.

In addition, a controversy continued as to the ideal energy to deliver per pulse and by which generator for optimal treatment. High energy generators (i.e., spark-gap) were expected to have higher efficacy in stone breakup but require significant anesthesia to allow pa-

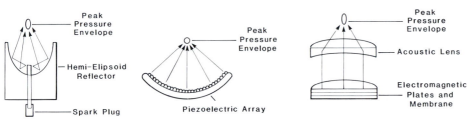

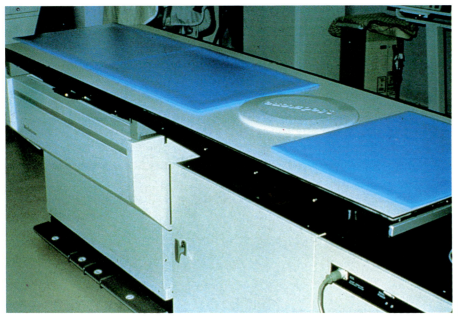

Figure 16-3
A. The different technological systems used for shock wave lithotripsy include a spark-gap system, a focused-reflector piezoelectric system with all emitters aimed at a single point, and an electromagnetic system with an acoustic lens to focus the wave. B. A typical extracorporeal shock wave lithotripsy unit used at Abbott Northwestern Hospital, Minneapolis, MN.

tient tolerance. Lower power generators (e.g., piezoelectric, electromagnetic) were predicted to have lower initial efficacy, but allow low or even no anesthesia. This controversy fueled a movement to drop general anesthesia for gallstone lithotripsy. Finally, renal lithotripters needed to be modified to allow ultrasound localization because the majority of gallstones are not calcified. Ultrasound generators were added to allow preoperative visualization of the gallbladder and were coupled to the generator to allow accurate aiming of the focused shock wave. In addition, body tissues with large air contents such as lung or gut will not readily transmit shock waves and must be avoided. Ultrasound imaging done in the path of the shock wave is generally used to assure exclusion of lung and gut in the pathway. While gut seems fairly resistant to damage by shock waves, lung is quite sensitive and must be carefully avoided.[33] Potential long-term renal effects remain at least of minor concern in both kidney and biliary lithotripsy.[34,35]

Ultrasound, as noted previously, has provided guidance for aiming the shock wave, monitoring progress during treatment, and for following patients postoperatively to assess clearance of fragments. Imaging during the ESWL treatment guides the aiming of the machine and assesses the adequacy of breakup of each stone. Because the gallbladder lumen often fills with a cloudlike swirl of debris as the treatment progresses, while the total number of small particles is increasing rapidly, it may be increasingly difficult to determine the level of success as treatment nears its finish.

The ultimate goal of ESWL is, of course, to rid the gallbladder of all stones and fragments and return the patient to the asymptomatic state. This needs to remain the gold standard in measuring successful treatment. There is growing agreement that clearance of all fragments postlithotripsy is directly correlated to the ability of the lithotripter to reduce fragment size to a very low level. Although fragments less than or equal to 4 mm are considered therapeutic, there is little question that optimal results are obtained when all fragments are 2 mm or less.[32,36–38] The cholesterol and calcium content of the stones may also affect fragmentation rates, although at least in vitro total stone volume seems to play a more important role.[27] If oral bile acid therapy is shown to be usually necessary for adequate clearance, calcium content could, of course, have a decidedly negative effect.[28]

In 1986, Sauerbruch et al. announced successful ESWL use in human beings with gallstones.[39] Sackmann et al. reported the first large successful series for gallstone lithotripsy in 1988.[32] They had concluded that if stones could be fragmented to <4-mm size fragments, the stones would be amenable to dissolution by oral agents. Therefore, only radiolucent stones were included and all patients received adjuvant litholytic therapy with bile acids. A combination of UDCA and CDCA was given postlithotripsy. Criteria used by Sackmann's group were as follows:

1. History of at least one recent episode of typical biliary pain.

2. Cholelithiasis confirmed by ultrasound.

3. Functional gallbladder as shown by OCG.

4. One to 3 stones that are nonopaque as shown by radiography.

5. Solitary radiolucent stone with a diameter up to 30 mm or up to 3 stones with similar total stone volume.

6. Shock wave path axis avoiding the lungs and gut.

7. Absence of complicated liver or biliary disease, need for anticoagulation, arrhythmia or pacemaker, or pregnancy.

8. Informed consent.

The results of Sackmann's study are shown in Fig. 16-4. It took 2 to 4 months until half of the patients were completely free of fragments. Eight to 12 months after ESWL, about 80 percent of the patients were free of stones. Adverse effects are charted in Table 16-1. Shock wave treatment was done under general anesthesia and was tolerated without serious adverse effects. There were no signs of tissue damage except cutaneous petechiae in 12 percent and transient hematuria in 3 percent. No signs of

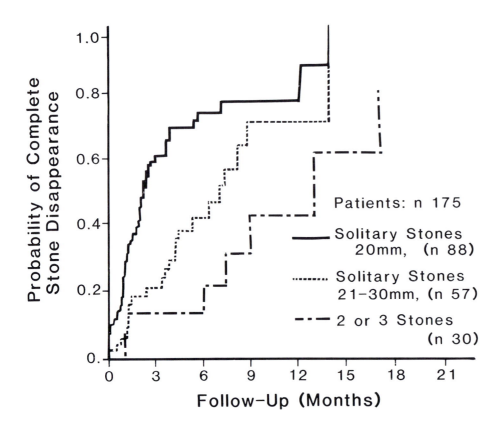

Figure 16-4
The probability of complete gallstone disappearance over time with extracorporeal shock wave lithotripsy (ESWL) depending upon the number of stones identified in the gallbladder at the start of the treatment. (Adapted from Sackmann et al.)[32]

hepatocellular damage or hepatobiliary dysfunction could be detected by laboratory tests. Approximately one-third of the patients experienced transient biliary pain related to stone fragments. It must, however, be noted that all patients had biliary pain prior to ESWL. About 2 percent of the patients developed mild pancreatitis between 2 and 6 months after treatment, and in only one patient was endoscopic sphincterotomy necessary. Elective cholecystectomy had been performed in about 1 percent of the patients because of insufficient stone fragmentation. No further operations were necessary.

The early success reported by Sackmann and other investigators in Europe fueled the rapid development of protocols and dissemination of machines into the United States in 1988. Several of the U.S. series still lack formal publication of results. Comparison of reports is difficult owing to variations in designing, inclusion criteria, and in presenting and stratifying the data on fragmentation. Most groups held fairly tightly to the inclusion criteria proposed by Sackmann's group. Several studies allowed inclusion of larger stone loads and occasionally some calcification. Satisfactory (largest fragment between 3 to 5 mm) fragmentation rates vary widely, from 22 to 78 percent. All studies tend to confirm that this is the single most important predictor of a successful outcome (stone-free gallbladder). In addition, all studies show that total stone load is a major factor in attaining satisfactory fragmentation. Further, in those patients who do not have adequate fragmentation, the chance of successful clearance falls dramatically.

The U.S. studies have not generally been able to equal the fragmentation results of the original German studies. Correspondingly more discouraging results were thus obtained. Finally, there seemed to be a fairly large site to site variation in fragmentation rates in the U.S. studies. The explanation did not seem merely

TABLE 16-1 Adverse Reactions Following Extracorporeal Shock Wave Lithotripsy (ESWL)

• Cutaneous petechiae	14%
• Biliary colic	35%
• Pancreatitis	1%
• Cholangitis or jaundice	1%
• Transient hematuria	3%

Source Adapted from Sackmann et al.[32]

to be related to experience but, again, correlated most strongly with adherence to inclusion criteria and in selection of total stone size and number.

It should be noted that Sackmann's group also had some difficulty equaling the results of the first 175 patients in their next 325.[40] The reasons for this have not been definitely stated, but concern has been raised about the changes in procedure that took place with the second generation machines. Bringing the patients out of the water bath necessitated the design of coupling mechanisms that may not deliver the same energy as earlier designs and might allow defects to occur in the coupling during treatment. These potential problems might be compounded by the fact that nearly all procedures using newer machines are now done with little or no anesthesia. Respiratory variation is less well controlled to allow possible aiming difficulties, and potential subtle movement by an awake patient may further confound coupling problems.

Schoenfield's study from this country confirmed that most patients require adjuvant bile acid therapy to obtain complete clearance of fragments.[41] The 6-month results showed that 35 percent of patients receiving posttreatment bile acids were free of stones, while only 18 percent of patients receiving posttreatment placebo were stone free. There are no studies comparing oral dissolution alone with oral dissolution following lithotripsy. The FDA asked for such studies before reconsidering approval of gallbladder stone lithotripsy in this country.[29] Thus, lithotripsy has largely retreated back to Europe for further studies.

Contact Dissolution

Because oral dissolution therapy even when successful requires considerable time, it is tempting to consider faster methods. This would require direct contact by a dissolving agent, infused or flushed around the stones via T-tube or nasobiliary catheter. The agent would have to be selected for stone composition (i.e., cholesterol versus calcium bilirubinate).

The only currently FDA approved dissolution agent is glyceryl 1-monooctanoate (monooctanoin). Monooctanoin is a normal digestive product of a medium chain triglyceride and has been shown to be an excellent solvent for cholesterol. Because of the long times required for dissolution, it has largely been used for common duct stones via T-tubes and nasobiliary catheters. Thistle et al. summarized the clinical experience with monooctanoin for dissolution of bile duct stones in 118 patients.[42]

In an effort to find a contact agent that would be faster than monooctanoin, Allen et al. began examining other candidates.[43] Very effective cholesterol solvents have been utilized in the laboratory for decades but have been too toxic or impractical for clinical use. Diethyl ether, for example, rapidly dissolves cholesterol but has a boiling point of 35°C, therefore expanding 225 fold to a gas when introduced into the body. Methyl tert-butyl ether (MTBE) is an aliphatic ether used as a gasoline additive that is a liquid at body temperature and has ether's high capacity for dissolving cholesterol. Thistle showed that MTBE administered topically or parenterally to several animal species had a toxicity similar to diethyl ether. In sufficient dosage, both can produce anesthesia and have the potential for inducing intravascular hemolysis. MTBE is absorbed through duodenal mucosa and has been reported to cause significant duodenitis. Intravascular infusion can cause massive hemolysis. However, the gallbladder mucosa seems to be resistant to any damaging effect. For these reasons, MTBE seems most useful for dissolution of gallbladder stones. Through meticulous attention to detail, the Mayo Clinic

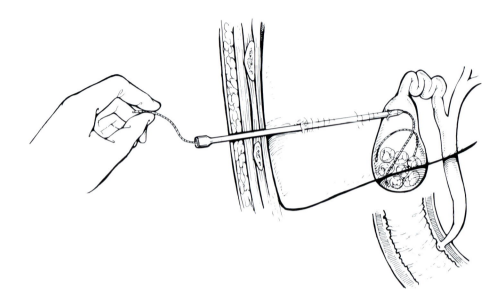

Figure 16-5
The technique of methyl tert-butyl ether (MTBE) infusion involves a percutaneous transhepatic puncture of the gallbladder, passage of a catheter, and repeated infusions and aspiration until the stones are dissolved. (Adapted from Thistle et al.)[44]

group has apparently avoided the serious potential pitfalls using MTBE.

Relatively safe access to the gallbladder can be accomplished via CT or ultrasound guided catherization. MTBE has been infused via a no. 5 French catheter, using local and intravenous analgesia (Fig. 16-5). Because MTBE normally floats on bile and good contact with the stone is desired, the catheter is curled around the stones in the gallbladder and as much bile as possible is aspirated. MTBE is then repeatedly instilled and aspirated until dissolution is complete. Progress is monitored fluoroscopically and overflow into the common duct and duodenum is avoided.

Thistle's results on his first 75 cases have been reported.[44] Of note is that a significant number of patients had at least some detectable debris still remaining in the gallbladder posttreatment. These fragments could well be the source of either further symptoms or early recurrence of stone formation. Five of 6 original patients had undergone cholecystectomy for residual or recurrent stones at the time of publication. However, only 1 of the subsequent 69 patients had surgery. The technique as described is extremely time-consuming and labor-intensive. There is some hope that autoinfusion pumps under development might speed dissolution times, lessen the labor-intensive nature of the procedure, and aid in flushing out residual debris.[45] Contact infusion therapy remains an experimental procedure, perhaps awaiting a safer and more effective dissolution agent.

Other percutaneous techniques for stone destruction and removal are also being studied. Miller, Kensey, and Nash have developed a percutaneously placed impeller device (lithotrite) that creates a vortex within the gallbladder, continuously recirculating the stones and their fragments through the impeller until they are reduced to tiny (< 1 mm) fragments.[46] Other laser mechanical or laser activated devices may hold some promise for the future as well.

Stone Recurrence

Recurrence has been a problem for all methods of stone removal in which the gallbladder is left intact. The best data are available from the numerous oral dissolution trials. Stones recur on average approximately 10 percent per year for 5 years.[47] Thereafter, the recurrence rate usually falls dramatically (Fig. 16-6). The overall recurrence rate, then, is usually between 50 and

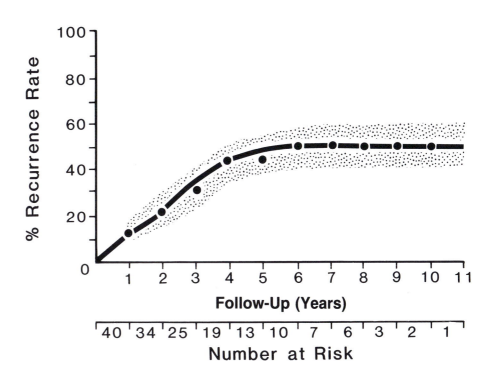

Figure 16-6
The gallstone recurrence rate after complete stone disappearance from the gallbladder following oral dissolution therapy. (Adapted from O'Donnell et al.)[47]

60 percent. Younger male patients, females of all ages, and those with a high number of stones before treatment seem to have higher recurrence rates. For those patients who recur and elect to have another course of treatment, their stones invariably dissolve.

One promising fact emerged from a large European gallstone dissolution trial. Retrospective questioning of subjects suggested that regular use of nonsteroidal anti-inflammatory agents reduced recurrence of gallstones. It was previously shown in a prairie dog model for stone formation that aspirin can inhibit formation of cholesterol gallstones.[48] Prostaglandins are believed to mediate secretion of the mucin gel layer on the gallbladder mucosa, and this gel layer may be the site of early cholesterol nucleation. Thus, the protective effect of aspirin and other nonsteroidal anti-inflammatory drugs (NSAIDs) may operate through inhibition of formation of the mucin gel layer. One study looked at trying to use this effect to prevent sludge and stone formation in massively obese patients on a rapid weight loss diet with variable results.[49]

Percutaneous Gallbladder Ablation

In an effort to solve the problem of stone recurrence, a number of authors have looked experimentally in animals at ways of ablating the gallbladder percutaneously.[50–52] Becker et al. have combined the technique of radio frequency cautery to close the cystic duct with a combination of 70 or 90 percent ethanol mixed and 1 or 3 percent sodium tetradecyl sulfate (STS) to ablate the gallbladder mucosa. Their first series was carried out fairly successfully in pigs.[53] This same group has recently reported this technique in a small series of eight human beings.[54] Cystic duct occlusion was first achieved with electrocautery. Within 1 to 4 weeks, gallbladder ablation with 95 percent ethanol and 3 percent STS was attempted. Three patients required one session of treatment, and 5 patients underwent multiple sessions. None of the patients had continued bilious drainage, suggesting that cystic duct occlusion was successful. Three patients had continued mucous discharge through the sinus tract despite repeat sclerotherapy. Biopsy samples of the gallbladder showed signs of mucosal regeneration. While preliminary and not entirely successful, such advanced percutaneous techniques may hold promise for the future.

The advance of nonsurgical approaches to the treatment of gallbladder disease has allowed for exciting new techniques and study. Along with the therapeutic research has come an increased understanding of the pathogenesis and natural history of cholelithiasis. The nonsurgical challenge has been met in the surgical community by the perhaps even more exciting and dramatic changes brought about by the embracing of laparoscopy and minimally invasive surgical techniques such as laporoscopic cholecystectomy. Both camps will undoubtedly find common ground with the growing experience in all the new and exciting techniques. Many of the nonsurgical techniques described here may eventually find their way into the laparoscopist's armamentarium for solving specialized problem cases. Way best summarized the current status of the treatment of cholelithiasis: "Surgery has advantages that the new techniques cannot match, but the reverse is also true. Consequently, a team is needed so [that] each patient receives the very best treatment, not simply the treatment performed by the first physician he or she encounters."[55]

References

1. Chen PN et al: Clinical analysis of therapeutic efficacy in 365 cases of gallstones treated by pressure over ear points. *Chin Acupuncture Mosibustion* 5:241–243, 1985.
2. Mayo WJ. "Innocent" gallstones. *JAMA* 56:1021–1024, 1911.
3. Godrey PJ et al: Gallstones and mortality: A study of all gallstone related deaths in a single health district. *Gut* 25:1029–1033, 1984.
4. Wetter LA, Way LW: Surgical therapy for gallstone disease. *Gastroenterol Clin North Am* 20:157–169, 1991.
5. Gracie WA, Ransohoff DF: The natural history of silent gallstones. *N Engl J Med* 307:798–800, 1982.
6. McSherry CK et al: The natural history of diagnosed gallstoned disease in symptomatic and asymptomatic patients. *Ann Surg* 202:59–63, 1985.
7. Way L, Altman D: Neoplasms of the gallbladder and bile ducts, in Schlesinger M, Fordtran J (eds), *Gastrointestinal Disease*, 3d ed. Philadelphia, Saunders, 1984, pp 1409–1413.
8. Newman HF: Complications of cholelithiasis. *Am J Gastroenterol* 50:476–496, 1968.
9. Ransohoff DF et al: Prophylactic cholecystectomy of expectant management for silent gallstones. *Ann Intern Med* 99:199–204, 1983.
10. Donaldson RM Jr: Advice for the patient with "silent" gallstones [editorial]. *N Engl J Med* 307:815–817, 1982.
11. Friedman LS et al: Management of asymptomatic gallstones in the diabetic patient. *Ann Intern Med* 109:913–919, 1988.
12. Bateson MC, Bouchier IAD: Prevalence of gallstones in Dundee: Necropsy study. *Br Med J* 4:4271–4275, 1975.
13. Bateson MC: Gallbladder disease and cholecystectomy rate are independently variable. *Lancet* 2:621–622, 1984.
14. Holzbach RT: Pathogenesis and medical treatment of gallstones, in Sleisenger MH, Fortran JS (eds), *Gastrointestinal Disease*, 4th ed. Philadelphia, Saunders, 1989, p 1668.
15. Wenckert A, Robertson B: The natural course of gallstone disease: Eleven-year review of 781 nonoperated cases. *Gastroenterology* 50(3):376–381, 1966.
16. Hickman MS et al: Computed tomographic analysis of gallstones: An in vetro study. *Arch Surg* 121:289–291, 1986.
17. Barakos JA, Ralls PW, Lapin SA: Cholelithiasis: Evaluation with CT. *Radiology* 162:415–418, 1987.
18. Baron RL et al: CT evaluation of gallstones in vitro: Correlation with chemical analysis. *Am J Roentgenol* 151:1123–1128, 1988.

19. Danzinger RG et al: Dissolution of cholesterol gallstones by chenodeoxycholic acid. *N Engl J Med* 286:1–8, 1972.

20. Schoenfield LJ, Lachin JM: Chenodiol (chenodyoxycholic acid) for dissolution of gallstones: The National Cooperative Gallstone Study. A controlled trial of efficiency and safety. *Ann Intern Med* 95:257–282, 1981.

21. Bateson MC: *Gallstone Disease and Its Management*. Norwell, CT, MTP Press Limited, 1986.

22. Stiehl A et al: Effects of biliary bile acid composition on biliary cholesterol saturation in gallstone patients treated with chenodeoxycholic acid and/or ursodeoxycholic acid. *Gastroenterology* 79:1192–1198, 1980.

23. Attilli AF et al: Effect of ursodeoxycholic acid on biliary lipid composition: A double blind study. *Ital J Gastroenterol* 12:177–180, 1980.

24. Podda M et al: A combination of cheno- and ursodeoxycholic acid is more effective than either alone in reducing bile cholesterol saturation. *Gastroenterology* 78:1316, 1980.

25. Salen G, Tint GS, Shefer S: Treatment of gallstones with ursodeoxycholic acid. *J Clin Gastroenterol* 10(suppl 2):s12–17, 1988.

26. Dolgin SM et al: *N Engl J Med* 304:808, 1981.

27. Salen G, Tint GS, Shefer S: Treatment of cholesterol gallstones with litholytc bile acids. *Gastroenterol Clin North Am* 20:171–182, 1991.

28. Drach GW et al: Report of the United States cooperative study of extracorporeal shock wave lithotripsy. *J Urol* 135:1127, 1986.

29. Anonymous: Meeting of the Food and Drug Administration gastroenterology-urology device section advisory panel on extracorporeal shock-wave lithotripsy for gallbladder stones. *Am J Gastroenterology* 85:238–240, 1989.

30. Hunter PT et al: Measurement of shock wave pressures used for lithotripsy. *J Urol* 136:733–788, 1986.

31. Chaussy D: *Extracorporeal Shock Wave Lithotripsy: New Aspects in the Treatment of Kidney Stone Disease*. Munich, S Karger, 1982, p 96.

32. Sackmann M, Delius M, Sauerbruch T: Shockwave lithotripsy of gallbladder stones: The first 175 patients. *N Engl J Med* 318:393, 1988.

33. Chaussy C: *Extracorporeal Shock Wave Lithotripsy: Technical Concepts, Experimental Research and Clinical Application*. Basel, S Karger, 1986.

34. Ruiz-Marcellan FJ, Ibarz-Servio L: Evaluation of renal damage in extracorporeal lithotripsy by shock waves. *Eur Urol* 12:73, 1986.

35. Williams CM et al: Extracorporeal shock-wave lithotripsy: Long-term complications. *Am J Roentgenol* 150:311–315, 1988.

36. Hood KA et al: Piezo-ceramic lithotripsy of gallbladder stones: Initial experience in 38 patients. *Lancet* 1:1322–1324, 1988.

37. Fromm H, Kalbert MB: Piezoelectric lithotripsy and adjuvant bile acid therapy of gallstones: Promising new data (selected summary). *Gastroenterology* 96:944–945, 1989.

38. Chapman WC et al: Preliminary biliary studies with an ultrasonic extracorporeal lithotripter, in Ferrucci JT, Delius M, Burhenne HJ (eds), *Biliary Lithotripsy*, 2d ed. Chicago, Year Book Medical, 1988, pp 155–175.

39. Sauerbruch T et al: Fragmentation of gallstones by extracorporeal shock waves. *N Engl J Med* 314:818–822, 1986.

40. Sauerbruch T et al: Technical considerations in performance of extracorporeal shock wave lithotripsy (ESWL) of gallstones, in Ferrucci JT, Delius M, Burhenne HJ (eds), *Biliary Lithotripsy*. Chicago, Year Book Medical, 1988, pp 69–78.

41. Schoenfield LJ et al: The effect of ursodial on the efficacy and safety of extracorporeal shockwave lithotripsy of gallstones. *New Engl J Med* 323:1239–1245, 1990.

42. Thistle JL et al: Monooctanoin, a dissolution agent for retained cholesterol bile duct stones: Physical properties and clinical application. *Gastroenterology* 78:1026–1022, 1980.

43. Allen MJ et al: Methyl tertiary butyl ether rapidly dissolves gallstones *in vitro* and *in vivo* (abstract). *Hepatology* 3:809, 1983.

44. Thistle JL et al: Dissolution of cholesterol gallbladder stones by methyl tert-butyl ether ad-

ministered by percutaneous transhepatic catheter. *New Engl J Med* 320:633–639, 1989.

45. Zakko SF et al: Percutaneous gallbladder stone dissolution using a microprocessor assisted solvent transfer (MAST) system (abstract). *Gastroenterology* 92:1794, 1987.

46. Miller FJ, Kensey KR, Nash JE: Experimental percutaneous gallstone lithotripsy: Results in swine. *Radiology* 170:985–987, 1989.

47. O'Donnell LDJ, Heaton KW: Recurrence and re-recurrence of gallstones after medical dissolution: A long-term follow-up. *Gut* 29:655–658, 1988.

48. Lee SP et al: Role of gallbladder mucus hypersecretion in the evolution of cholesterol gallstones: Studies in the prairie dog. *J Clin Invest* 67:1712, 1981.

49. Broomfield PH et al: Effects of ursodeoxycholic acid and aspirin on the formation of lithogenic bile and gallstones during loss of weight. *New Engl J Med* 319:1567–1572, 1988.

50. Getrajdman GI et al: Cystic duct occlusion and transcatheter sclerosis of the gallbladder in the rabbit. *Invest Radiol* 21:400–403, 1986.

51. Remley KB et al: Systemic absorption of gallbladder sclerosing agents in the rabbit: A preliminary study. *Invest Radiol* 21:396–399, 1986.

52. Stein EF et al: Percutaneous ablation of the gallbladder in pigs. *Radiology* 153(P):194, 1984.

53. Becker CD, Quenville NF, Burhenne HJ: Gallbladder ablation through radiologic intervention: An experimental alternative to cholecystectomy. *Radiology* 171:235–240, 1989.

54. Becker CD et al: Ablation of the cystic duct and gallbladder: Clinical observations. *Radiology* 176:687–690, 1990.

55. Way LW: Trends in the treatment of gallstone disease: Putting the options into context. *Am J Surg* 158:251–253, 1989.

17

Complications of Laparoscopic Cholecystectomy

John N. Graber

Prevention of complications of laparoscopic cholecystectomy is of utmost importance. The initial skepticism that was seen in 1989 when the first laparoscopic gallbladder procedures were being performed was based upon the belief that these operations would not be safe. The concept of operating while watching the anatomy on television rather than holding the organ in the surgeon's hand meant increased risk to many surgeons. A review of the reports from early experiences[1-3] suggests that these concerns were not unreasonable.

At first there were only anecdotal reports of disastrous problems, even deaths associated with the new procedure. Eventually papers were given at national meetings[1] and reports began to appear in journals[2] detailing a variety of serious problems that would likely not have occurred if the operation had been done in the open setting. Injuries such as common bile duct transections, portal vein bleeding, intestinal perforations, and deaths have now been detailed in the literature (Table 17-1). Knowing of the actual incidence of these injuries and how to avoid them is the major issue for any responsible surgeon. The ability to diagnose and carry out a plan to manage these complications should be expected of any surgeon performing laparoscopic cholecystectomy.

A review of the literature shows that the complication rates in initial series has been somewhat higher than what might be expected with incisional cholecystectomy.[3,4] Also, a learning curve is evident.[5,6] The more typical complications are bile duct injuries and leaks, bleeding requiring transfusion or reoperation, and intestinal injuries. Death has been reported rarely; however, anecdotally death has occurred in many centers and usually it is the result of a massive bleeding complication, intestinal injury, myocardial infarction, or pulmonary embolus.[3,8]

Minor complications are detailed in Table 17-2. These can be controlled mostly by changes in protocol. Nausea is mostly a function of the anesthetic. Right rib margin pain is usually the result of putting punctures too close to the costal margin.

One concept that is universal and needs to

TABLE 17-1   Major Complications of Laparoscopic Cholecystectomy: A Review of the Literature

Author	Graber[5]	Hawaslim[6]	Peters[2]	Spaw[7]	Wolfe[3]	Larson[8]
N	100	50	283	500	381	1983
Death	0	0	0	0	3	2
Bleeding (transfusion)	1	—	—	—	1	5
Bleeding (reoperate)	0	2	1	1	—	2
Bile duct injury	2	1	1	0	—	5
Intraabdominal abscess	2	—	—	—	—	—
Bile leak	0	1	3	1	5	7
Undetected common bile duct (CBD) stones	2	—	2	—	—	6
Gas embolism	0	—	—	—	—	—
Deep vein thrombosis	0	—	—	—	—	—
Myocardial infarction	0	—	—	1	—	1*
Intestinal injury	0	—	—	2	2*	1
Pneumonia	0	—	—	—	5	2
Pulmonary embolus	0	—	—	—	—	1*
Stroke	0	—	—	—	2*	—
Wound infection	1	—	3	—	2	5

* Mortalities were from these groups.

be understood by all surgeons is that to convert to an open laparotomy is not a complication. Instead, it is an exercise of good surgical judgment. If this is clearly understood by all who are involved in these surgeries (i.e., surgeons, staff, reviewers, and patients), there will be a greater ability to resist the surgical momentum that leads to complications.

Table 17-3 reviews typical reasons for surgeons to convert to an open laparotomy. Difficult exposure leading to a lack of understanding of the anatomy is most common. By converting to an incisional approach, the surgeon's overall orientation is returned. A three-dimensional view of the anatomy is restored. More information can be obtained by touching tissues directly. As a consequence of these factors and others, making an incision in tough cases can lead to prevention of complications.

Bile Duct Transection

Of all likely complications, bile duct injuries are the most severe. The incidence of these injuries in the early reports has been around 1 percent.[2,5,6,8] Often, the injuries including transections are not recognized at the time of operation. If bile duct injury is recognized, immediate repair is warranted. This repair usually requires conversion to open laparotomy. Bile duct transection or obstruction caused at surgery but not recognized is associated with severe postoperative pain that keeps the patient awake all night after surgery.[17] The pain may resolve or become more tolerable after 24 h, and the patient may be discharged. After 3 to 5 days, the patient will notice the onset of scleral icterus in addition to poor return of bowel function and ongoing right upper quadrant abdominal pain. The bilirubin level will be elevated to between 5 and 10 g/dl. The differential diagnosis at this time may include an obstructing retained common duct stone that might pass. When the patient presents with this picture in the early postoperative period, an endoscopic retrograde cholangiopancreatography (ERCP) should be obtained.

In the setting of bile duct transection, the ERCP will show only the clipped end of the distal common bile duct (Fig. 17-1A). A transhepatic cholangiogram in this setting will offer little therapeutic advantage (Fig. 17-1B). Urgent open operative repair by a surgeon well versed in this type of surgery is warranted.

TABLE 17-2 Minor Complications of Laparoscopic Cholecystectomy Adapted from a Series of 100 Initial Cases[5]

Nausea lasting more than 12 hours	20%
Right shoulder pain (diaphragmatic etiology)	29%
Right costal margin pain	12%
Puncture site complications	
Infection requiring I & D	1%
Infection requiring antibiotics only	0
Prolonged site pain	1%
Excessive scarring	0
Hematoma (minor)	1%
Subcutaneous emphysema (lasting <24 hours)	1%
Instrument fracture (fragment retrieved without laparotomy)	2%

TABLE 17-3 Reasons for Converting Laparoscopic Cholecystectomy to an Open Procedure (N = 1983)

Marked inflammation	26	1.3%
Difficult adhesions	20	1.0%
Unclear anatomy	10	0.5%
Bleeding	6	0.3%
Technical/instrument problems	2	0.1%
Bile duct injury	4	0.2%
Need to perform open CBD exploration	15	0.8%
Unexpected cancer	2	0.1%
Biliary-enteric fistula	3	0.2%
Total	88	(4.5%)

Source: Adapted from Larson et al.[8]

The reason that the common bile duct may be inadvertently transected during laparoscopic surgery is not usually an accidental laceration or excessive retraction. Instead, it is the result of a misinterpretation of the anatomy—a misidentification in which the common duct is thought to be the cystic duct and purposefully divided in the routine process of cholecystectomy.

There are several reasons for this. First, there is reluctance to dissect the cystic/common duct junction clearly for fear of bleeding or other injury. The extent of the dissection down the cystic duct relates to the confidence that a surgeon has that it can be done safely. The amount of experience one has with laparoscopic technique is a major factor. Not visualizing the cystic/common duct junction takes away a major landmark in anatomical identification.

The second factor is that forceful anterior retraction on the gallbladder, as is done laparoscopically in order to view the cystic duct, distorts the normal angle of the cystic common duct junction by straightening it out (Fig. 17-2). This can falsely make the cystic and common duct appear as one continuous cystic duct, and the dissection is carried past the junction without recognizing it. This seems to be the most common mechanism of misidentification. In conjunction with a concern that further dissection is more risky and that a "long enough" segment of duct has been exposed, absolute identification of the cystic/common duct junction is abandoned and the wrong duct is transected.

Thirdly, the field of view generated by the 0° viewing laparoscope is limited in that it may allow only one perspective. As a consequence, the common hepatic duct, which extends from the other side of the cystic/common duct junction into the liver, may not be seen. Not visualizing the common hepatic duct can only confirm a mistaken impression that the common duct is the cystic duct.

Overriding all of these technical considerations is the special anatomical configuration that makes the occurrence of one of these errors more likely. This is the absent or very short cystic duct (Fig. 17-3). Awareness of this potential trap is necessary so that the surgeon always goes through the necessary steps to be certain not to misidentify the common bile duct.[2]

TABLE 17-4 Rules to Avoid Common Bile Duct Injuries

- Always begin cystic duct dissection on the gallbladder.
- Encircle the cystic duct 360° at the gallbladder and then proceed toward the common duct.
- Use a laparoscope that views at 30° or 45° to the side and grasp the neck of the gallbladder to retract it side to side so as to identify clearly any structures that may be hidden behind the duct.
- Obtain a cholangiogram in all cases where possible before dividing the cystic duct.

It is necessary to adhere to several principles in order to minimize the chance of bile duct injury (Table 17-4). First, when dissecting the cystic duct, begin on the neck of the gallbladder and encircle the duct 360°. There is a tendency to begin dissection at an obvious and a convenient site distal to the gallbladder, but there is a chance that the structure encircled at this site may be the common duct regardless of initial impressions. This is especially true in the cases with a short cystic duct. Once the duct is encircled at the neck of the gallbladder, progressive distal dissection can be continued.

Secondly, using a laparoscope that views at 30 or 45° to the side is very helpful for allowing visualization around the backside of the duct (Fig. 17-4).[16] By rotating the scope 180°, a look at one side and then the other can be obtained. Also, grasp the gallbladder neck and retract it from side to side to expose this area clearly. In this way, the often errant common hepatic duct can be identified behind the cystic/common

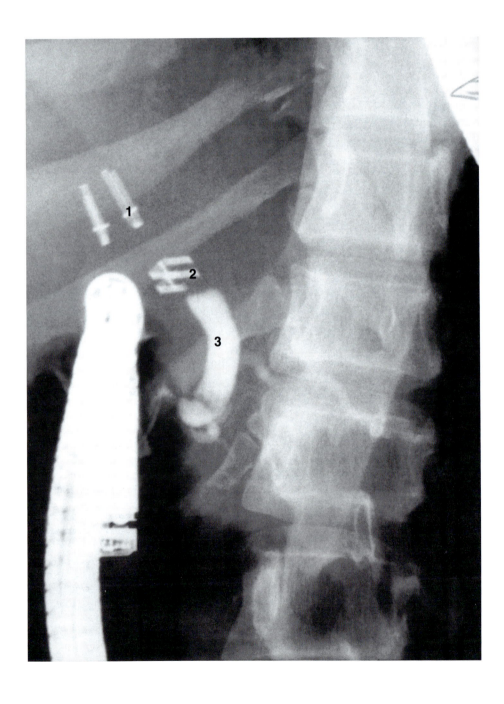

Figure 17-1
A. ERCP in a case of a common bile duct transection showing only the clipped distal end of the common duct.
1 = Occluding clips on common hepatic duct.
2 = Occluding clips on proximal common bile duct.
3 = Distal common bile duct.

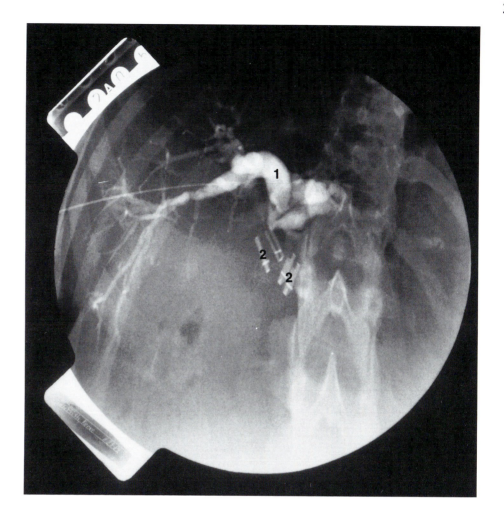

Figure 17-1
B. Little more information is obtained from a transhepatic cholangiogram. 1 = Dilated intrahepatic ducts. 2 = Clips on common duct.

duct junction. A clear understanding of the triangle formed by the cystic duct, the liver, and the common hepatic duct is mandatory.

Thirdly, cholangiography should be considered in all cases. There are two methods of cholangiography, and each offers assistance in avoiding ductal injuries. A cholecystcholangiogram offers a look at the anatomy before dissection of the cystic duct is begun[9] but does not confirm that there is no injury after dissection. A cystic duct cholangiogram is done through a small ductotomy and would identify any errors that can then be corrected without serious injury.

Lastly, dissection to the common duct junction offers the most convincing evidence of correct anatomical identification. This should be accomplished to the extent that it is technically possible.

Management of bile duct injuries depends upon the severity of the event (Fig. 17-5). A small tear or cut in the common duct may be safely treated by placing a small drain into the rent and suturing the defect laparoscopically. Repair of common duct transections and, as is typical of laparoscopic injuries, concomitant common hepatic injuries requires more surgery than can be done through the scope, and an open laparotomy is warranted. In the open setting, the pertinent anatomy must first be dissected out and the extent of the injury determined. Then a biliary drainage procedure must be done. Since these ducts are not dilated, the anastomosis is extremely difficult. For simple common duct transections, an end to end repair of the duct might be considered, but it is not generally recommended because the incidence of stricture formation is very high. On the other hand, if it does stricture, it will cause a gradual dilation of the upper duct and make a later cho-

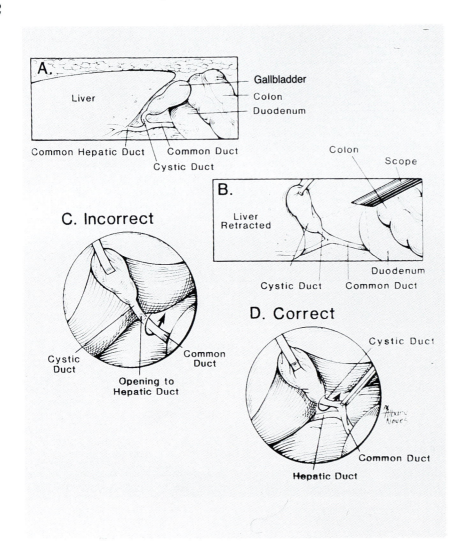

Figure 17-2
Mechanism of misidentification of bile ducts. **A.** Sagittal view of normal gallbladder and ductal anatomy. **B.** Distorted view of cystic/common duct junction due to forceful anterior retraction on the gallbladder. **C.** Anatomy as viewed through a laparoscope; common bile duct is misidentified as a long cystic duct and incorrectly encircled. **D.** Beginning dissection on the gallbladder, identifying the actual cystic/common duct junction, and viewing from different angles with a side viewing laparoscope ensure correct identification of the cystic duct. (Reprinted with permission from Graber et al: *Las Surg Med* 12:92–96, 1992.)

ledochoenterostomy technically easier. For common hepatic transections a direct anastomosis to a Roux-en-Y limb is necessary. A surgeon who cannot perform these difficult procedures should not schedule a laparoscopic cholecystectomy.

Bile Leaks and Bilomas

The incidence of bile duct leaks and bilomas has been shown in some series to be 0.5 to 2 percent.[6,8] The most common cause appears to be inadequate cystic duct closure[10] but may also be the consequence of undetected bile duct injury or liver laceration. We have seen a case where contrast was seen to leak through the cystic duct when injected via ERCP even though the clips appeared to be in appropriate position and were placed normally.

A bile duct leak may present as unusually severe right upper quadrant pain but not always. The most common presenting symptom is bloating and poor return of bowel function. White blood cell count may be normal but usually is mildly elevated as may be alkaline phosphatase and bilirubin. An ultrasound or CT scan will reveal the collection (Fig. 17-6). Some surgeons have suggested that biliary scintigraphy (HIDA scan) is helpful to diagnose an ongoing leak.[2] If the bile is localized, it can be drained percutaneously.[10] Then, if the drainage stops and the collection resolves on repeat studies, the drain can be removed and the patient will likely do well. If the drainage continues or if the bile appears to be freely dispersed in the peritoneal cavity, an ERCP is warranted to determine the site and nature of the leakage (Fig. 17-7). Also, this study will delineate other problems such as bile duct injuries or the presence of common duct stones that may have obstructed the duct and prevented spontaneous closure of the leak (Fig. 17-8). If there are stones, they can be removed and the sphincter cut to reduce back pressure in the duct and enhance closure of the leak. In this regard, a stent may be helpful. If these measures fail, the patient should be explored with an open laparotomy and the leak closed or controlled as needed.

Other Organ Injuries

Intestinal injuries are rare and not seen in most reports. Potential causes of such injuries include monopolar electrocautery and laser burns or traction tearing of the colon and duodenum.[3,11] These injuries can be avoided in all cases by careful attention to technique. The surgeon must always know that the uninsulated segments of cautery equipment do not inadvertently contact other tissue when in use (Fig. 17-9). Duodenal injuries are most likely when cauterizing the cystic artery with a grasping device with a 1- to 2-cm exposed metal tip or by past pointing with a free beam laser or laser of a combination free beam and contact nature.

This type of burn injury usually does not result in direct perforation but may result in necrosis of the duodenal or colonic wall and leak as late as 3 to 5 days later. Of course, even this is unlikely, but when a burn injury occurs it should always be treated by placement of a Lembert suture. In this regard, the suturing technique must be of adequate quality to avoid further bowel injury. Avoid use of heavy gut suture and knot-tying technique that requires extensive pulling of the suture through the tissue. These techniques are reviewed in Chap. 1.

Solid organ injuries such as splenic or renal lacerations are rare and are usually the result of poor laparoscopic technique rather than strictly related to cholecystectomy. Liver lacerations on the other hand can be caused by accidental puncture with an instrument, by excessive retracting force with an instrument, by too vigorous retraction on the gallbladder, or by tearing scarred and adherent tissue from its attachment to the liver margin.

Clearly these injuries can be avoided by strictly controlling the amount of pressure applied against the liver capsule. Puncture injuries are the most common and occur early in the surgeon's experience when he or she has lost video site of an instrument. In an attempt to bring the instrument into the field of view, it is pushed superiorly straight into the liver without appearing on the monitor. Many of the instruments employed laparoscopically are rather pointed and can penetrate the liver without much resistance. Other sites of liver laceration can occur when purposefully pushing on the liver capsule to move the liver aside when aspirating fluid from the right subphrenic space or by lifting the liver margin to examine the gallbladder bed.

Management of these injuries usually involves obtaining hemostasis and possibly placing a drain that can be removed 24 h later if no bile is seen. Suturing such lacerations is not recommended for fear of causing hematobilia. Some surgeons suggest use of topical hemostatic agents, such as Avitene Powder, Surgicel, or Gelfoam-Thrombin, that can be applied laparoscopically. If there is uncontrollable bleeding from a liver laceration, the operation should be converted to an open laparotomy and the laceration explored for specific control of the bleeding points.

Vascular Injuries

Vascular injuries range from oozing from the liver bed to portal vein lacerations. Control of typical intraoperative bleeding during cholecystectomy is reviewed in Chap. 13. More serious bleeding usually involves larger vessels such as the portal vein or the hepatic artery. Portal vein injuries generally are the result of

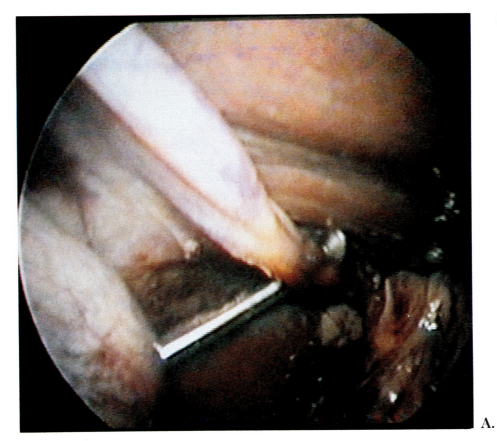

Figure 17-3
The short cystic duct. **A.** The dissector has been incorrectly inserted behind what appears to be the cystic duct.

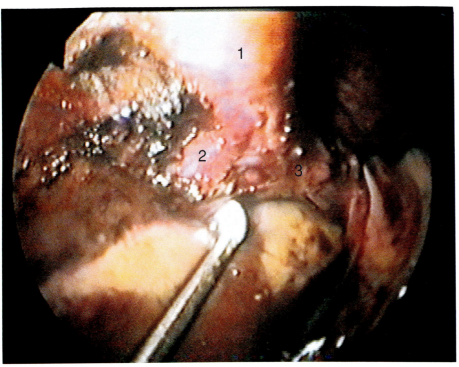

Figure 17-3
B. Retraction of the gallbladder fundus and use of a 45° viewing scope reveal the short cystic duct (1), the common hepatic duct (2), and the common bile duct (3).

**Figure 17-3
C.** Dissection on the gallbladder allows correct identification and control of the cystic duct **(D)**.

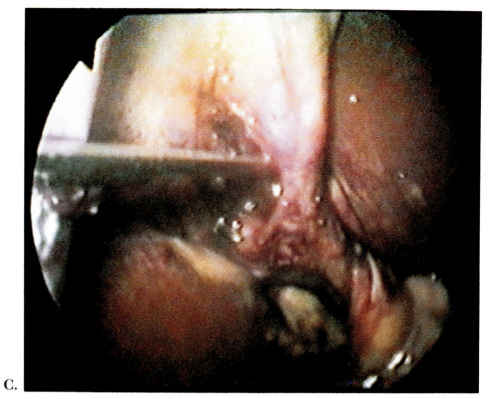

C.

D.

dissection in the wrong area. If dissection is begun on the cystic duct at the neck of the gallbladder and progressed centrally from there, the portal vein should not be seen. Serious bleeding from behind the common bile duct should be treated by pushing the gallbladder gently with the graspers already in place down into the porta hepatis so as to tamponade the bleeding while an incision is made and immediate compression of the portal triad is accomplished by placing a finger into the foramen of Winslow (Pringle maneuver).

Abscess Formation

The major issue in preventing an abscess is to minimize any residual debris or bilious fluid collections. Although sterile gallstones left in the peritoneal cavity have been shown not to cause infection in animals or human beings[12,13] and many times stones escape the surgeon both incisionally and laparoscopically without consequence, any such residual debris theoretically enhances the chance of infection. Improved techniques for removing the gallbladder and gallstones from the abdominal cavity will be developed, but meticulous attention to the removal of all debris and fluid will always be important. A silastic drain did not prevent one of the abscesses from forming in our series. It is unclear that prophylactic antibiotics or antibiotic irrigation will have any effect on the rate of abscess formation. Copious irrigation of the right upper quadrant visceral surfaces followed by complete aspiration of all free fluid at the conclusion of the procedure are always recommended.

If an abscess occurs following cholecystectomy, it will present over 5 to 7 days as poor return of bowel function, fever at first low grade and later spiking in nature, and pain. White blood cell count will be elevated and liver function tests may be abnormal. A CT scan or an ultrasound will reveal a collection, most commonly in the subhepatic space (Fig. 17-10) or in the right lower quadrant. The scan may also identify gallstone debris.

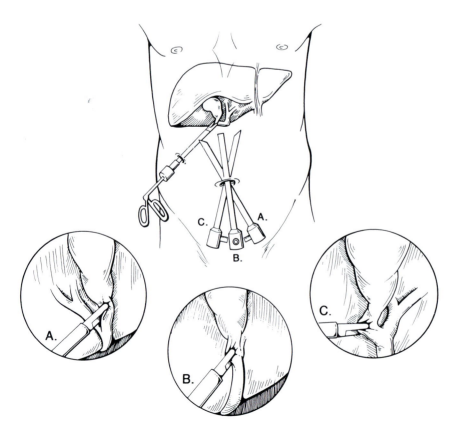

Figure 17-4
A 45° or 30° viewing scope allows visualization behind the duct from both sides, often exposing a hidden common hepatic duct.

Chapter 17 Complications of Laparoscopic Cholecystectomy

Figure 17-5
An ERCP showing a clip partially obstructing the common hepatic duct. This clip was removed at laparotomy and a T-tube placed into the duct at this site. The patient has done well for over 3 years.
1 = Clip partially occluding common hepatic duct.

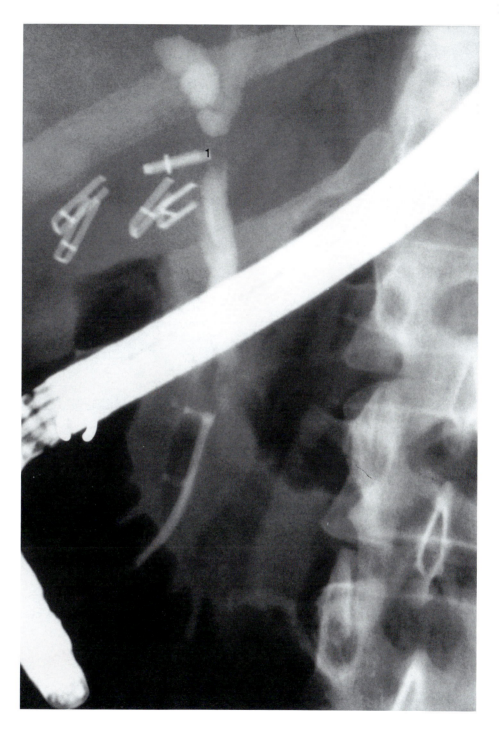

The treatment is drainage. This often can be accomplished percutaneously with CT guidance, and when the drainage stops and the collection is seen to resolve on repeat studies, the drain can be removed. If the abscess cannot be drained percutaneously, open drainage is necessary.

Retained Common Bile Duct Stones

When laparoscopic cholecystectomy was initiated in 1989 there was no well-described technique for laparoscopic removal of common duct

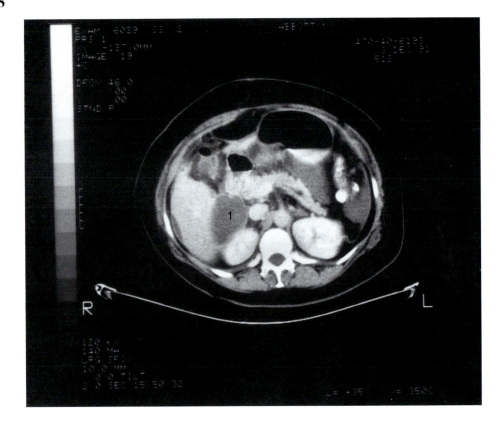

Figure 17-6
CT scan showing a postoperative bile collection (biloma) in the right hepatorenal fossa.
1 = Postoperative bile collection.

stones. Consequently, when stones were identified on routine cholangiography, the operation was completed without removal of the stones and the patient referred for ERCP extraction in the postoperative period.[14] These "retained" stones cannot be considered a complication. However, when a patient has recurrent right upper abdominal pain "just like the pain I had before you took out my gallbladder" and has an elevated bilirubin and alkaline phosphatase, the patient often needs urgent investigation and intervention. In this setting, the previously unrecognized retained stones should be considered a complication. We recommend obtaining liver function studies on any postoperative patient who has recurrent biliary tract symptoms and, if elevated, proceeding to ERCP. In good hands, the success rate of removing the stones should be 85 percent with relatively low morbidity.[15]

The major issue is identification of these common duct stones intraoperatively so that a treatment plan can be applied. For this and other reasons, a cholangiogram is warranted in all cases. If the common duct is not visualized with a cholecystcholangiogram, a cystic duct study should be done.

Abdominal Wall Problems

In general, problems associated with the abdominal wall are related to basic laparoscopic technique (Chap. 7). There are some matters that are relevant to laparoscopic cholecystectomy. Removing the gallbladder or large stones from the abdominal cavity remains a challenge (Chap. 13). As techniques of morcellation and stone emulsification improve, these problems will be minimized, but for now the gallbladder and stones must often be forcibly pulled through the fascia and skin. At times, this technique leaves particulate matter in the puncture tract and can lead to inflammation and infection. We have found that immediate irrigation of the tract with the laparoscopic irrigation device is very efficient at removing this debris (Fig. 17-11). Because of the pressure of the pneumoperito-

Figure 17-7
ERCP study showing an uncontrolled bile leak from an injury to the right hepatic duct, from which the aberrant cystic duct originated. This leak was drained successfully percutaneously; however, the injury resulted in a stricture in 4 months.
1 = Right hepatic duct leak.

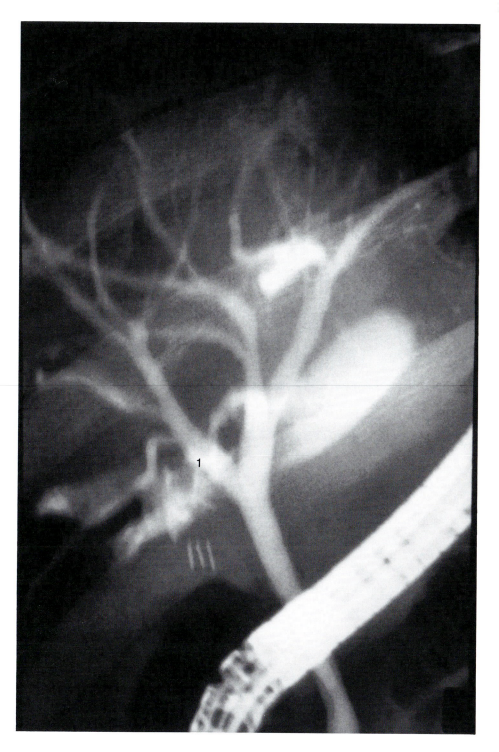

neum, CO_2 gas escapes from the puncture site after the gallbladder and cannula have been removed. When the irrigation fluid is instilled into the tract, it is immediately blown out and the debris is carried with it.

Herniation can occur through the puncture sites.[8] At the end of the procedure, placing a finger through the puncture tract into the abdomen will at least assure you that no bowel or omentum has become trapped as you let out the pneumoperitoneum. The larger the trocar used, the more likely these complications will

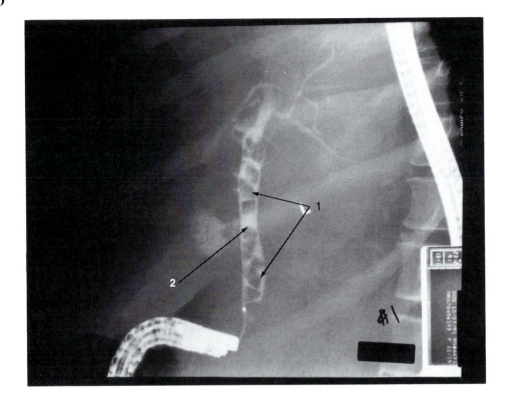

Figure 17-8
A postoperative ERCP in a patient who had presented with acute cholecystitis and a small cystic duct. An intraoperative cholangiogram was not done. Postoperatively, she developed a bile leak through the cystic duct stump and was found to have multiple common duct stones. A sphincterotomy and stone extraction was successful.
1 = Retained CBD stones. 2 = Cystic duct stump bile leak.

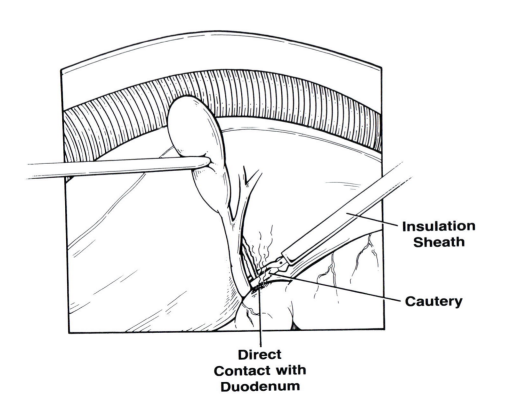

Figure 17-9
Monopolar cauter devices can cause burns of adjacent organs, such as the duodenum, when cauterizing bleeding vessels near the cystic artery.

Figure 17-10
Postoperative CT scan showing an abscess in the right hepatorenal fossa. At laparotomy, gallstones were identified in the abscess. 1 = Subhepatic abscess.

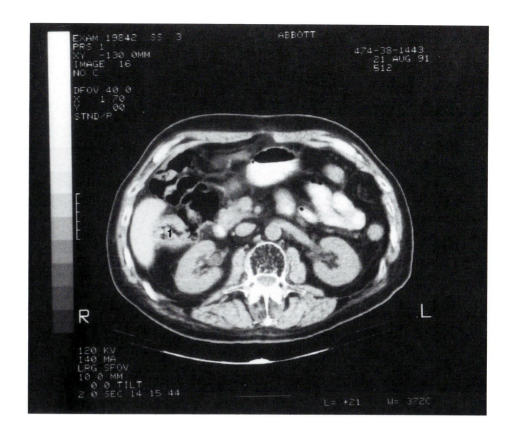

Figure 17-11
After pulling the gallbladder through a puncture site, the surgeon often finds debris left in the tract, and this can be removed by instilling irrigation fluid into the tract, letting the escaping CO_2 gas blow the irrigant and debris out of the tract.

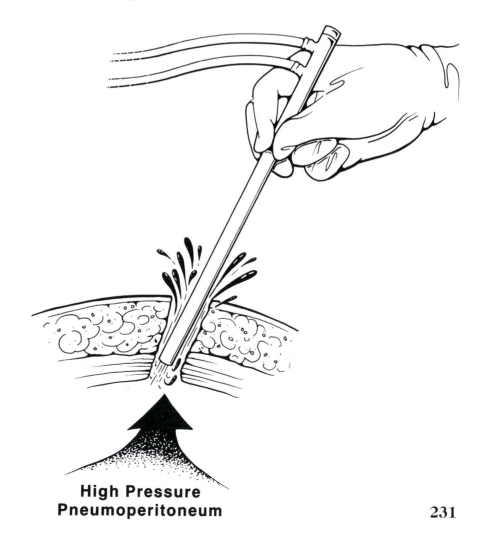

be. If an incision is made in the fascia to remove a large gallbladder or stone, a suture must be placed in the fascia to prevent herniation. Also keep in mind that if a cannula is inserted into an obese patient directed into the pelvis, it can cause tearing of the abdominal wall fascia with bleeding when it is rotated toward the upper abdomen. In large patients, the cannulas will need to be inserted more in the direction that they will be needed during the procedure in order to avoid this.

Discussion

A review of the complications reported in the literature helps to make changes in an individual surgeon's technique and procedure that can result in a dramatic improvement in the incidence of subsequent complications. Bile duct injuries are the most severe problems, and with observation of specific principles, their occurrence can be minimized. Laparoscopic cholecystectomy is clearly a safe procedure in experienced hands. Thorough review of the problems others have had will lead to improved outcomes for all surgeons.

References

1. Graber JN et al: Complications of laparoscopic cholecystectomy. *Lasers Surg Med* (supplement 3), 1991.
2. Peters JH et al: Complications of laparoscopic cholecystectomy. *Surgery* 110(4):769–778, 1991.
3. Wolfe BM et al: Endoscopic cholecystectomy, an analysis of complications. *Arch Surg* 126:1192–1198, 1991.
4. Morgenstern L, Wong L, Berci G: Twelve hundred open cholecystectomies before the laparoscopic era. *Arch Surg* 127:400–403, 1992.
5. Graber JN et al: Complications of laparoscopic cholecystectomy: A prospective review of an initial 100 consecutive cases. *Lasers Surg and Med* 12(1):92–97, 1992.
6. Hawaslim A, Lloyd LR: Laparoscopic cholecystectomy, the learning curve. *Am Surg* 57(8):542–545, 1991.
7. Spaw AT, Reddick EJ, Olsen DO: Laparoscopic laser cholecystectomy: Analysis of 500 procedures. *Surg Laparosc Endosc* 1(1):2–7, 1991.
8. Larson GM et al: Multipractice analysis of laparoscopic cholecystectomy in 1983 patients. *Am J Surg* 163:221–226, 1992.
9. Pietrafitta J et al: Cholangiography during laparoscopic cholecystectomy: Cholecyst-cholangiography or cystic duct cholangiography. *J Laparoendosc Surg* 1:197–206, 1991.
10. Ralph-Edwards T, Himal HS: Bile leak after laparoscopic cholecystectomy. *Surg Endosc* 6:33–35, 1992.
11. Saye WB, Miller W, Hertzmann P: Electrosurgery thermal injury, myth or misconception? *Surg Laparosc Endosc* 1(4):223–228, 1991.
12. Schultz LS et al: Laser laparoscopic cholecystectomy—a clinical trial. *Lasers Surg Med* (supplement 2), p 21, 1990.
13. Welch N et al: Gallstones in the peritoneal cavity. *Surg Laparosc Endosc* 1(4):246–247, 1991.
14. Arregui ME et al: Laparoscopic cholecystectomy combined with endoscopic sphincterotomy and stone extraction. *Surg Endosc* 6:10–15, 1992.
15. Morrissey JF, Reichelderfer M: Gastrointestinal endoscopy, second of two parts. *N Engl J Med* 325(17):1214–1222, 1991.
16. Hunter JG: Avoidance of bile duct injury during laparoscopic cholecystectomy *Am J Surg* 162:71–76, 1991.
17. Ferguson CM, Rottner DW, Warshaw AL: Bile duct injury in laparoscopic cholecystectomy. *Surg Laparosc Endosc* 2(1):1–7, 1992.

18

Laparoscopic Peptic Ulcer Surgery

Joseph J. Pietrafitta

The ability of the general surgeon to perform acid reducing operations through the laparoscope has become a reality. Prior to this development, the open operations that were available to treat peptic ulcer disease had significant short term sequelae. The discomfort associated with these open operations was of a magnitude that discouraged patients from seeking this treatment course. In addition, the recovery period was relatively prolonged. As the field of laparoscopic surgery develops, it appears that further changes will occur.

This chapter will present only the techniques that are a clinical reality. It should also be understood that active investigation is underway to advance the techniques of laparoscopic peptic ulcer surgery. The ultimate goal will be to develop the technical expertise to perform all open peptic ulcer operations laparoscopically in a safe, efficient, and expeditious manner.

The major procedures that have been developed include plication of a perforated peptic ulcer (laparoscopic and endoscopically assisted laparoscopic) and various forms of vagotomy including: (1) posterior truncal with anterior highly selective vagotomy, (2) posterior truncal vagotomy with anterior seromyotomy, and (3) anterior and posterior highly selective vagotomy. Bilateral truncal vagotomy with drainage has also become a reality. This has been made possible through the development of a pyloroplasty/hemipylorectomy stapling device.

Plication of a Perforated Peptic Ulcer

Perforated peptic ulcers continue to occur with surprising regularity. The standard treatment is closure of the ulcer either directly if possible or with plication in varying forms using omentum. This is a relatively simple surgical procedure that is very amenable to laparoscopic techniques.[1-4] The procedure can be performed totally laparoscopically or with endoscopic assistance. The decision to perform this procedure laparoscopically is determined by the extent of intraabdominal contamination (the time between actual perforation and operative intervention) and the ability of the surgeon to irrigate and "clean out" the abdominal cavity adequately.

The first step is to create a pneumoperitoneum followed by placement of an umbilical trocar. Once this trocar is introduced, the patient is placed in the reverse Trendelenburg position in order to displace the bowel from the upper abdomen. A general survey of the abdominal cavity is then undertaken to assess the pathologic process. If a perforated ulcer is identified, either still open and leaking or loosely covered by omentum, then laparoscopic closure can be performed. Once the process is identified as a perforated ulcer, additional trocars are introduced. Two additional trocars, one on the left and another on the right side of the abdomen at the level of the umbilicus that are 10/11 mm in size are inserted (Fig. 18-1). Placement of these larger trocars will allow utilization of a ligaclip applier and an introducer sleeve for needle and suture introduction. This trocar placement will also allow easy suture placement and intracorporeal knot tying.

Laparoscopic Technique

All of the modalities that are available to perform laparoscopic closure involve the place-

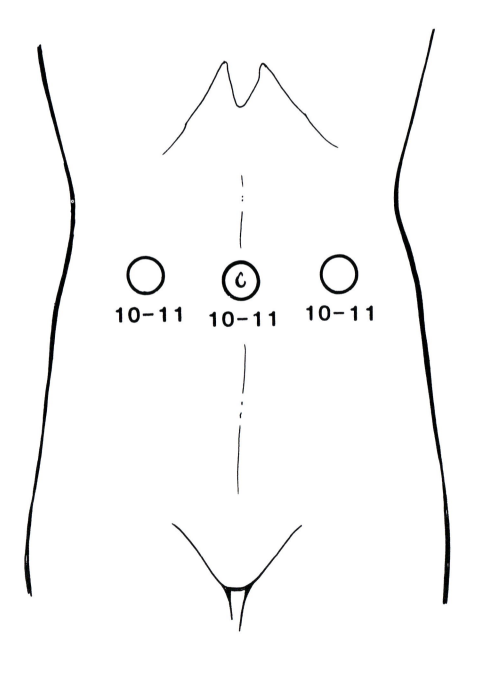

Figure 18-1
Trocar placement for plication of a perforated duodenal ulcer. A 10-mm trocar is placed at the umbilicus. Two additional trocars 10/11 mm in size are placed one to the left and the other to the right of the umbilicus.

ment of sutures. Two to three sutures are placed either into the ulcer (depending on the extent of induration) or through normal tissue adjacent to the ulcer (Fig. 18-2A, B, and C).

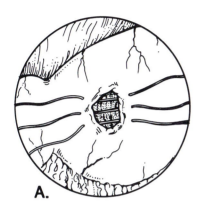

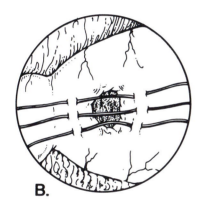

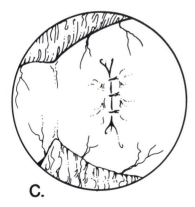

Figure 18-2
A. Three sutures placed through the ulcer. Minimal induration present. **B.** Three sutures placed adjacent to the ulcer. Moderate induration present.
C. Extracorporeal or intracorporeal knot-tying technique can be used.

The knots can be tied either intracorporeally or extracorporeally, using a knot pusher to advance the knot into the peritoneal cavity (Fig. 18-3A and B). Omentum can also be tied into the sutures over the ulcer. If this is done, the omentum can be held in position with a grasper placed through the right-sided trocar as the suture is tied through the left-sided trocar (Fig. 18-3C).

Endoscopically Assisted Technique
In this technique the omentum is mobilized laparoscopically. The surgeon then places the omentum near the open ulcer. The endoscopist pulls the omentum through the ulcer and holds it in place while it is being sutured in position by the laparoscopist (Fig. 18-4A, B, and C).

Truncal Vagotomy and Hemipylorectomy/ Pyloroplasty

Until recently, laparoscopic truncal vagotomy was not considered feasible because of a relative lack of ability on the part of the surgeon to be able to perform a drainage procedure other than a pyloromyotomy[9] or a hand-sewn pyloroplasty. With introduction of a pyloroplasty/hemipylorectomy device this ability should change dramatically.[10]

Truncal as well as selective vagotomies and seromyotomies can all be performed using a four-trocar technique. The initial trocar is placed at the umbilicus in a short-waisted patient or above the umbilicus in the midline in a longer-waisted patient. Once the initial trocar is inserted, the patient is placed in the reverse Trendelenburg position. One additional trocar is placed on the patient's right side. The size of this trocar depends on the size of the liver retractor that is being used. Two additional trocars are placed on the patient's left side for the operator. These are used for two-handed operating. These trocars should both be 10/11 mm in size, allowing the use of a Babcock clamp, a laparoscopic clip applier, and regular grasping and dissecting instruments (Fig. 18-5).

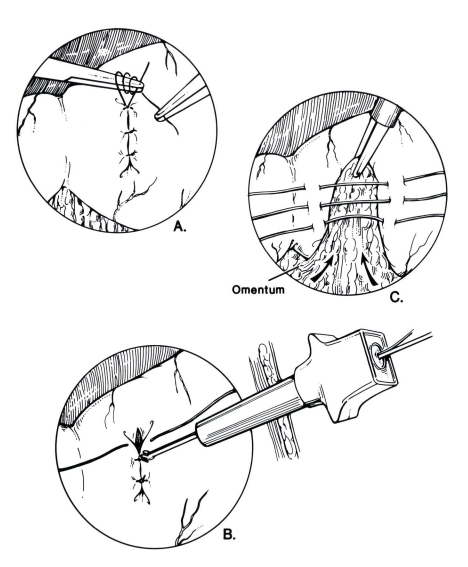

Figure 18-3 **A.** Suture being tied using an intracorporeal technique. **B.** Suture being tied using an extracorporeal knot pusher. **C.** Omentum being tied into the sutured closure.

Liver retraction is accomplished first. It should be noted that the left lobe of the liver should not be mobilized by incising its attachments to the diaphragm. If this is done, the lobe becomes "floppy" and difficult to control. The instrument that is used for liver retraction is simply placed under the left lobe of the liver and slid up the diaphragm, raising the liver above the area of dissection.

Once the liver is adequately mobilized, the operating surgeon begins to work anterior to the esophagus, using grasping and dissecting instruments. The peritoneum is incised longitudinally and the anterior vagus nerve is identified (Fig. 18-6A and B). The esophagus and anterior vagus are then retracted to the patient's left. If necessary, a dilator (nos. 32–40 French) is placed in the esophagus to help identify that structure. The dilator should be removed prior to actual manipulation and traction of the esophagus.

The posterior vagus nerve is then identified (Fig. 18-7A). It is grasped and retracted into the field by the operating surgeon (Fig. 18-7B). The nerve is transected above and below the grasper, using clips and scissors or hook cautery or cautery scissors alone without actually clipping the nerve (Fig. 18-7C). The specimen is removed for analysis.

The anterior vagus nerve is then either transected as a truncal vagotomy, or a highly selective vagotomy or seromyotomy is performed.

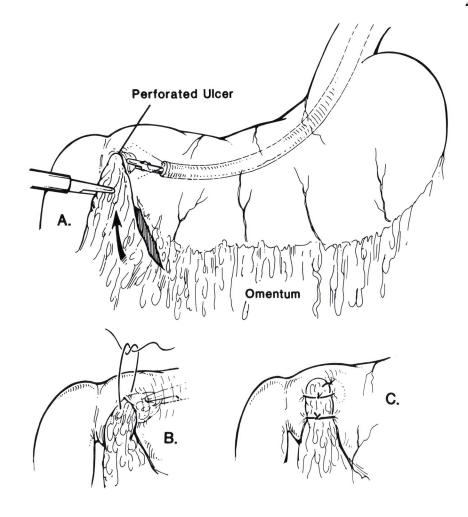

Figure 18-4
A. Omentum held by laparoscopist.
B. Endoscopic grasper grasps the omentum and pulls it into the ulcer.
C. Omentum sutured in place while being held in position by the endoscopist.

If a truncal vagotomy is performed, it is necessary to perform a pyloroplasty as a drainage procedure. This can be done using either suture or stapling techniques. Suture techniques are extremely cumbersome and impractical for the average surgeon. Use of the new hemipylorectomy/pyloroplasty stapling device will facilitate this procedure. This device excises the anterior half of the pyloric muscle (hemipylorectomy) while fashioning a gastroduodenostomy (pyloroplasty) with minimal enlargement of the size of the gastric outlet (Fig. 18-8A, B, and C).

A gastrotomy is first performed using laser or cautery. The lateral most trocar on the left is then exchanged for a larger one (i.e., 25- or 29-mm trocar) (Fig. 18-9A). The stapling device is introduced through this trocar into the gastric lumen, opened slowly, and advanced into the pylorus. The apex of the gastrotomy is held with a Babcock placed through the other left-sided trocar as the stapler is being advanced into position (Fig. 18-9B). The anterior wall of the pylorus is invaginated into the stapler, using a special invaginating device. The stapler is closed and fired excising an elliptical segment of tissue while fashioning a gastroduodenostomy (Fig. 18-9C and D). After the hemipylorectomy/pyloroplasty is completed, the gastrotomy incision is closed using a linear stapling device.

Highly Selective Vagotomy (Anterior Trunk)

A highly selective anterior trunk vagotomy can also be performed.[5,6] After the posterior nerve

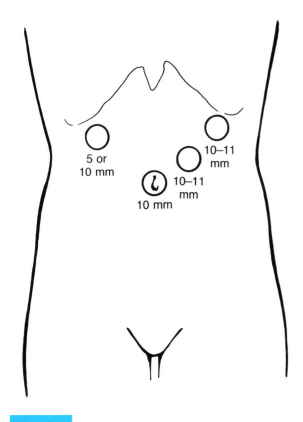

Figure 18-5
Trocar placement for vagotomy regardless of type. The first trocar is placed at the umbilicus for the 45° telescope. A higher position can be used for a longer-waisted patient. A second trocar is placed on the patient's right side. This trocar size depends upon liver retractor being used. The third and fourth trocars are placed on the left side of the abdomen. These two are used by the operating surgeon.

has been transected (described earlier), the anterior nerve is placed on traction toward the midline (Fig. 18-10A). The nerve is dissected off the lesser curve of the stomach. All the vessels and their accompanying nerves are transected, using clips and cautery. The entire lesser curvature is skeletonized (Fig. 18-10B). The dissection is continued to within 6 cm of the pylorus and 8 cm up the esophagus. It is important to note that on occasion (in 35 percent of cases) there will be mediastinal emphysema and on occasion carbon dioxide can be seen in the subcutaneous tissues of the head and neck. This is generally of no consequence and disappears rapidly.

Anterior Seromyotomy

As an alternative to anterior highly selective vagotomy, a seromyotomy can be performed.[7,8] In this procedure, the seromuscular layer is incised down to the mucosa of the stomach. This can be performed using a unipolar or bipolar hook cautery contact laser or a newly designed seromyotomy scissors. The seromyotomy is begun on the esophagus above its junction with the greater curve of the stomach. It is then extended onto the anterior wall of the stomach staying 1 cm left lateral to the lesser curvature vessels. If the seromyotomy incision is placed farther than 1 cm away from the lesser curvature of the stomach, the nerves will not be transected before reaching the submucosal layer of the stomach and the effectiveness of the operation will be greatly diminished. The seromyotomy is extended to within 6 cm of the pylorus (Fig. 18-11).

If the hook cautery is used, it is important to elevate the seromuscular layer of the stomach away from the mucosa as it is incised (Fig. 18-12A). This will prevent development of a transmural mucosal burn. If the seromyotomy scissors is used, a mucosal hole may be less likely to occur. The back of the scissors is insulated preventing the delivery of electrical current to the mucosal side of the incision (Fig. 18-12B).

There is a technique that is used to ensure mucosal integrity at the completion of the procedure. The stomach is filled with methylene blue after the posterior truncal vagotomy has been performed. The blue color can be seen through the mucosa as the seromuscular layer is cut. If even a small hole is made in the mucosa, the blue dye can be seen leaking at the site of the perforation and steps can be taken immediately to suture the hole.

This technique does not ensure against delayed perforations due to transmural burns that would perforate at 3 to 5 days after completion of the procedure. If the surgeon wants to ensure mucosal integrity and protect against delayed perforation from a transmural burn, the seromuscular layer can be closed at the completion

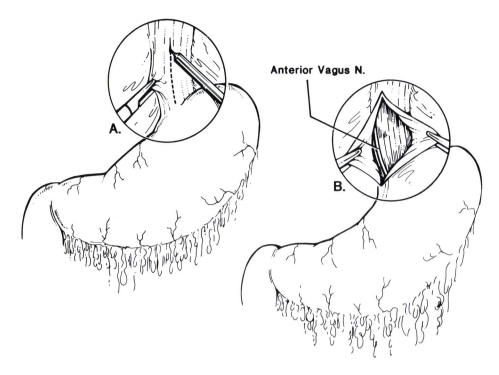

Figure 18-6
A. The peritoneum over the esophagus is incised.
B. The anterior vagus nerve can be seen.

of the seromyotomy. This can be done using the hernia stapler or a running suture (Fig. 18-13).

There is a theoretical concern that nerve regeneration will occur. In order to prevent this from occurring, the seromuscular layer can be closed in an overlapping fashion so that the nerves are not "lined up" and the likelihood of reinnervation is greatly diminished (Fig. 18-14*A* and *B*).

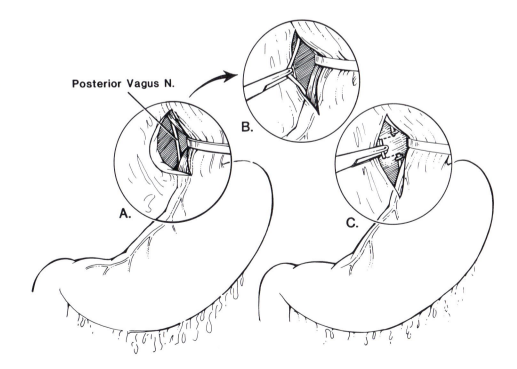

Figure 18-7
A. The posterior vagus nerve is identified.
B. The nerve is grasped and pulled up into the field. **C.** The nerve is transected and the specimen removed.

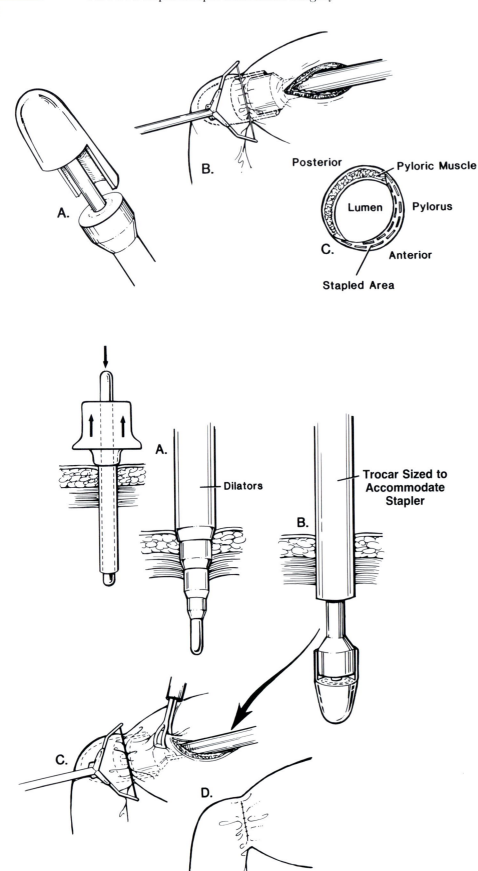

Figure 18-8
Diagrammatic representation of the hemipylorectomy/pyloroplasty stapling device: **A.** A posterior shield attached to the stapler head prevents the posterior wall of the pylorus from entering the open stapler when it is placed into the pyloric channel. **B.** Stapler in position, the anterior wall of the pylorus is invaginated into the open stapler. **C.** The stapler is closed and fired, resulting in excision of the pyloric musculature and anastomosis (shown in cross section) of stomach to duodenum.

Figure 18-9
A. Exchange of a 10/11-mm trocar for a 25- or 29-mm trocar. The actual size depends upon the size of the pyloroplasty stapler that will be used. **B.** The open stapler advanced through the gastrotomy into the pylorus. **C.** The pylorus being invaginated. The stapler is closed and fired. **D.** The resulting partial pyloric excision and anterior duodenogastric anastomosis.

Chapter 18 Laparoscopic Peptic Ulcer Surgery

Figure 18-10
A. To perform a highly selective vagotomy, the surgeon places the anterior vagus nerve on traction toward the midline. **B.** The vessels and nerves are dissected off the lesser curvature of the stomach, using clips and cautery scissors.

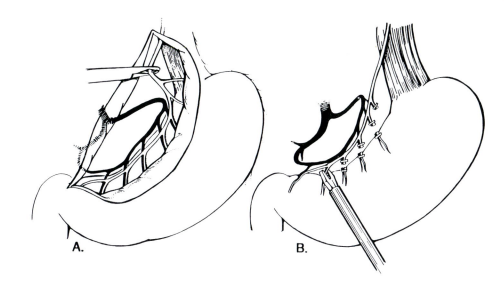

Figure 18-11
Diagram showing placement of the seromyotomy, which extends from the esophagus to within 6 cm of the pylorus and is placed 1 cm left of the lesser curvature vessels in order to transect the nerve as it passes into the muscle (shown in cross section).

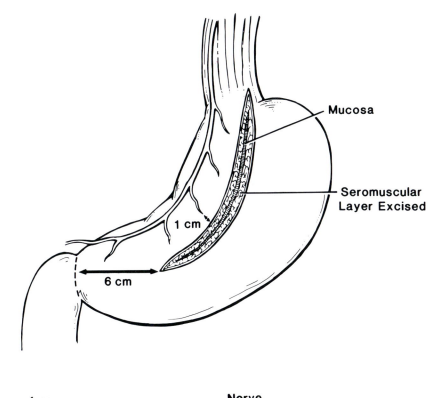

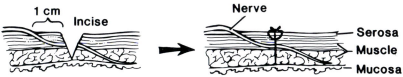

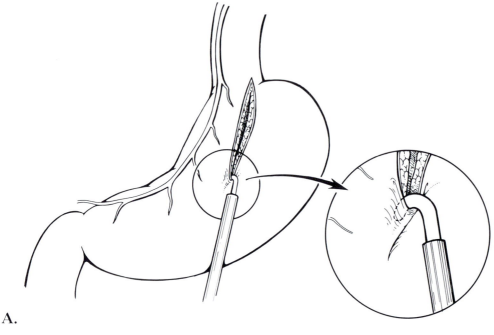

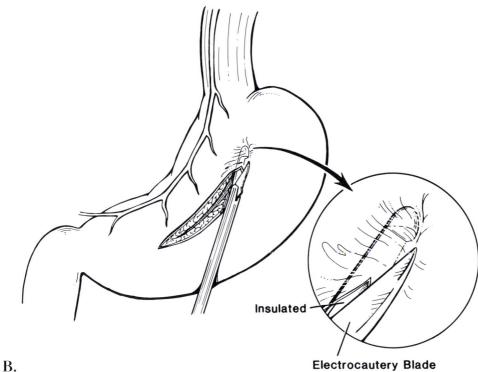

Figure 18-12
A. Seromyotomy being performed using a hook cautery. Note elevation of the seromuscular layer away from the mucosa.
B. Seromyotomy being performed using a specially designed seromyotomy scissors. Note that the back jaw of the scissors is insulated.

Highly Selective Vagotomy of the Posterior Trunk

A highly selective vagotomy of both trunks can be performed. A highly selective vagotomy of the posterior trunk is somewhat difficult to perform. The additional time required and potential risk involved are probably not warranted. The additional risk consists of the potential bleeding that can occur. Bleeding in this area may be extremely difficult to control and may

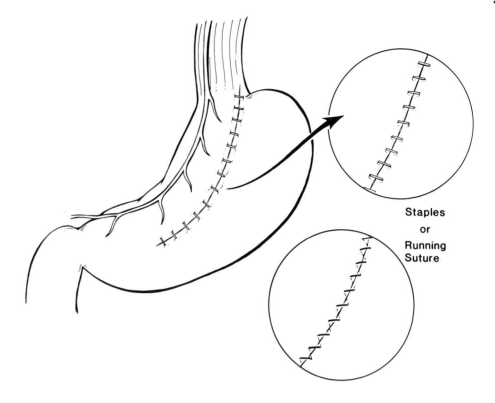

Figure 18-13
Closure of the seromuscular layer can be accomplished using hernia staples or by using a running suture.

result in the need to perform an emergency laparotomy. Leaving innervation to the antrum from the anterior nerve alone is more than adequate to ensure normal function of the antral pump mechanism and adequate gastric drainage.

The development of the hemipylorectomy/pyloroplasty stapler may be the key component in the success of laparoscopic peptic ulcer surgery. It will allow the surgeon to perform a drainage procedure in association with bilateral truncal vagotomy. It will also allow a drainage procedure to be performed in the patient undergoing a highly selective vagotomy when there is a question concerning integrity of the distal anterior nerve trunk.

If a laparoscopic approach to treating peptic symptoms is shown to be effective, routinely safe, and associated with minimal morbidity, then it will be an extremely important advance in medicine. An outpatient procedure with only 2 or 3 days off work and little pain or discomfort

Figure 18-14
Overlapping closure performed. **A.** Using hernia clips. **B.** Using a running suture.

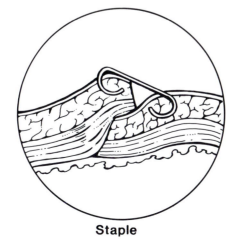
Staple

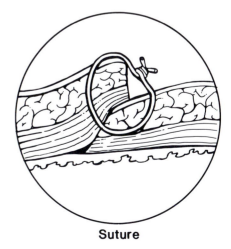
Suture

would surely be a viable option for people who have frequent recurrent episodes of peptic pain. The potential cost savings in avoiding lifelong antacid and H_2 blocker medication by such an operation are also attractive. Further controlled studies will determine which of the procedures described here will produce this outcome.

References

1. Nathanson LK, Easter DW, Cushieri A: Laparoscopic repair/peritoneal toilet of perforated ulcer. *Surg Endosc* 4(4):232–233, 1990.

2. Mouret P et al: Laparoscopic treatment of perforated peptic ulcer. *Br J Surg* 77(9):1006, 1990.

3. Costalat G et al: Coelioscopic treatment of perforated gastroduodenal ulcer using the ligamentum teres hepatis. *Surg Endosc* 5(3):154–155, 1991.

4. Fletcher DR, Jones RM: Perforated peptic ulcer. A further application of laparoscopic surgery. *Aust N Z J Surg* 62(4):323–324, 1992.

5. Bailey RW, Flowers JL, Graham SM: Combined laparoscopic cholecystectomy and selective vagotomy. *Surg Laparosc Endosc* 1(1):45–49, 1991.

6. Katkhouda N, Mouiel J: A new technique of surgical treatment of chronic duodenal ulcer without laparotomy by videocoelioscopy. *Am J Surg* 161(3):361–364, 1991.

7. Shapiro S et al: Development of laparoscopic anterior seromyotomy and right posterior truncal vagotomy for ulcer prophylaxis. *J Laparoendosc Surg* 1(5):279–286, 1991.

8. Voeller GR, Pridgen WL, Mangiante EC: Laparoscopic posterior truncal vagotomy and anterior seromyotomy: A porcine model. *J Laparoendosc Surg* 1(6):375–378, 1991.

9. Pietrafitta JJ et al: Laser laparoscopic vagotomy and pyloromyotomy. *Gastrointest Endosc* 37(3):338–343, 1991.

10. Pietrafitta JJ et al: Experimental transperitoneal laparoscopic pyloroplasty. *Surg Laparosc Endosc* 2(2):104–110, 1992.

19

Laparoscopic Treatment of Gastroesophageal Reflux

Joseph J. Pietrafitta
Ronald A. Hinder

Laparoscopic antireflux surgery is one of the most recent additions to the surgeon's armamentarium of laparoscopic gastrointestinal procedures.[1-3] It represents a major advancement in the technical ability of the surgeon to perform laparoscopic general surgery. The standard open procedure that had routine success is the Nissen fundoplication. The operation that has been performed laparoscopically has been a reproduction of the open procedure that was refined and is currently being performed by Demeester.

The procedure includes a 360° wrap of stomach around and attached to the esophagus. It is 1 to 1½ cm long, employing a U stitch that is reinforced with Teflon pledgets. The wrap is performed over a no. 58 French Maloney dilator. This is the wrap that was performed open by the surgeons who are currently recommending this laparoscopic technique and does not in any way represent a surgical compromise in order to allow its performance laparoscopically.

The results of this technique have been studied in great detail by Hinder and associates. All of their patients have undergone both preoperative and postoperative assessment including manometry as well as 24-h ambulatory Ph monitoring. The results of this laparoscopic procedure have been shown to be as effective as the open technique from both the laboratory as well as the clinical standpoint. The technique of laparoscopic Nissen fundoplication will be described in detail.

In addition to performing the Nissen fundoplication, others have looked at performing the Toupe procedure. In this operation, the greater curvature of the stomach is wrapped around the esophagus 270°. This procedure will also be described.

Trocar placement in this procedure is determined by the need to retract the liver, mobilize the esophagus and proximal stomach, and suture the wrap, using either intracorporeal or extracorporeal knot tying. Trocar placement is also dependent on whether the procedure is done in the lithotomy or supine position, with the surgeon standing either between the patient's legs or on the patient's right side. A total of 4 or 5 trocars are used.

The first trocar, 10/11 mm in size, is inserted in the supraumbilical area for placement of the telescope. A 30 or 45° telescope is extremely helpful in the performance of this procedure. The second trocar is placed in the right subcostal area. Its size is dependent upon the liver retractor that is being used. If a liver retractor is not available, then a 10-mm spoon forceps serves as an extremely useful instrument for elevation of the liver. Two or three additional trocars are placed. Their location depends on the position of the surgeon and the difficulty mobilizing the esophagus, crura, and the proximal stomach and whether or not additional stomach retraction is necessary (Fig. 19-1A and B).

Once the pneumoperitoneum is obtained and the initial trocars (nos. 1 or 1a and 2) are inserted, the patient is placed in the reverse Trendelenburg position. This allows displacement of the bowel from the upper abdomen. The other trocars are then placed. The initial step is to retract the liver. The liver retractor is placed under the left lobe, and the tip of the retractor is placed up against the diaphragm. It is then slid upward (anteriorly), lifting the liver off of the esophagus. The ligamentous attachments of the liver are not necessarily transected. If they

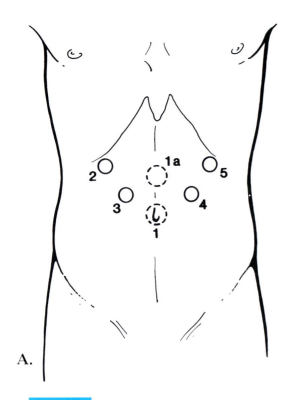
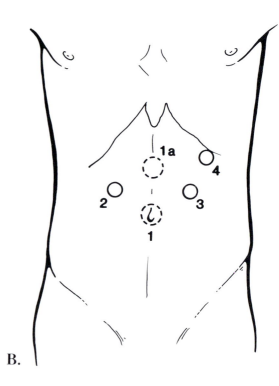

Figure 19-1
A. Trocar placement with the patient in the lithotomy position: Trocar no. 1–10/11-mm trocar at the umbilicus for telescope placement. Note optional position (no. 1a) for the long-waisted individual. Trocar no. 2 is 5 mm or 10/11 mm in size, depending upon the liver retractor that is being used. Trocars no. 3 and 4 are 10/11 mm in size for the operating surgeon and are used for dissecting instruments as well as clip appliers. An optional trocar no. 5 is placed if gastric retraction is necessary. **B.** Trocar placement with the patient in the supine position and the operating surgeon on the left side of the table: Trocars no. 1, 1a, and 2 are placed in the same position as with the patient in the lithotomy position. Trocars no. 3 and 4 are placed on the left side of the abdomen above the level of the umbilicus. These two trocars should be at least 3 in. apart.

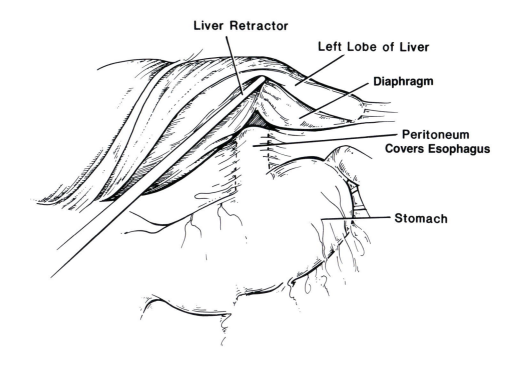

Figure 19-2
Liver retractor in position elevating the left lobe. The hepatic ligaments are not transected.

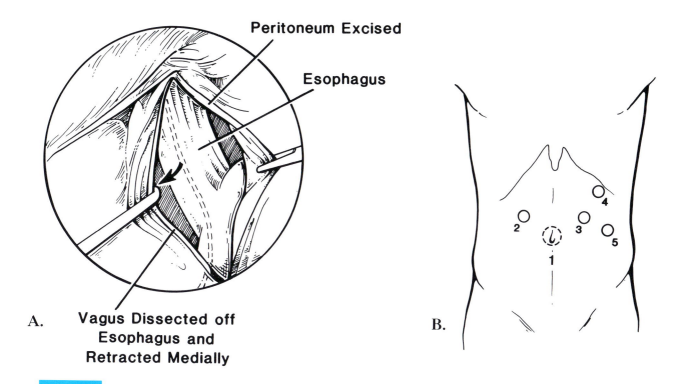

Figure 19-3
A. Peritoneum incised, anterior vagus nerve identified, dissected off the esophagus and proximal stomach, and retracted medially. **B.** A fifth trocar can be placed if necessary. This should be 10/11 mm in size in order to allow use of a Babcock grasper.

are, the lobe becomes somewhat floppy and difficult to retract (Fig. 19-2). Once this is accomplished, the actual procedure can begin.

The esophagus is identified. If this identification is difficult, an esophageal dilator (38–42 French) can be introduced into the stomach by mouth and moved by the anesthesiologist. This will aid in the identification of the esophagus. The peritoneum over the esophagus is incised vertically over the esophagus. The anterior vagus nerve is identified, retracted toward the midline, and dissected off the esophagus and proximal stomach and protected. This can be done with scissors or cautery (Fig. 19-3A).

At this point, if additional retraction of the stomach is necessary an additional (fifth) trocar can be placed (Fig. 19-3B).

Once the esophagus has been identified and mobilized, it may be necessary to maintain esophageal retraction. An umbilical tape can be placed around the esophagus, grasped with a locking grasper, and then used to retract the esophagus to the patient's left. This is done through the fifth trocar.

With the esophagus retracted, the next step becomes evaluation of the esophageal hiatus. This is done by identifying the crura of the diaphragm. The right crura is identified first. It is then completely mobilized from all surrounding tissue. This is accomplished by working down the crura from its apex, using hook cautery, cautery, or laser. If necessary, ligating clips are used (Fig. 19-4).

After the right crura has been mobilized, the left crura is similarly dissected free of all surrounding tissue. This is performed with the esophagus retracted to the patient's right. The left crura is mobilized beginning at its apex, working inferiorly (Fig. 19-5). Once the crura disappears from view behind the greater curvature of the stomach, the mobilization is continued beneath the esophagus, which is elevated and retracted to the patient's left.

There is often an abundance of periesophageal fat beneath the esophagus on the greater curvature side. It may be necessary to excise the fat pad. This will allow easy passage of the greater curvature of the stomach behind the esophagus so that the surgeon can perform the wrap (Fig. 19-6A).

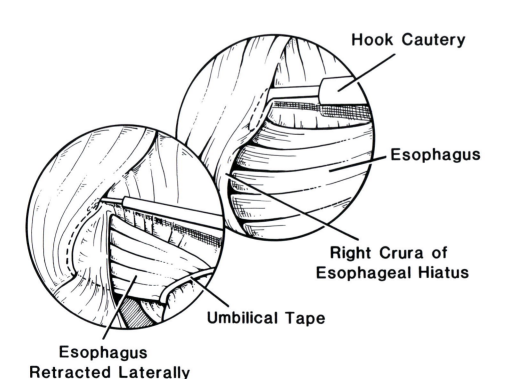

Figure 19-4
Identification and mobilization of the right crura of the diaphragm.

Chapter 19 Laparoscopic Treatment of Gastroesophageal Reflux

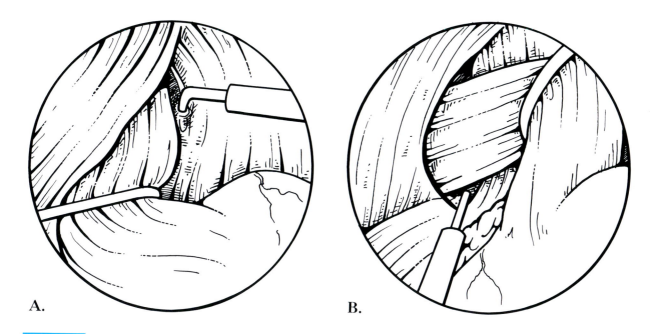

Figure 19-5
A. Mobilization of the left crura beginning at its apex. The left crura disappears behind the greater curvature of the stomach. **B.** Continued mobilization of the left crura is accomplished with the esophagus retracted to the patient's left and elevated.

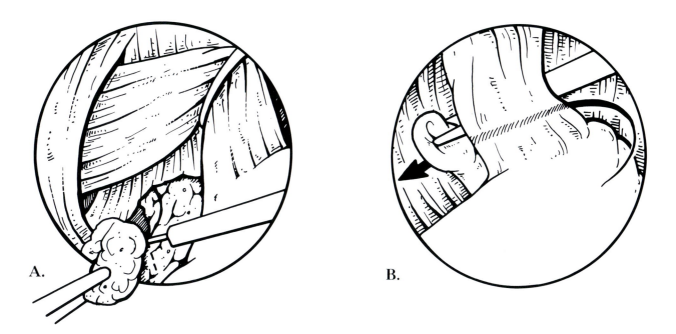

Figure 19-6
A. Periesophageal fat pad being excised. **B.** The greater curvature of the stomach can then be passed beneath the stomach.

Part Two Laparoscopic Abdominal Surgery

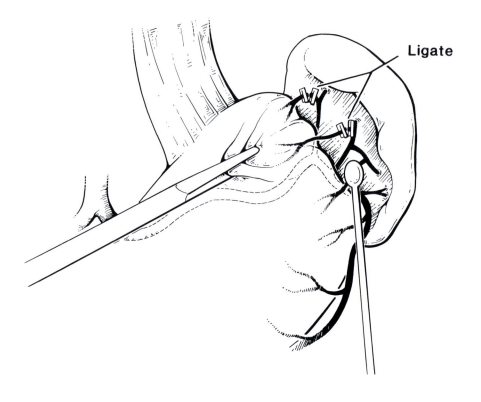

Figure 19-7
Further mobilization of the stomach by division of the short gastric vessels. Although clips are shown in the figure, it is more appropriate to ligate these vessels.

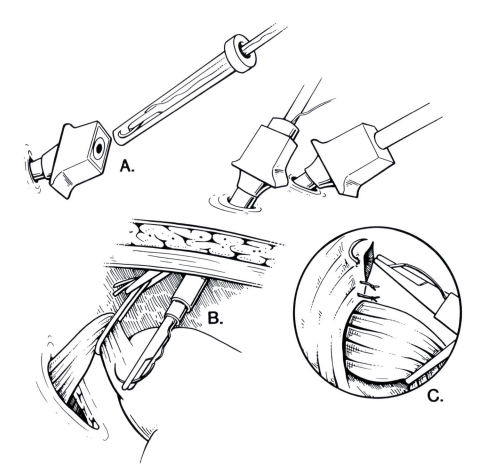

Figure 19-8
A. The suture is preloaded in an extractor sleeve.
B. Extractor sleeve is placed down the 10/11 mm trocar.
C. Approximation of the crura is shown with two sutures in place and a third suture being placed. Intracorporeal or extracorporeal knot-tying techniques can be employed.

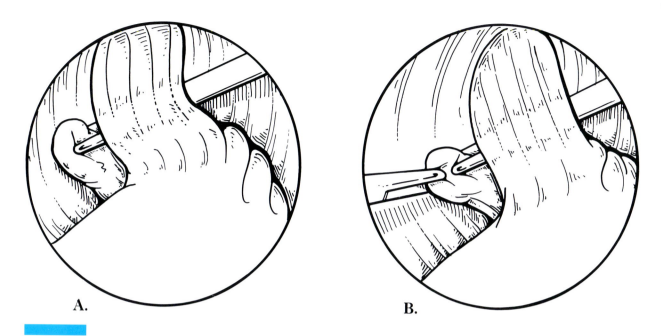

Figure 19-9
A. The stomach is passed behind the esophagus. **B.** The stomach can then be grasped from the opposite side.

Figure 19-10
A. A single suture is placed, and it is reinforced with PTFE pledgets. **B.** The suture is tied down to complete the wrap.

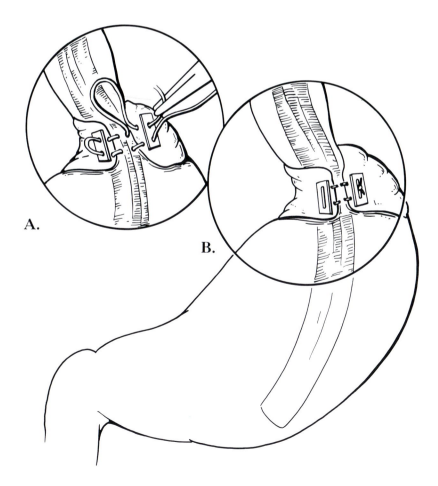

At this point, it must be determined whether or not it will be necessary to mobilize the greater curvature of the stomach further by ligating any of the short gastric vessels. An attempt should be made to pass the greater curvature of the stomach beneath the esophagus (Fig. 19-6B).

If there is tension on the stomach when this maneuver is attempted, further mobilization of the greater curvature is necessary. The short gastric vessels should be ligated with suture ties. The use of clips should be discouraged because of the possibility of dislodgment (Fig. 19-7).

At this point, closure of the esophageal hiatus with approximation of the crura should be performed. This can be done using a 0 or 2–0 nonabsorbable suture. Curved needles that have been partially straightened to fit down a 10-mm extractor sleeve are used. The needle and suture are preloaded into the extractor sleeve and then passed down the 10/11-mm trocar (Fig. 19-8A, B, and C). Either intracorporeal or extracorporeal knot-tying techniques can be used. Two to three sutures are usually placed.

Once the diaphragmatic hiatus is repaired, the wrap can be performed. The greater curvature of the stomach is passed behind the esophagus. The stomach is then grasped on the opposite side (Fig. 19-9A and B).

At this point, a no. 58 French dilator is introduced into the stomach. The wrap is then completed with a single U stitch reinforced with polytetrafluoroethylene (PTFE) (Teflon) pledgets (Fig. 19-10A and B).

An alternative method is to perform a 270° wrap—the so-called Toupe procedure. The esophagus and stomach are mobilized in a similar manner. It is not necessary, however, to take the short gastrics because the wrap is incomplete. The posterior wall of the stomach

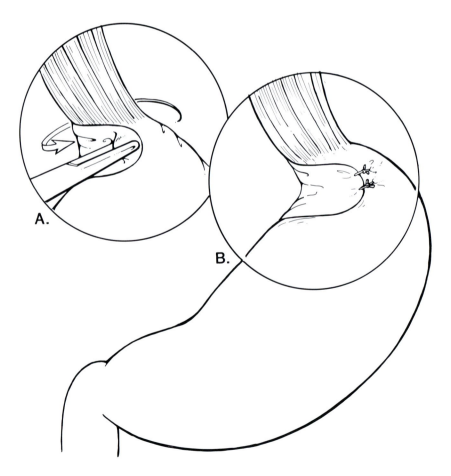

Figure 19-11
A. A 270° wrap is made by passing the stomach behind the esophagus where it is then grasped and **(B)** sutured to the anterior wall of the stomach.

near the greater curvature is sutured to the anterior wall of the stomach (Fig. 19-11).

References

1. Berguer R et al: Minimal access surgery for gastroesophageal reflux: Laparoscopic placement of the Angelchik prosthesis in pigs. *Surg Endosc* 5(3):123–126, 1991.

2. Nathanson LK, Shimi S, Cushieri A: Laparoscopic ligamentum teres (round ligament) cardiopexy. *Br J Surg* 78(8):947–951, 1991.

3. Albrink MH et al: Laparoscopic fundoplication. *Surg Rounds* (6):520–526, 1992.

20

Laparoscopic Inguinal Herniorrhaphy

Leonard S. Schultz

Introduction

It has been slightly more than 5 years since therapeutic laparoscopic techniques were introduced to general surgeons, initially in the form of laparoscopic cholecystectomy.[1,2] Since then, surgeons have developed laparoscopic approaches to other commonly performed open abdominal and chest cavity procedures. One area of intense interest has involved laparoscopic inguinal herniorrhaphy.[3-6]

Variations in the repair techniques are currently based upon the stable fixation of prosthetic mesh (polypropylene or polytetrafluoroethylene [PTFE]) over the defect(s) in the inguinal femoral region. Although no official classification of methods has yet been adopted, the efforts of investigators can be divided into three approaches: (1) Transabdominal preperitoneal repair in which the peritoneum covering the inguinal area is incised and the mesh then introduced through a cannula and positioned against the musculofascial tissue in the preperitoneal space and stapled in place. Once the mesh is in place, the peritoneum is then reapproximated with staples. (2) Extraabdominal preperitoneal repair in which all dissection takes place in the preperitoneal space following CO_2 insufflation of this fascial plane under reduced pressure. The mesh is introduced through access cannulas that remain extraperitoneal and is then positioned over the weakened inguinal area and fixated with staples. This technique, which closely resembles the open method of preperitoneal repair, eliminates the need for peritoneal incision and staple closure. (3) Intraabdominal peritoneal onlay patch repair in which mesh (all available types have been used) is introduced through a transabdominal cannula and is then stapled in place over the peritoneum that covers the involved inguinal area. A recent modification requires opening the peritoneum over Cooper's ligament so that the mesh can be stapled directly to this inferomedial margin of the inguinal region. As with the extraabdominal method, a peritoneal incision is avoided, but peritoneal stapling is not. Peculiar to this repair is the potential for direct exposure of mesh to small bowel surfaces.

Common to all these methods is the dictum that fixation of the mesh that is placed directly between the weakened muscle layer and the peritoneum will prevent reherniation so long as the mesh is not dislodged and that its total area more than covers the entire inguinal surface.

Our own group has defined the dimensions

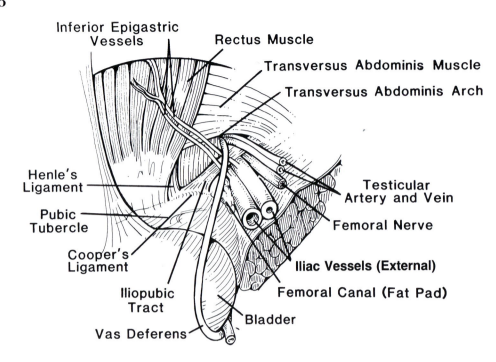

Figure 20-1
Preperitoneal exposure of the inguinal area; a dissection required to ensure proper mesh placement and fixation.

of this weakened tissue as extending from just beyond the midline, lateral to the internal ring, just inferior to the semilunar line of Douglas (termination of the posterior rectus fascia) and extending caudad, just below Cooper's ligament and the superior ramus of the pubic bone as it passes beneath the iliac vessels (Fig. 20-1). These anatomic boundaries must be defined by the surgeon prior to mesh placement in order to prevent recurrence. This is true whether the peritoneum is in place or is incised to allow dissection of structures within the preperitoneal space.

Because the ideal method is still evolving, the reader should be aware that controversies regarding this operation (all variations) certainly exist and include such topics as the necessity of dissection of the sac, the proper composition of the prosthetic device and the site of its ideal placement, and even the real value of this procedure. Available data can attest to laparoscopic herniorrhaphy's main advantages: that of allowing the patient to return to full and unrestricted activity within days rather than weeks while experiencing considerably less pain during early convalescence.[7] It is for these reasons alone that laparoscopic inguinal herniorrhaphy should be studied carefully.

Historical Review

Repair of the inguinal hernia within the preperitoneal space using tissue apposition was first introduced by G.L. Cheatle (1920)[8] and A.K. Henry (1936)[9] and later expanded upon by Lloyd Nyhus and colleagues in their classic article published in 1959.[10] Nyhus and his group described the procedure as an iliopubic tract repair. The reliance upon mesh instead of tissue apposition for long-term strength was originally described by Rene Stoppa in 1975[11] and later expanded upon in 1984.[12] These innovative "open" methods are in concert with the important work of Lichtenstein, who pointed out that polypropylene mesh applied to the anterior surface of the muscle defect offers the advantages of reduced pain and early ambulation.[13,14] Despite these advances, prolonged convalescence to achieve unrestricted activity was the rule.

In 1990, R. Ger focused the surgeon's attention on laparoscopy as a method of access for repair of the indirect inguinal hernia.[3] In 1990 we described a laparoscopic preperitoneal mesh repair (known as "plug and patch") that allowed return to full employment within 4 to 5 days (same as for laparoscopic cholecystectomy).[5] We first performed this procedure on December 22, 1989. The first published report of this method occurred in the German literature about 9 months later by L. Popp, who successfully repaired a female hernia with this method.[4]

Since these early reports, a number of investigators have emerged, who have described ingenious variations of the preperitoneal repair as described earlier. The proponents of the extraabdominal approach are B. McKernan and H. Laws[15] and E. Phillips (Fig. 20-2); those developing the peritoneal onlay patch technique include R. Fitzgibbons and C. Filipi[16] and R. Toy and F. Smoot[6] (Fig. 20-3). Those surgeons exploring the various aspects of the transabdominal approach include L. Schultz, J. Graber, H. Olgin, T. Dong, M. Arregui, R. Rodriguez, R. Lauderdale, and M. Gazayerli.

Rodriguez and Lauderdale deserve special mention for their popularization of the mesh "butterfly." Two notches were cut on opposite sides of the mesh that was then placed beneath the inferior epigastric vessels. This maneuver proved very helpful in fixating the mesh prior to the introduction of the endostapling device. Gazayerli attempted a primary tissue repair[17] modeled after the Nyhus iliopubic tract method utilizing suture but concluded that polypropylene mesh was an indispensable aspect of a successful repair. As a result of that effort, a specialized abdominal wall retractor and extracorporeal knot tier were developed.[18]

The technique with the greatest longevity and surgical experience to date has been the transabdominal preperitoneal repair with polypropylene mesh. It was originally conceived as a "plug and patch" technique where, after incising the peritoneum, dissecting out the dilated internal ring of an indirect hernia, and excising the peritoneal sac, a roll plug of mesh was fitted into the inguinal canal. Placement of the plug was followed by an overlay of a flat patch of mesh over the internal ring. High recurrence rates at 1 year of follow-up were noted.[19]

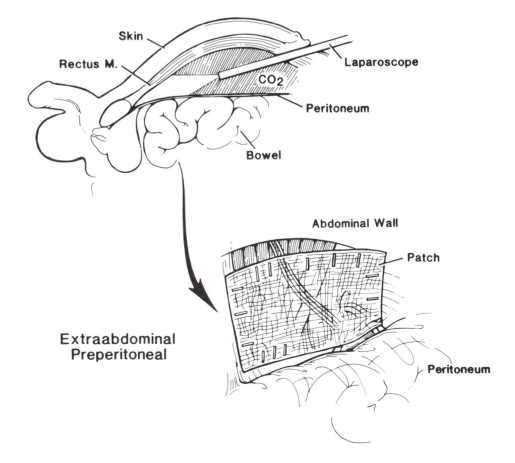

Figure 20-2
Extraabdominal preperitoneal laparoscopic approach for inguinal hernia repair. Note CO_2 gas insufflation is completed outside the abdomen and the peritoneum is not incised. Fixation of the mesh is the same as with the transabdominal preperitoneal method.

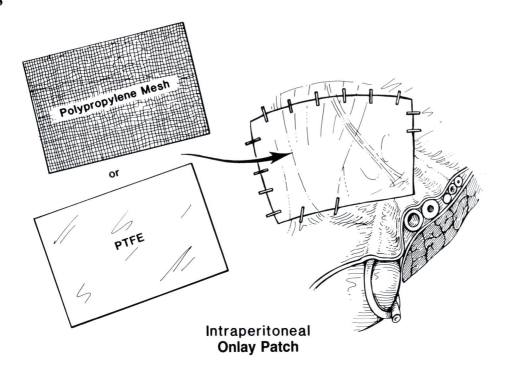

Figure 20-3
Intraabdominal peritoneal onlay patch technique for laparoscopic inguinal herniorrhaphy. Here, identification of inguinal area landmarks are made with the peritoneum in place. Both PTFE and polypropylene mesh have been used in this method along with staple fixation.

Direct space hernias developed in those with indirect repairs, and indirect hernias developed in those with direct space repairs. Consequently, it was learned that the entire inguinal area needs to be covered with mesh at the first operation to prevent frequent herniation of adjacent potentially weak areas. It was apparent that a surgeon could not determine the likelihood of future herniation despite direct observation with the laparoscope. Although an obvious fascial defect could be identified as a "hole," weakened tissue without a visual anatomic alteration could not be evaluated for future integrity. And thus the need to dissect, define, and cover direct, indirect, and femoral spaces with mesh evolved (this change was initiated on October 18, 1990). More recently, staple fixation of the mesh to the musculofascial edges of the defect has been added to the procedure. This refined approach promises to eliminate recurrence of inguinal hernias, even those presenting as large scrotal masses.

Anatomy

Inguinal anatomy has long been seen as confusing by many surgeons. Viewing the same structures from the peritoneal side may only enhance the confusion. For example, an attempt to delineate the inguinal ligament from the iliopubic tract as these structures appear laparoscopically on a video monitor will be quite difficult for the surgeon new to this approach because the inguinal ligament cannot be seen from the abdominal side of the muscle wall.

To help dispel this confusion, I have relied upon the contributions of a number of authors concerned with inguinal anatomy[20-24] and have integrated their descriptions into Fig. 20-4, which I feel best serves as an adequate guide to identification of inguinal structures. This is seen laparoscopically as Fig. 20-5, while Fig. 20-6 represents a diagram that has helped solidify my thinking of important anatomy in an easy-to-recall simplistic image.

Indications and Contraindications

In general, the following material pertains to the adult physique where adolescents are treated as adults if there is proportional height and weight. No pediatric patients are included, nor is it recommended that these techniques

Chapter 20 Laparoscopic Inguinal Herniorrhaphy

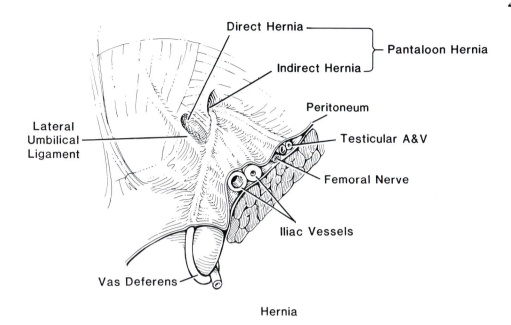

Figure 20-4
Diagrammatic appearance of the inguinal area depicting pertinent landmark structures with intact peritoneum. A pantaloon hernia has been included for perspective.

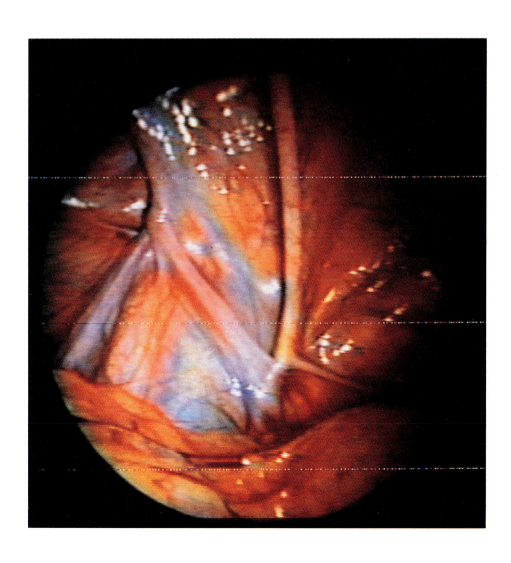

Figure 20-5
A left indirect inguinal hernia as seen through a 45° laparoscope. Clearly seen are the lateral umbilical ligament, the vas and testicular vessels as they join to form the spermatic cord at the caudad edge of the dilated internal inguinal ring, and the iliac artery and vein between the vas and testicular vessels. Lastly, one can see the inferior epigastric vessels coming toward the rectus muscle along the medial margin of the internal inguinal ring.

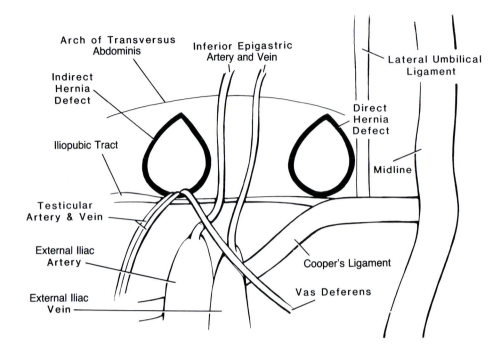

Figure 20-6
A schematic representation of the inguinal area. All pertinent structures are labeled and are in proper anatomic relationship to each other.

be used on infants or children until their usefulness is evaluated by pediatric surgeons.

All patients selected for surgery must be symptomatic from a clinically diagnosed inguinal hernia. Ordinarily, femoral hernia patients if identified preoperatively are not done laparoscopically because results with the "plug" repair done under local anesthesia have been excellent and have yielded prompt return to employment. If noted during laparoscopic evaluation, the femoral hernias are fixed in the same manner as other inguinal hernias.

Conventional "open" repairs under local anesthesia with or without intravenous sedation is reserved for those considered to be at too great a risk for general anesthesia. Patients with coagulopathies and especially those with stigmata of esophageal varices are also done "open" with local anesthesia.

Patients are normally advised by the surgeon of the relative newness of this procedure at the initial office visit. A general discussion of different forms of treatment for inguinal hernia with description of the relative benefits and disadvantages of each approach is important. A young, healthy patient who is very interested in returning to work as soon as possible may be more suited to the advantages of a laparoscopic repair. An older, retired individual who has had some previous heart trouble may choose the advantages of a local anesthetic and an incisional approach.

Preoperative Preparation

A videotape of the laparoscopic procedure is shown to the patient, any questions answered, an informed consent signed, and a physical examination performed. Preoperative insurance company authorization for surgery and professional payment is obtained before the initial office visit (see Chap. 26) so that often an appointment for surgery is made for the patient at the time of the initial office visit.

On the day of surgery, the patient presents usually to our office surgery suite or to a hospital outpatient surgery admissions office. Other than being kept nothing by mouth (NPO), nothing specific is requested of the patient except that he or she be escorted home.[25]

Operative Protocol

The patient is brought to the operating room (OR) after intravenous (IV) fluids have been started. A prophylactic IV antibiotic is administered and a small dose of IV midazolam hydrochloride (Versed) is given to allay anxiety. General anesthesia is usually accomplished with IV droperidol. The patient is shaved and prepped in an area cephalad to the umbilicus and extending to below both groins (Fig. 20-7). The genitals are prepped along with the abdomen and proximal thighs. This allows an adequate exposure in case external manipulation is required. A nasogastric tube is inserted for intraoperative gastrointestinal decompression and removed at the end of the surgery. A Foley bladder catheter is used to decompress the bladder during the operation, and it is removed at the end of the procedure. Keeping the bladder empty during the operation is also helpful to prevent postoperative urinary retention. In addition, IV antiemetics are given (20 mg of metoclopramide hydrochloride [Reglan] and 1 mg of midazolam hydrochloride [Versed]) to reduce the chance of postoperative nausea and/or vomiting, and 60 mg of ketorolac tromethamine (Toradol) is administered intramuscularly to reduce postoperative pain. After insertion of trocars, the patient is then placed in the Trendelenburg position for the remainder of the surgery.

The surgeon stands on the left-hand side of the patient facing the pelvis. This position serves well for the surgeon to repair a single or bilateral hernia no matter which side is involved. The assistant stands opposite the surgeon and is responsible for instruments and camera holding. The video monitor is placed at the foot of the table (Fig. 20-7).

Once the CO_2 pneumoperitoneum is established, a standard 10-mm trocar is placed cephalad to the umbilicus for insertion of a laparoscope. Further, two 10- to 11-mm trocars are placed at the same level approximately 5 cm on either side of the umbilicus (Fig. 20-8). A larger cannula may be used to accommodate a reusable stapling device.

Procedure

Initial survey of the pelvis will usually reveal an obvious "hole" that indicates the presence of either a direct or an indirect hernia, as well as the anatomic landmarks as previously described. Once the cannulas are in place, 5-mm reducers are placed over the cannula orifices to allow standard use of instruments for dissection purposes. The procedure usually begins just lateral and cephalad to the internal ring (Fig. 20-9). A short curvilinear incision is made in a caudad direction just lateral to the ring, which is then extended as a transverse incision just below the semilunar line of Douglas or approximately 1 cm above the hernia defect. Incision of the peritoneum and dissection can be done with laser, cautery, or scissors (Fig. 20-10). We have found that the laser cuts with less bleeding or injury to surrounding tissues, but it is costly and may not be appropriate. The posterior peritoneal flap is developed and then dissection is continued to identify the inferior epigastric vessels that divide the inguinal area into direct and indirect spaces (Fig. 20-1). The internal inguinal ring is identified and the sac dissected from surrounding tissue as well as from the components of the spermatic cord that enter along the caudad edge of the internal ring (Fig. 20-11). Medially, the rectus muscle is identified and followed down to the pubic tubercle and Cooper's ligament, which overlies the superior ramus of the pubic bone. The iliopubic tract can be identified attached to the pubic tubercle and Cooper's ligament and continuing laterally to form the medial edge of the femoral canal, as well as the lower margin of the internal ring. This is not to be confused with the inguinal ligament, which cannot be visualized from this laparoscopic approach. When all the structures have been dissected and defined, a rolled piece of polypropylene mesh measuring 10 × 8 cm is placed into a 10-mm reducing sleeve (Fig. 20-12) by grasping one end of the rolled mesh with a nontoothed grasper and bringing it into the extractor, which now serves as a cartridge. This is then placed down the 10- to 11-mm trocar on the side of the hernia and passed under direct

262 Part Two Laparoscopic Abdominal Surgery

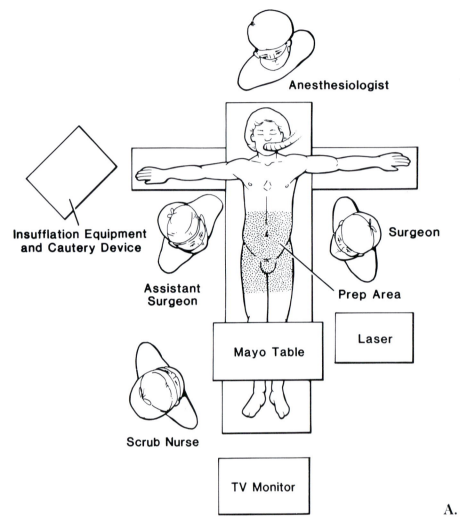

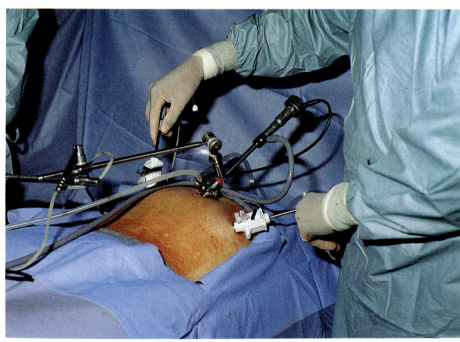

Figure 20-7
A and **B.** Standard operative environment for laparoscopic hernia repair. Of note is that the assistant surgeon, present early in the series, has been replaced by the scrub nurse, who is now replaced as an assistant by a self-retaining retractor seen below (Omni-Tract).

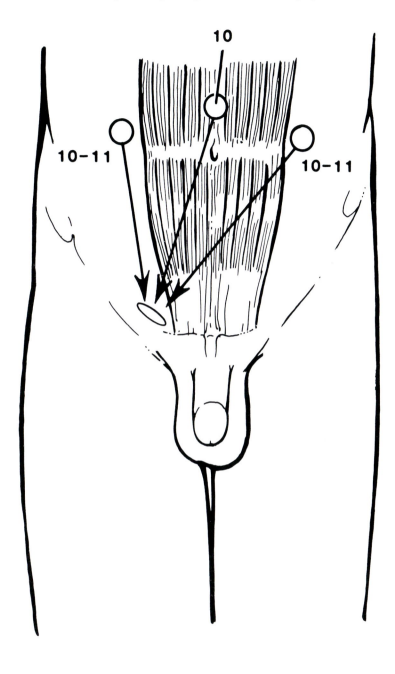

Figure 20-8
Sites for trocar placement. Uniformly wide trocars (10- to 11-mm diameter) allow for easy access to bilateral hernias (20 percent of patients). Placement should never be any lower than umbilical level to prevent optical disadvantage in the short torso individual.

vision into the hernial defect. It is prudent to insert the mesh through the ipsilateral cannula under direct vision so as to avoid possibly losing it among coils of intestine as it traverses the abdomen if it is inserted from the side opposite the hernia. At that point, two nontoothed graspers are used to unroll the mesh and to place it up against the entire inguinal musculofascial tissue with the inguinal area extending from just past the midline down to and over Cooper's ligament extending over the inferior epigastric vessels and beyond lateral to the internal ring.

The mesh covering should also extend from below the semilunar line of Douglas to below Cooper's ligament. More than one piece of mesh of the same size may be needed to ensure adequate coverage.

The stapling device is utilized to place staples along the peripheral margins of the mesh beyond the previously defined margins of the inguinal area (Fig. 20-13).

The staple should be driven well into Cooper's ligament. Postoperative pain from these staples has not been seen in our series. Staples

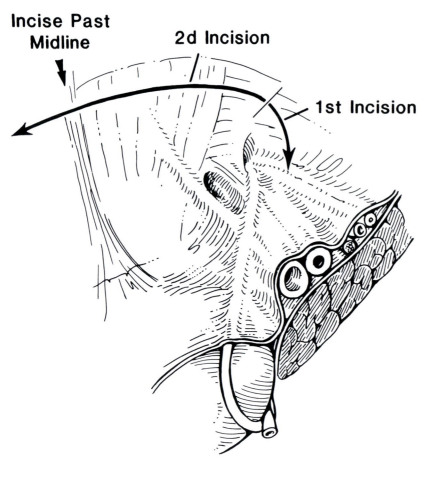

Figure 20-9
Typical curvilinear incision made in two parts. The first starts the dissection in a "safe" avascular area and allows for adequate caudad flap mobility. The second transverse component provides entry to the preperitoneal space at a level cephalad to the inguinal area.

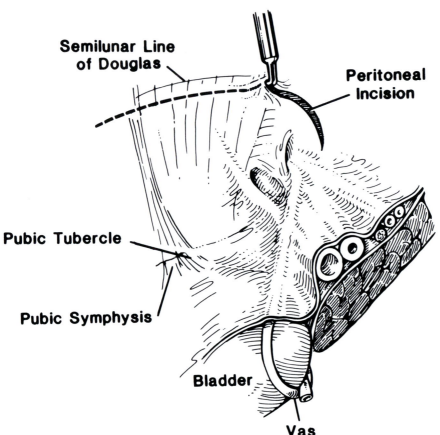

Figure 20-10
The peritoneal incision and subsequent dissection of preperitoneal tissue has been successfully done with bipolar forceps (as seen in this diagram), contact Nd:YAG laser, or monopolar cautery.

Figure 20-11
Dissection of the hernia sac is accomplished by use of traction–countertraction provided by use of a toothed grasper pulling the apex of the sac toward the abdominal cavity while pushing tissue attached to the sac back toward the inguinal canal. This maneuver is done on the anteromedial side of the sac so as to avoid spermatic cord injury.

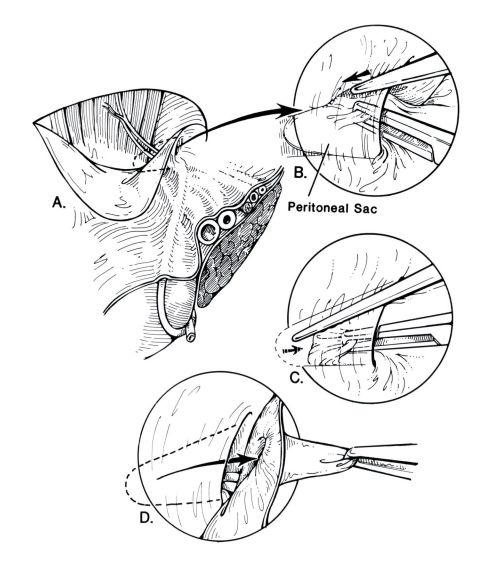

Figure 20-12
The large polypropylene mesh patch is curled tightly and then drawn up into a 10-mm reducing sleeve prior to placement down the trocar.

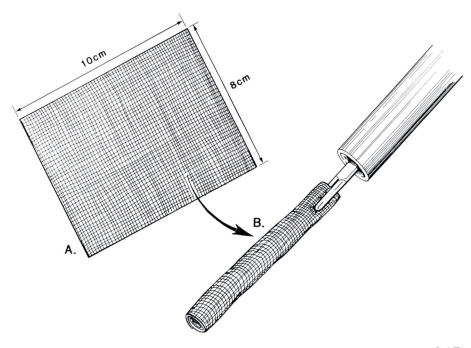

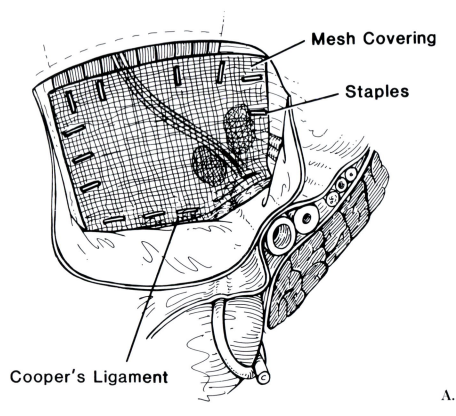

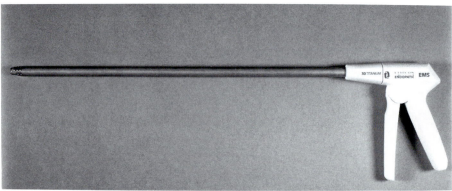

Figure 20-13
A. Staple fixation on the mesh. Except in cases of large scrotal hernias where maximal fixation would be desirable, we have found staple placement that avoids the lateral and inferior margins of the internal ring sufficient to secure the mesh while avoiding transient postoperative neuralgias.
B. The multifire endoscopic "tacker" is seen below (Ethicon).

should not be placed over the spermatic cord or iliac vessels because the potential for vessel disruption or nerve damage is real. Except when maximum fixation is required as in the case of large scrotal hernias, we do not recommend routine placement of staples just below or lateral to the internal ring. If staples are needed in these areas, the iliopubic tract should be carefully dissected and separated from the underlying femoral nerve. The staples may be placed gently through the mesh and the feet of the staples allowed to engage the iliopubic tract with an instrument between the tract and the underlying femoral nerve. This will prevent postoperative neuralgias that have been reported. Usually, 15 to 20 staples suffice to fixate the mesh adequately.

With this completed, the leaves of peritoneum are reapproximated after reducing the intraabdominal pressure to 5 to 8 mmHg. The edges of the peritoneum are held together with a toothed forceps and staples are placed to cover the mesh completely with peritoneum (Fig. 20-14). All instruments are then removed and the CO_2 gas allowed to escape through open valves in the cannulas. Finally, the cannulas are re-

Figure 20-14
Edges of peritoneum are reapproximated with staples to ensure separation of gut from mesh. To accomplish this maneuver, intraabdominal pressure should first be reduced to 5 to 8 mmHg to allow easier apposition of the edges.

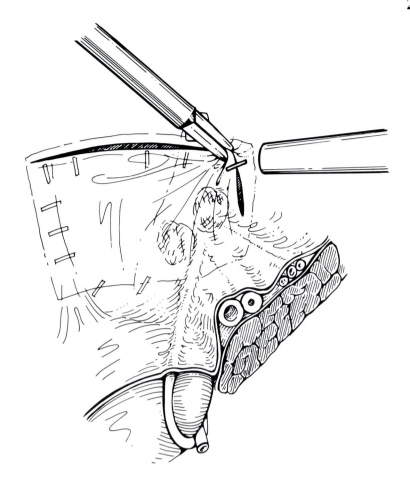

moved and the skin overlying the puncture sites closed with interrupted 4–0 disposable subcuticular suture and ½ in. surgical strips. No attempt is routinely made to close fascial defects of puncture sites of less than 10 to 11 mm. It is certainly recommended that puncture holes larger than that size, resulting from trocars, should be closed with suture material.

The patient is then brought out of the Trendelenburg position and the procedure terminated with removal of the Foley catheter and nasogastric tube. The patient is taken to outpatient recovery and is usually discharged within 2 to 3 h after the procedure is completed. Postoperative medication prescribed is 10 tablets of acetaminophen with ½ gr of codeine.

Results and Complications

The outcome data of the first 200 inguinal hernias repaired by our group covered the interval from December 1989 through February 1992. This involved a 97 percent follow-up of 160 patients of which 149 were male. The average age of this group was 45.7 years, ranging from 15 to 90 years of age. Of the 200 hernias repaired, 20 percent were bilateral. Most hernias were indirect, (121) while others were direct (77) or femoral (2) in type.

Eight percent of our patients experienced nausea that lasted longer than 4 to 6 h. This particular problem is important because we do not discharge patients who are retching or who have profound nausea. Early in our experience, nausea was the reason for a few hospital admissions. The preoperative drug protocols described earlier have kept the incidence of nausea to a minimum.

Patients complain of pain, often in the shoulder strap area, but most commonly at the puncture sites especially when associated with abdominal distension, which is common with all laparoscopic procedures (Table 20-1). Testicular or groin pain has been very uncommon in

TABLE 20-1	Postoperative Pain Location
Description	Incidence (%)
Shoulder Strap Pain	12%
Puncture Site	29%
Testicular/Groin	3%

TABLE 20-2 Postoperative Pain Medication

93 patients required an average of 4.7 pain tablets.
35 patients required no medication.
32 patients could not recall.
10 tablets of acetaminophen with ½ gr of codeine dispensed to all patients upon discharge.

this series. The presence of testicular or groin pain usually signifies hematoma formation or perhaps, at a slightly later time, hydrocele formation. Usually, these problems resolve spontaneously.

Table 20-2 indicates that a number of patients require no medication postoperatively and those patients who do take a minimum number of acetaminophen and ½ gr of codeine tablets for approximately 24 to 48 h. A reasonable evaluation of pain requirements was obtained in our series because only 10 tablets were prescribed for patients following discharge from the outpatient clinic.

Most significantly, patients were back to activities of daily living within 2.4 days, and the 68 percent of patients who were employed returned to work with unrestricted activity on an average of 4.5 days. Interestingly, patients who had bilateral laparoscopic hernia repairs averaged return to activities of daily living in the same 2.3 days but required 1 additional day of convalescence (5.7 days) before return to work.

There were 14 hospital admissions in this series, mostly for minor complications, such as urinary retention and nausea. We now use a no. 14 French Foley catheter following induction of anesthesia with removal at the end of the operation. This has eliminated urinary retention in subsequent patients.

There were two wound hematomas in the series that did not require hospitalization. Two patients had puncture site bleeding that resulted in overnight admissions and observation. This problem should be eliminated by checking the puncture sites prior to removal of the cannulas. Two additional patients were admitted for adult apnea and cardiac monitoring and discharged the next day.

The only serious complications were two small bowel obstructions. One of these was due to a Richter's type hernia through a 12-mm puncture site that occurred 4 days postoperatively. This was reduced and repaired under local anesthesia and the patient went home the next day. We no longer use 12-mm trocars, limiting our trocar size to 10/11 mm, and we still do not routinely suture the fascia.

The second obstruction occurred following complete breakdown of bilateral laparoscopic repair in association with mesh that was not fixated to the musculofascial boundaries of the hernia defect (performed prior to the advent of staples). The obstruction was due to a small bowel adhesion to mesh exposed after dehiscence of the overlying peritoneum when clips were used to reapproximate the peritoneum. This hernia recurrence was repaired with a conventional anterior incision 1 week after the original procedure.

After evaluation of the initial 25 patients revealed the need to provide mesh support for the entire inguinal area, the protocol was revised to use larger pieces of mesh (Fig. 20-15). This change, which began October 18, 1990, now includes over 150 patients. Of the initial 135 patients within this group, there have been 4 recurrences resulting in a drop in the early recurrence rate from almost 30 percent in the first 25 patients to 3 percent. Of these 4 recurrences, 1 was due to placement of too small a piece of mesh that was inadequately fixated by a new member of the team, and the other 3 were in patients with large scrotal hernias. These recurrences then served as a basis for the latest change in protocol that provides staple fixation of the peripheral margins of the mesh. Such fixation has been found to prevent migration of mesh through the dilated external ring seen in larger-sized hernias.

RECURRENCE RATE
1st 25 Patients – 8 Recurrences
From Dec. 89 to Dec. 90

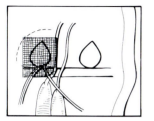

(6) Direct Space Recurrences

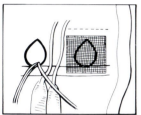

(2) Indirect Space Recurrences

Figure 20-15
Evaluation of recurrences indicated that it was the unprotected portion of the inguinal area that caused the new hernia. Such data led to the use of larger pieces of mesh at the original surgery that covered all four potential weak spots: direct and indirect spaces as well as suprapubic and femoral canal areas.

Discussion and Future Considerations

Currently, all inguinal hernia repairs are done by placing a large sheet of mesh over direct, indirect, and femoral spaces that are then stapled to adjacent fascial and ligamentous structures. No recurrences have occurred in this continuing group of patients despite the inclusion of several patients so treated with large scrotal hernias. The long-term outcome of the patients treated with mesh fixation will be the subject of subsequent reports.

Data are emerging that detail the real benefits of laparoscopic inguinal herniorrhaphy. Reduced patient discomfort and prompt return to employment are both humane and economic advantages of major importance, especially when multiplied for hundreds of thousands of patients. As with the results of other frequently performed laparoscopic procedures, such outcomes translate into billions of dollars saved when viewed on a national scale.

This is only the beginning of the story, however, because the lessons learned for inguinal herniorrhaphy can be directly transferred to the treatment of umbilical and ventral hernias. Certain differences should be noted. Although these other hernias often have peritoneum that can cover polypropylene mesh, there will be situations where this is not possible, leaving the mesh exposed to direct intestinal contact. Consequently, less adherent materials are now being developed. Whether or not this is necessary may be determined by a national trial led by R.J. Fitzgibbons of the Department of Surgery of Creighton University and F.R. Toy and R.T. Smoot, Jr., of Seaford, Delaware.

Finally, evaluation of the sequelae of peritoneal injury in laparoscopic inguinal hernia repair will help to determine which of the three basic approaches is superior. Future developments in instrumentation will further this effort.

References

1. Reddick EJ: Laparoscopic laser cholecystectomy. *Clin Laser Monthly* 6:400–401, 1988.
2. Schultz L, Graber J, Hickok D: Laparoscopic laser cholecystectomy. *Lasers Surg Med* (abstract) (supplement 1):14, 1989.
3. Ger R et al: Management of indirect inguinal hernia by laparoscopic closure of the neck of the sac. *Am J Surg* 159:371–373, 1990.
4. Popp LW: Endoscopic patch repair of inguinal hernia in a female patient. *Surg Endosc* 4:10–12, 1990.
5. Schultz LS et al: Laser laparoscopic herniorrhaphy: A clinical trial preliminary results. *J Laparoendosc Surg* 1:41–45, 1990.
6. Toy FR, Smoot RT Jr: Toy–Smoot Laparoscopic hernioplasty. *Surg Laparosc Endosc* 1:151–155, 1991.
7. Schultz LS et al: Laser laparoscopic inguinal herniorrhaphy: Analysis of initial 100 cases. *Laser Surg Med* (abstract) (supplement 4):27, 1992.

8. Cheatle GL: An operation for the radical cure of inguinal and femoral hernia. *Br Med J* 2:68–69, 1920.

9. Henry AK: Operation for femoral hernia by a midline extraperitoneal approach. *Lancet* 1:531–533, 1936.

10. Nyhus LM et al: Preperitoneal herniorrhaphy. A preliminary report in 50 patients. *West J Surg* 67:48–53, 1959.

11. Stoppa R, Petit J, Henry X: Unsutured Dacron prosthesis in groin hernias. *Int Surg* 60:411–415, 1975.

12. Stoppa R et al: The use of Dacron in the repair of hernias of the groin. *Surg Clin North Am* 64:269–281, 1984.

13. Lichtenstein IL, Shore JM: Simplified repair of femoral and recurrent inguinal hernias by a plug technique. *Am J Surg* 128:439–443, 1974.

14. Lichtenstein IL, Shulman AG: Ambulatory outpatient hernia surgery, including a new concept, introducing tension free repair. *Int Surg* 71:1–6, 1986.

15. McKernan JB, Laws HL: Laparoscopic preperitoneal prosthetic repair of inguinal hernias. *Surg Rounds* 7:597–610, 1992.

16. Fitzgibbons RJ, Filipi CJ: Laparoscopic inguinal hernia, in Green FL, Pousky JL, eds. *Endoscopic Surgery* 1992 (in press).

17. Gazayerli MM: Anatomical laparoscopic hernia repair of direct or indirect inguinal hernias using the transversalis fascia and iliopubic tract. *Surg Laparosc Endosc* 2:49–51, 1992.

18. Gazayerli MM: The Gazayerli knot-tying instrument or ligator for use in diverse laparoscopic surgical procedures. *Surg Laparosc Endosc* 1:254–257, 1992.

19. Schultz LS: Nd:YAG offers advances to laparoscopic inguinal herniorrhaphy. *Clin Laser Monthly* 10:77–78, 1992.

20. Condon RE: The anatomy of the inguinal region and its relation to groin hernia, in Nyhus LM, Condon RE (eds): *Hernia*. Philadelphia, Lippincott, 1989, pp 18–64.

21. Anson BJ, Morgan EA, McVay CB: Surgical anatomy of the inguinal region based upon the study of 500 body halves. *Surg Gynecol Obstet* 111:707–715, 1960.

22. Lichtenstein IL: *Hernia Repair without Disability: A Surgical Atlas Illustrating the Anatomy, Technique, and Physiologic Rationale of the "One Day" Hernia*. St. Louis, Mosby, 1970, pp 106–116.

23. Spaw AT, Ennis BN, Spaw LP: Laparoscopic hernia repair: The anatomic basis. *J Laparoendosc Surg* 1:269–277, 1991.

24. McVay CB: Inguinal and femoral hernioplasty, anatomic repair. *Arch Surg* 57:524–530, 1948.

25. Reavis WJ, Schultz LS: Laser laparoscopic cholecystectomy: Initial patient contact. *Laser Surg Med* (abstract) (supplement 3):24, 1991.

21

Laparoscopic Pelvic Lymphadenectomy

John C. Hulbert

Carcinoma of the prostate is common. In 1991, approximately 28,000 deaths were attributed to this disease in the United States alone, and more than 70,000 new cases were diagnosed. Current therapy for localized disease includes radical prostatectomy or radiation treatment, either in the form of external beam radiation or intrinsic radioactive seeds; therapy for disease that has spread to the regional lymph nodes and beyond is in the form of hormonal manipulation—currently this is in the form of either a luteinizing hormone-releasing hormone (LH-RH) agonist, such as leuprolide, or bilateral orchiectomy.

Recent methods of determining whether or not the disease has spread beyond the prostate prior to treatment include a radionuclide bone scan to evaluate for skeletal metastases, computed tomography (CT), magnetic resonance imaging (MRI), and lymphangiography;[1-4] none of these noninvasive techniques is accurate in indicating the presence of metastatic disease in the regional lymph nodes; even fine needle biopsy of a lymph node may be performed only if the lymph node is significantly enlarged on CT scan.[5] The tumor marker prostate specific antigen (PSA) is much more sensitive than the marker, prostatic acid phosphatase (PAP), and may be of assistance in diagnosing the disease; it is certainly of use in evaluating the success and course of treatment.[6] Gross elevation of the PSA may indicate the presence of lymphatic involvement or indeed bone involvement, but it is not absolutely predictable.[7] The only accurate technique for evaluation of regional lymph nodes for metastatic disease has been pelvic lymphadenectomy, which is usually performed as part of a radical prostatectomy, although it also may be done prior to radiation treatment to stage the disease more accurately. This has been an invasive technique, requiring a prolonged hospital stay and convalescence because it has been done through a long incision in the abdomen.[8]

The laparoscope that has been embraced widely by gynecologists and general surgeons is now being used by urologists to perform pelvic lymphadenectomy without the need for a major

Part Two Laparoscopic Abdominal Surgery

incision. Following is a discussion of the technique and its proposed place in the management of urologic malignancies.

Informed Consent and Patient Preparation

Informed consent for laparoscopic pelvic lymphadenectomy should include a discussion of the rationale for performing the procedure, the dangers of laparoscopy, and the need for consent for laparotomy in case of injury to bowel or blood vessels during the procedure. The patient should be aware of the novel nature of this procedure. Relative contraindications would include patients with extensive prior pelvic surgery or those who are markedly obese. Absolute contraindications include bleeding disorders and medical inability to withstand a general anesthetic or pneumoperitoneum. The patient needs to be prepared with a light bowel preparation (Go-Litely). A standard history is taken and a physical examination is performed as for all such procedures, and the routine investigations are made in accordance with the patient's age and general condition.

Technique

After induction of general anesthesia and endotracheal intubation, a nasogastric tube is placed in the stomach and a catheter in the bladder. The patient is positioned supine on the operating table with the arms at the sides, and the abdomen and genital area are shaved, prepped, and draped as is customary. A pneumoperitoneum is established as is standard for any laparoscopic procedure with the use of a Verres needle placed at the base of the umbilicus. Alternatively a Hasson cannula may be

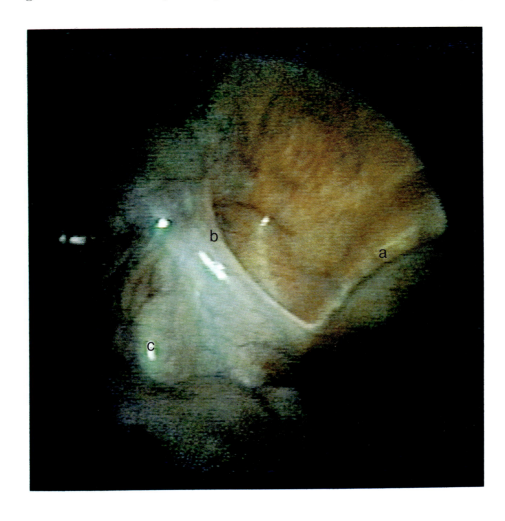

Figure 21-1
The key landmarks for dissection in this view of the left inguinal region are (*a*) the obliterated umbilical artery (or lateral umbilical ligament), (*b*) the vas deferens, and (*c*) the external iliac artery. (See also Fig. 20-5.)

used in patients with previous surgery or otherwise at the discretion of the surgeon. A 10-mm port is inserted through the base of the umbilicus, the laparoscope inserted through it into the abdominal cavity, and initial inspection of the entire abdominal cavity is performed.

The key anatomical landmarks for the dissection are the obliterated umbilical artery medially, the external iliac artery laterally, and the vas deferens, which can be seen running across from the inguinal canal in a medial direction (Fig. 21-1). Accessory ports are inserted in a position that may vary from operator to operator, but the placement of a 5-mm or 10-mm port in the region of McBurney's point is most appropriate with another such port at the corresponding position on the contralateral side and a third port midway between the umbilicus and the pubic symphysis (Fig. 21-2A). The instruments required are scissors, such as Endoshears (U.S. Surgical Corporation), which enable cutting and coagulating simultaneously; grasping instruments; and of particular use, a suction irrigation instrument that also is extremely useful for blunt dissection (Fig. 21-2B).

The targeted lymph node chains are the obturator nodes lying medial to the iliac vessels and around the obturator nerve and vessels in the obturator fossa; it is not usually advocated to do an extensive dissection of the external and common iliac nodes. The dissection commences by the surgeon opening the peritoneum

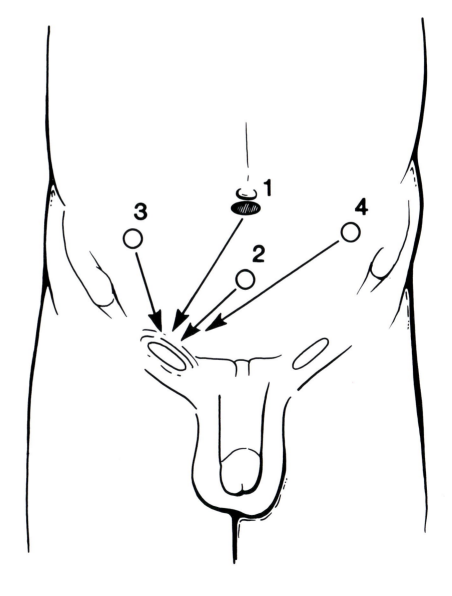

Figure 21-2
A. Position of laparoscopic ports for pelvic lymphadenectomy. This port placement will allow access to pelvic nodes on both the left and right sides.

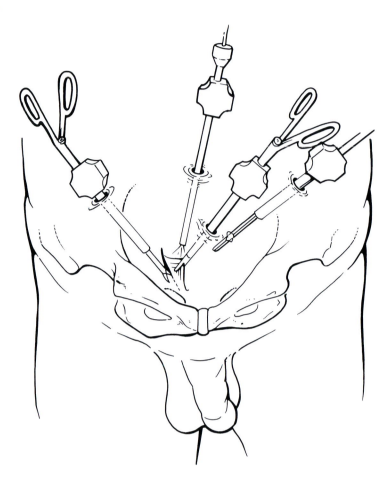

Figure 21-2
B. The ports allow the placement of multiple instruments as well as the laparoscope for dissection in the region of the pelvic lymph nodes.

immediately medial to the external iliac artery and lateral to the obliterated umbilical artery (Fig. 21-3); this opening is extended superiorly for a distance of approximately 3 cm and inferiorly down across the iliac vessels as far as the bifurcation of the hypogastric and external iliac arteries (Fig. 21-4A). If the incision in the peritoneum is to be extended further, identify the ureter as it crosses the common iliac vessels at this point. By gentle sharp and blunt dissection by the surgeon, the lymphatic tissue immediately medial to the external iliac vein can be dissected free from the vein at its most caudad point so that the pubic ramus can be seen and the periosteum will glisten white underneath at this point (Fig. 21-4B and C). Tributaries of the external iliac vein may be identified during the course of this dissection; if they are small, they can be coagulated and divided. If they are of any significant size, they should be clipped with Endoclips and then divided. The lymphatic channels of the obturator node package can be seen crossing the pubic ramus. These should be coagulated and divided as they cross this bony structure. The obturator node package then can be lifted and slowly dissected up out of the obturator fossa from the obturator nerve and vessels, and at this point the obturator nerve can be seen coming into view (Fig. 21-5); the entire node package can then be gradually mobilized back to the bifurcation of the hypogastric and external iliac vessels. It is useful to use the suction irrigation cannula to dissect the node package bluntly out of the pelvis, utilizing sharp dissection with coagulation for lymphatics and small vessels. The last portion of the node package at the bifurcation of the hypogastric and common iliac vessels is difficult to remove and is easily left behind (Fig. 21-6).

The node package can usually be removed in its entirety through a 10-mm port. If the nodes are enlarged a small lap sack may aid the removal by the surgeon's placing the nodes in the sack and then removing them through one of the port sites.

The external iliac nodes are frequently

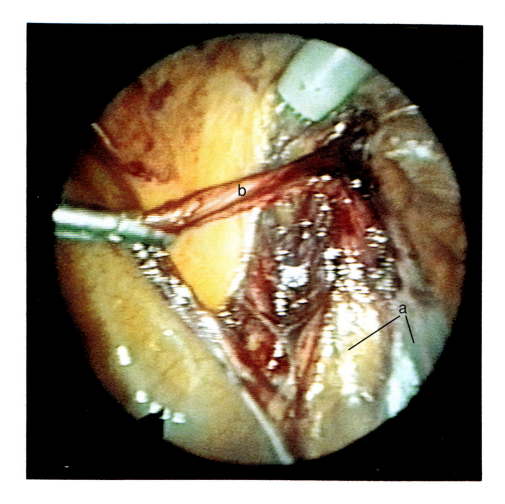

Figure 21-3
Initial dissection after opening the posterior peritoneum over the external iliac vessels (*a*). The vas deferens (*b*) shown retracted, is clipped prior to its division (right side).

spared because aggressive removal of all the external iliac nodes, particularly those lateral to the iliac vessels, may give rise to postoperative lymphedema. The incidence of postoperative sterility and impotence is not precisely known. Concentration on the nodes medial and over the iliac vessels and in the obturator fossa is usually adequate in patients with prostate and bladder cancer because these seem to represent the first landing site for metastatic deposits.

When the right side is completed, attention can be turned to the equivalent anatomical area on the left; here there are frequently adhesions between the sigmoid colon and the anterior wall of the abdomen even in the absence of previous surgery, and these need to be taken down in order to reveal the external iliac vessels pulsating through the peritoneum. The identical procedure is carried out on the left side as on the right.

Results

In our own series of 32 patients who have undergone laparoscopic lymphadenectomy, 31 for prostate cancer and 1 for bladder cancer, the average number of nodes removed was 16. This compares favorably with the number of nodes removed at open lymphadenectomy. The operating time initially was 4 h but now averages 1 h and 45 min. Complications have included scrotal lymphedema in 2 patients, abdominal wall hematomas in 3 patients, and a trocar perforation of the bladder that had to be repaired in 1 patient. No major vascular injuries or injuries to the bowel have been recorded. Hospital stay has averaged 1.2 days, with most of the patients now leaving the hospital within 24 h. Of the 32 patients, 10 had positive nodes and prostate specific antigen levels over 20, with

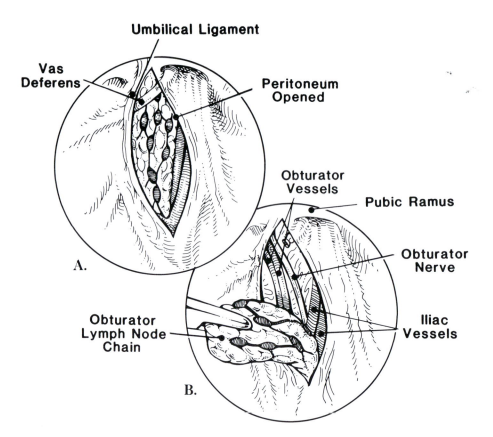

Figure 21-4
A. The initial incision in the peritoneum showing the vas deferens crossing the field with the external iliac artery and vein laterally.

Figure 21-4
B. Indicates a partial excision of the obturator lymph node chain from around the obturator vessels and from the medial aspects to the external iliac vessels.

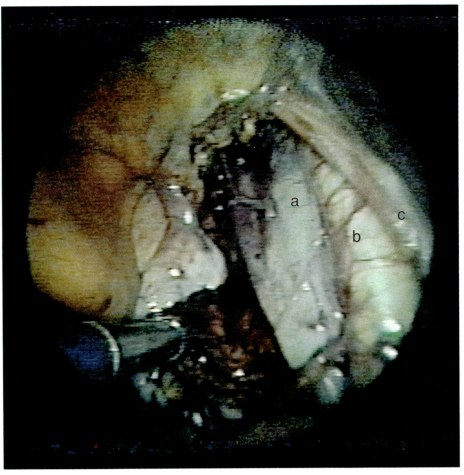

Figure 21-4
C. View of the obturator lymph node chain being separated from the external iliac vein (*a*) and artery (*b*). Note the testicular vessels (*c*) crossing the caudad aspect of the external iliac artery (right side).

Figure 21-5
The obturator nodes are dissected up and out of the obturator fossa. The obturator nerve (*a*) glistens as a brilliant white cordlike structure deep in the pelvis. The nodes are dissected from around the obturator nerve, artery, and vein (left side).

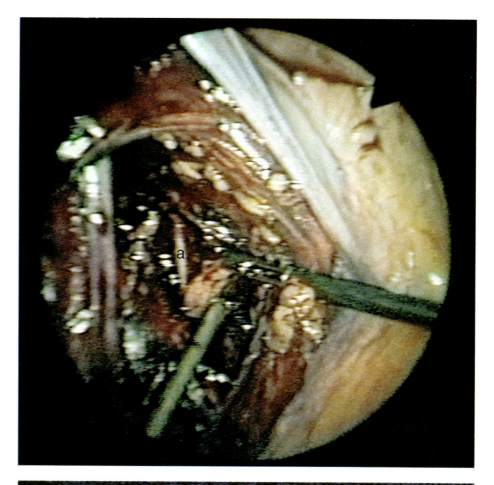

Figure 21-6
Completed dissection showing the glistening periosteum of the pubic ramus (*a*). The obturator nerve (*b*) can be seen crossing the obturator fossa, and the external iliac artery and vein (*c* and *d*) are seen laterally. The obturator node package has been completely removed, and the external iliac nodes have been partially removed (left side).

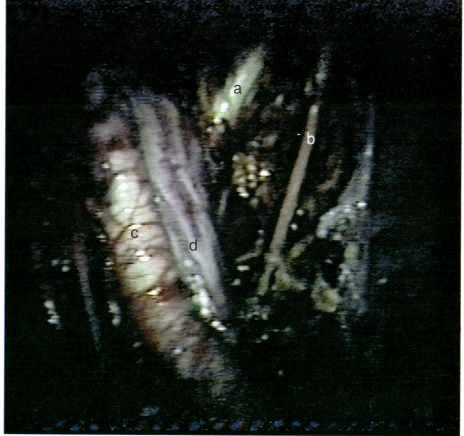

Gleason scores of their prostatic histology in excess of 6.

Conclusions

Laparoscopic pelvic lymphadenectomy is a useful addition for our capabilities of staging prostate and bladder cancer with a much lower morbidity than in the past. It is not a therapeutic procedure, but increasing the accuracy of staging of the disease and a precise knowledge therefore of the status of the regional lymph nodes may significantly influence treatment.

This technique should not be advocated as a separate procedure unless there is a significant likelihood of the nodes being positive. Our results and the literature support the contention that higher Gleason scores in the prostatic histology (i.e., more poorly differentiate cell types associated with a prostate specific antigen level over 20) have an incidence of positive lymph nodes greater than 50 percent and would therefore better be treated by hormonal manipulation. In the past, many patients unknowingly went through open surgery only to discover positive nodes or went through radiation treatment for prostate cancer in the presence of positive nodes that were not detected. These patients may have been better treated by hormone therapy with its much lower morbidity and cost. Laparoscopic lymphadenectomy can be performed with a view to proceeding immediately to suprapubic prostatectomy should the nodes be negative based on frozen sections or the procedures can be performed separately.

The current trend is for radical prostatectomy to be performed by the radical retropubic route through a lower abdominal incision. Indeed, radical perineal prostatectomy that is less invasive and done through a small incision in the perineum fell out of favor because of the inability of this technique to allow sampling of the regional nodes without another operation through an incision. With the surgeon's capability now of performing laparoscopic lymphadenectomy, the radical perineal prostatectomy may once again become acceptable for removing the prostate in patients with localized prostate cancer.

In conclusion, laparoscopic pelvic lymphadenectomy is a useful addition to our methods of staging prostate and bladder cancer and may be used selectively to influence treatment with much lower morbidity than in the past, but its full role is yet to be defined accurately.

References

1. Golimbu M et al: CAT scanning in staging of prostatic cancer. *Urology* 18:305, 1981.

2. Levine MS et al: Detecting lymphatic metastases from prostatic carcinoma: Superiority of CT. *AJR Am J Roentgenol* 137:207, 1981.

3. Emory TH et al: Use of CT to reduce understaging in prostatic cancer: Comparison with conventional staging techniques. *AJR Am J Roentgenol* 141:351, 1983.

4. Resnick MI, Kursh ED, Bryan PJ: Magnetic resonance imaging of the prostate, in Murphy GP et al (eds): *Prostate Cancer, Part B. Imaging Techniques, Radiotherapy, Chemotherapy, and Management Issues.* New York, Alan R. Liss, 1987, pp 89–96.

5. Dan SJ et al: Lymphography and percutaneous lymph node biopsy in clinically localized carcinoma of the prostate. *J Urol* 127:695, 1982.

6. Brawer MK, Lange PH: Prostate specific antigen in management of prostatic carcinoma. *Urology* 33:11, 1989.

7. Greskovich FJ et al: Prostate specific antigen in patients with clinical Stage C prostate cancer: Relation to lymph node status and grade. *J Urol* 145:798–801, 1991.

8. McDowell GC et al: Pelvic lymphadenectomy for staging clinically localized prostate cancer: Indications, complications and results in 217 cases. *Urology* 35:476, 1990.

22

Laparoscopic Varicocelectomy

Keith W. Kaye
Deborah J. Lightner
Leonard S. Schultz

A varicocele is an abnormal tortuosity and dilatation of the spermatic veins within the spermatic cord. This was first noted by Celsus in the first century. Celsus also described the presence of testicular atrophy on the affected side. In 1929, Macomber and Sanders reported improvement in semen quality and pregnancy following repair of a varicocele.[1] Since then, numerous reports indicate that approximately 30 to 40 percent of infertile men have a clinical varicocele as a major contributing factor. About 60 to 70 percent will obtain improvement in semen quality with correction of the varicocele, with an overall pregnancy rate of up to 40 to 50 percent.[2-4]

In many patients, the varicocele can clearly be seen above the testicle and may be palpated with its classical "bag of worms" appearance. These clinical varicoceles were said to be present on the left side in 90 percent of cases. Recent studies, however, using Doppler and spermatic venography, have demonstrated that subclinical varicoceles are much more common and may be present in up to 80 percent of infertile men, 60 percent of these being bilateral.[5,6] The lack of size or symptoms from a subclinical varicocele does not mean that it can be ignored in evaluating subfertile men because the size of the varicocele does not correlate with the extent of testicular and epididymal dysfunction.[7] Overlooking a right-sided or subclinical varicocele may be the cause of failure to obtain clinical improvement following left varicocelectomy.[6]

The major pathologic abnormality is an absence or inadequacy of the valves in the spermatic veins (Fig. 22-1). With man's incomplete adaptation to the upright posture, blood flows in a retrograde manner from the renal vein on the left side and the inferior vena cava on the right. The result is an increased hydrostatic pressure at the level of the spermatic cord and testicles. The most accepted theory as to why this causes reduced fertility is that the retrograde flow of blood increases the intratesticular temperature by 0.5 to 0.9 °C (1.0 to 1.5 °F).

279

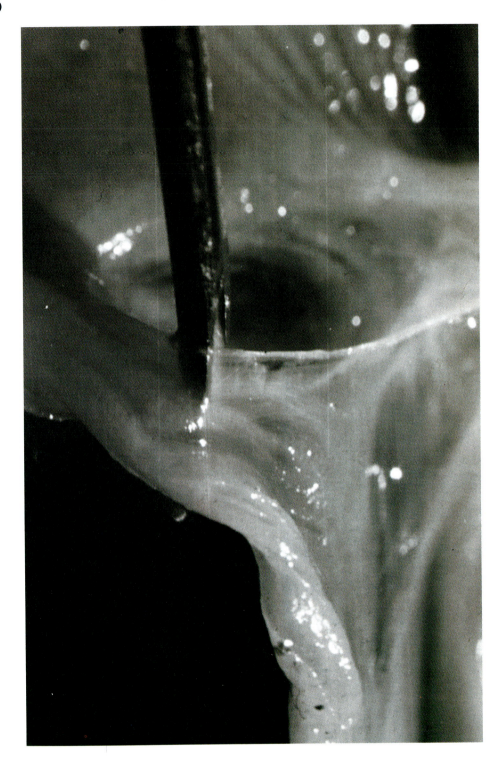

Figure 22-1
Prominent valve at origin of spermatic vein.

Normal intratesticular temperature is 1.2 to 1.9 °C (2 to 3 °F) cooler than intraabdominal temperature.[8]

Using microsurgical techniques, it has been found that at the level of the deep inguinal ring, there may be two distinct venous complexes that make up the varicocele. There are either one or two main internal spermatic veins that are situated somewhat more medial and posterior to the testicular artery, and in 26 percent of males, there may be one to three large veins that are intimately associated with the testicular artery. These are the venae commitantes of the testicular artery.[9]

Standard Approach

Until recently, varicoceles could be ablated either by open surgical operation or by venographic occlusion. The open techniques either involved opening the inguinal canal or a high retroperitoneal approach. A recent modification has been to use a microsurgical technique.[9] This has the advantage of permitting exact identification and ligation of the main spermatic veins and, in addition, the venae commitantes should they be involved. Also, the magnification permits the testicular artery and lymphatics to be identified and left intact, thus preventing the not uncommon complication of hydrocele or testicular atrophy following varicocelectomy. The disadvantage, however, of all open techniques is that although virtually all of them are performed on an outpatient basis under either local or general anesthesia, the patients still require several weeks, if not months, for complete recovery.

Venographic occlusion is particularly advantageous for defining and treating small subclinical or recurrent varicoceles.[10] The disadvantage, however, is that this usually takes up to several hours to perform with the patient awake, requires a high degree of radiologic expertise, and may not be as effective as surgical occlusion for larger clinical varicoceles.

Development of Laparoscopic Approach

Laparoscopic approach to varicocelectomy was first reported by Sanchez-de Bedajoz et al. in 1988.[11] Further reports appeared in 1990 and early 1992.[12-14] With the development of laparoscopic herniorrhaphy and the clear visualization that could be obtained of the deep inguinal ring, vas deferens, and spermatic vessels, it became apparent to us that a laparoscopic approach to varicocele correction should be a fairly simple laparoscopic endeavor (Fig. 22-2A and B).[15] Consequently, in December 1990, the clinical trials on laparoscopic varicocelectomy were commenced at our institution with the major objective being to achieve similar, if not better, clinical results with less complications and primarily with less surgical morbidity.

Procedure

Patient Selection

Patients undergoing varicocelectomy are often ideal for laparoscopic surgery. They are generally young, fit, and not obese. For that reason, this procedure is an excellent initial laparoscopic case for the surgeon and for developing a team for laparoscopic surgery. Contraindications, especially when beginning laparoscopic surgery, would be significant obesity, previous abdominal incisions (especially in the lower quadrants), and any coagulation defects. Patients who have had previous hernia repairs can undergo laparoscopic varicocelectomy without much difficulty. The procedure is also particularly advantageous for patients undergoing bilateral varicocelectomy.

Patient Preparation

The procedure, alternatives, advantages, disadvantages, and risks of each approach are fully discussed with the patient. Risks of laparoscopy in general and the relatively slight specific risks of laparoscopic varicocelectomy are addressed in particular. Each patient is given an informed consent form that is required to be signed prior to surgery (Fig. 22-3). Patients are requested to shave their abdomen prior to surgery, be off aspirin or aspirin products for one week, have a history taken and physical performed, and have nothing orally from midnight the night before surgery.

In the operating room, patients are placed under general anesthesia in the supine position with arms at their sides. A Foley catheter is inserted to reduce the risk of bladder perforation. The abdomen is then prepped from costal margin to symphysis pubis in case immediate laparotomy is needed. A nasogastric tube is not used routinely; however, should there be any

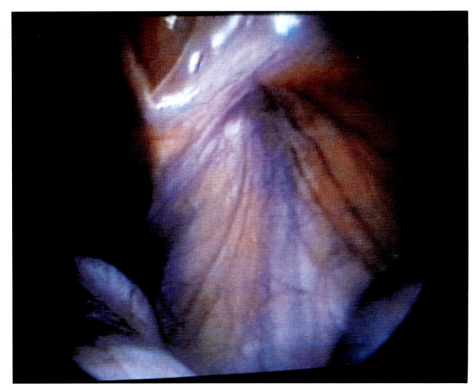

A.

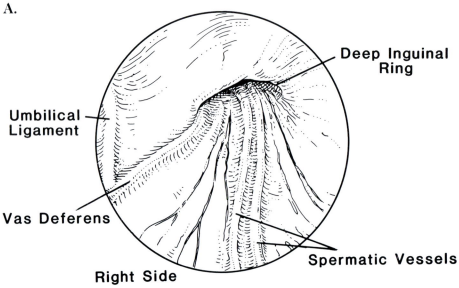

B.

Figure 22-2
A and **B.** Normal laparoscopic anatomy of right deep inguinal ring region.

question of gastric distension after induction of anesthesia, the tube should be used without hesitation. One dose of parenteral cephalosporin is given.

Placement of Trocars

It is our preference when establishing the pneumoperitoneum to have two towel clips placed through the umbilicus, one on either side in order to retract the umbilicus and anterior abdominal wall as far anteriorly as possible. The Verres needle is then inserted immediately ABOVE the umbilicus and angled inferiorly approximately 15° to enter at the maximum convexity of the umbilicus. The abdominal wall is kept in this tented-up position during initial carbon dioxide insufflation. This technique has given least trouble with misplacement of the

Figure 22-3 Informed consent form for laparoscopic varicocelectomy.

This operative procedure has been developed to lessen pain after your operation as well as to lessen the convalescent period and your absence from work now associated with the standard surgical correction of a varicocele.

Although all methods used in this procedure have already been approved by the Food and Drug Administration and the proposed method of laparoscopy are part of standard surgical practice, their application to correction of a varicocele is unique.

We anticipate that we can avoid the standard incisions with their resultant pain and discomfort by substituting three or four one-half inch incisions through which the instruments will be passed that will allow for cutting of the enlarged veins (spermatic veins) from the testicle. This procedure should take about the same time as the standard techniques but should result in less need for pain medications and a more rapid return to regular activity and work.

The risks of the proposed surgery are the same as with the standard approach: postoperative bleeding and wound infection as well as the less commonly observed complications. The only specific complication for laparoscopic varicocelectomy is bleeding from the vein should one of the ligatures become dislodged. The most serious complication is bowel or a major vessel injury that might require opening of the abdomen for repair. As opposed to open surgical repair, there is rarely a decrease in testicular size, fluid collection around the testicle, or a decreased sperm count.

The alternative treatment for varicocelectomy remains the same: i.e., removal by formal incision. In fact, during the same operation, this treatment may be necessary if it is the opinion of Dr. _____. The use of the proposed methodology might lead to an increased risk and/or postoperative complications.

_____
DATE

_____
SIGNATURE OF PATIENT

_____
SIGNATURE OF WITNESS

The above has been explained to and it appears that he understands it.

_____
NAME OF PATIENT

_____
SIGNATURE OF SURGEON   DATE

Part Two Laparoscopic Abdominal Surgery

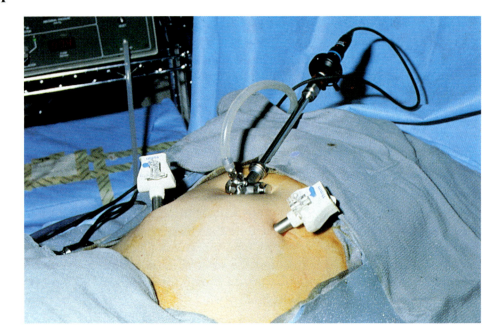

Figure 22-4
Position of 10-mm subumbilical and 11-mm abdominal ports.

Verres needle and least difficulty with insufflation because of omentum or bowel obstructing the needle.

A 10-mm trocar is placed in the subumbilical position, using standard techniques. One 11-mm working port is then established on either side. These are situated 2 cm lateral to the midpoint between anterior-superior iliac spine and midline about 2 cm below the umbilicus (Fig. 22-4). These three ports are all that is required for either uni- or bilateral procedures. The reason for using 11-mm trocars is that this permits a wide choice of instrumentation and accommodates both the clip applier and laparoscopic dissection and hemostatic device from either side. Once the trocars are established, the patient is placed in 30° Trendelenburg position in order to move the viscera out of the pelvis so the area of the deep inguinal ring can clearly be seen. The patient may also be rotated laterally away from the side being operated.

Instrumentation

The beauty of this operation, especially for those starting out in laparoscopic surgery, is that the whole procedure can be performed with only six basic instruments. Three others, although not essential, often really help (Tables 22-1 and 22-2) (Fig. 22-5). The essential instruments are the needle-tip grasper to elevate the posterior peritoneum adjacent to the veins, insulated disposable coagulating scissors and

TABLE 22-1   Essential Instruments

Name	Manufacturer	Size	Use
Needle-tip grasper	Storz	5.5 mm	Elevate peritoneum adjacent to vein.
Endoshears	U.S. Surgical Corp.	5.5 mm	Cut peritoneum; transect veins. Combines cutting with cautery.
Endodissector	U.S. Surgical Corp.	5.5 mm	Dissect and isolate veins. Can use with cautery.
Wave dissector	Storz	5.5 mm	To apply countertraction to vascular complex.
Fallopian tube ring	Storz	5.5 mm	To grasp isolated vein so that clips can be applied.
Clip applier	U.S. Surgical Corp.	10.5 mm	Hemoclip ligation of veins.

Chapter 22 Laparoscopic Varicocelectomy

TABLE 22-2 Advisable Instruments

Name	Manufacturer	Size	Use
Doppler	Meadox Surgimed	5.5 mm	Identify the testicular artery.
Hemostat and dissector	Cook Urology	11.0 mm	Tamponade bleeding vessel; dissects; mobilize bowel. Has peanut pads or Kittner dissectors.
Suction-irrigator device	Weck	5.5 mm	Irrigate heparin saline. Instill papaverine, aspirate blood and fluid, hydrodissection.

dissectors, a wave grasper, a fallopian tube ring to grasp the isolated vein, and a clip applier. Other helpful instruments include a laparoscopic Doppler for easy venous and arterial identification, a laparoscopic hemostat and dissector, an irrigation suction device for irrigation with heparinized saline (7500 units per liter), and papaverine to help identify the artery or to aspirate fluid or blood. The latter can also be used for hydrodissection.

Surgical Technique

The procedure is performed by the surgeon, who stands on the left side of the operating table throughout, whether for a uni- or a bilateral varicocelectomy. The assistant remains on the right side. It is helpful to have two video monitors, one on either side, although a single monitor at the foot of the operating table would also suffice. The surgeon uses the left port only, whereas the assistant holds the laparoscope and camera with the left hand and uses the right port for instrumentation (Fig. 22-6).

The first stage involves carefully defining the anatomy of the deep inguinal ring. It may be necessary to move bowel out of the way, and the laparoscopic hemostat and dissector has been found to be particularly helpful in this

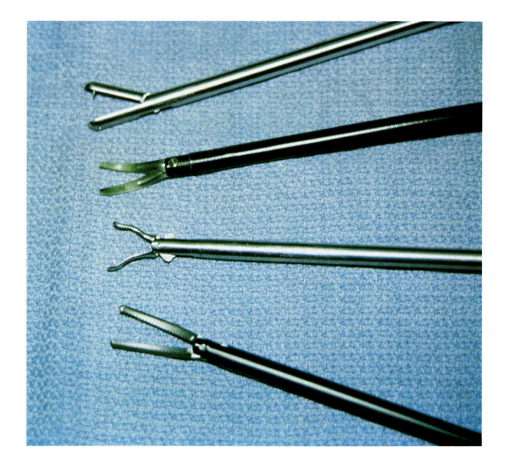

Figure 22-5
Basic instruments for laparoscopic varicocelectomy. From above: needle-tip grasper, Endoshears, wave grasper, Endodissector.

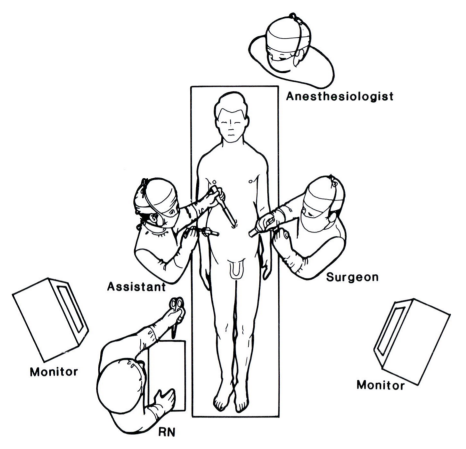

Figure 22-6
Position of surgeon and assistant for right or left varicocelectomy. Surgeon may use one or both hands to work through left port while the assistant steadies the camera with left hand and applies counter-traction with the right hand through right port.

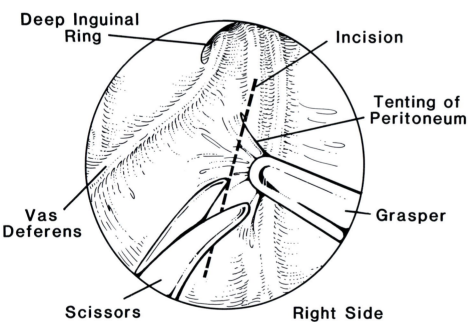

Figure 22-7
A. Needle-tip grasper placed immediately medial to spermatic vessels and tenting it so that the surgeon can made initial peritoneal incision. Note that on right side, initial incision is MEDIAL and parallel to spermatic vessels.

regard. The vas deferens passing over the obliterated umbilical artery (lateral umbilical ligament) and down the side wall of the pelvis is identified, as are the spermatic vessels passing into the internal inguinal ring. In bilateral cases, the dissection commences on the right-hand side. Initially, the assistant passes the needle-tip grasper through the right port and grasps

Figure 22-7
B. The spermatic vessels are exposed after incising the peritoneum.

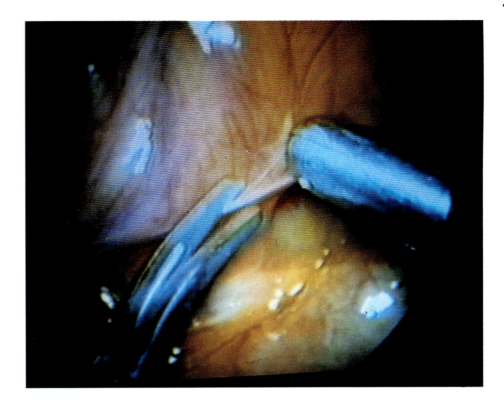

Figure 22-7
C. Making the T incision in the posterior peritoneum on the right over the spermatic vessels.

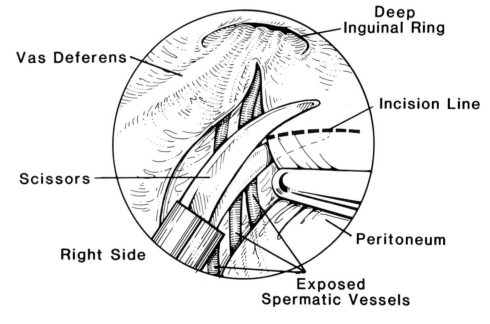

the peritoneum immediately MEDIAL to the vessels, about 3 cm above the deep ring. Using the curved coagulating scissors through the left port, the surgeon then makes a 5-cm peritoneal incision parallel and MEDIAL to the spermatic vessels (Fig. 22-7A and B). This is done by a combination of cutting and cautery. Care is taken not to get too close to the vas deferens distally. With the assistant continuing to retract the peritoneum, the surgeon uses the rotating knob on the scissors to position the curved end better and then frees up the peritoneum distally and laterally over the spermatic vessels. At this stage with the assistant retracting the lateral cut edge of peritoneum anteriorly, the surgeon makes a second cut in the posterior peritoneum to produce a T incision (Fig. 22-7C). The scissors are then rotated so that the curve faces posteriorly and the medial and lateral borders of the spermatic vessel package are roughly defined. It is not necessary to separate the vascular packet completely from the underlying psoas muscle or to isolate it completely.

Next, the assistant replaces the needle-tip grasper with the wave grasper and gently grasps the very lateral edge of the alveolar tissue of the vascular packet. Meanwhile, the surgeon replaces the scissors with the Endodissectors and

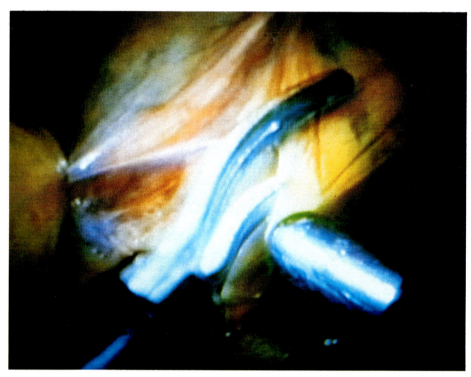

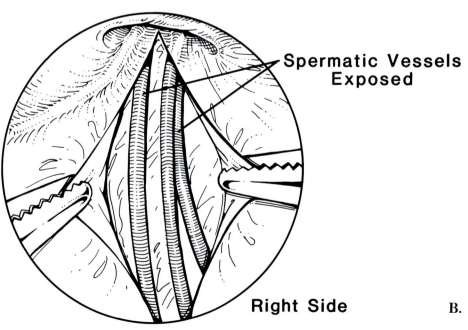

Figure 22-8
A and **B.** Defining spermatic veins. Assistant applies traction laterally with surgeon retracting medially, identifying veins on right side.

grasps the medial edge of the vascular package. By gentle traction and countertraction, the surgeon spreads the package apart (Fig. 22-8A and B). Usually at this stage, one or two large obvious veins are seen. The vein is then carefully dissected, with the surgeon staying close to the vein wall and making sure there is no attached artery, other vessels, or lymphatics. The surgeon then places the curved dissector beneath the vein and is helped by the assistant who depresses the tissue lateral to the vein posteriorly with the wave grasper.

Usually, the first large vein is easily identifiable and there is no concern that it could be

Figure 22-9
A and B. Isolated main right spermatic vein in ring grasper.

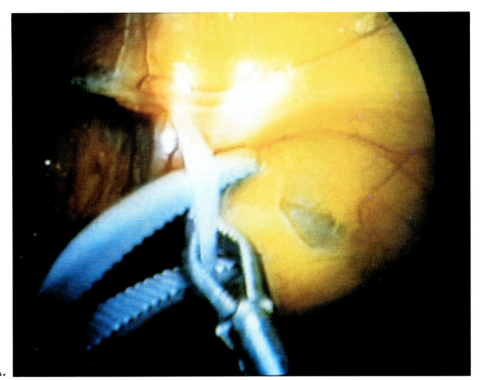

A.

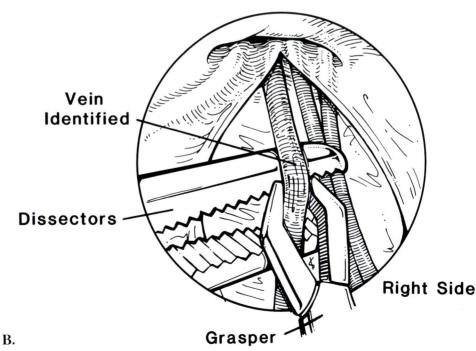

B.

the artery. At times, however, it may be very difficult to differentiate artery from vein. In these cases, one of two maneuvers or both may be performed. The irrigation suction device can be passed and a few mL of papaverine solution instilled on the vessel. With patience, if this is an artery, pulsations can be seen as the vascular spasm relaxes. More recently, we have begun using the laparoscopic Doppler, which clearly defines artery from vein.

Once the vein is isolated with the surgeon's curved dissector beneath it, the assistant removes the wave dissector and replaces it with the fallopian tube ring grasper (Fig. 22-9A and B). The surgeon removes the dissector, replaces the 5.5 reducer on the 11-mm port with a 10-mm reducer, and passes the clip applier (Fig. 22-10A and B). With its rotating head, four clips are easily applied, two proximally and two distally. The scissors are replaced and the vessel transected between clips.

The process is then repeated with the assistant giving countertraction using the wave and the surgeon retracting and dissecting using the curved dissector.

At times, it may be difficult to dissect or separate the vessels. It may then be very helpful to perform hydrodissection by placing the end of the suction irrigation device within the tissues of the vascular package and forcefully injecting a few mL of irrigant. This opens up the tissues and facilitates further dissection. Once all the veins have been transected, the site is reexamined. Bleeding may be tamponaded using the hemostatic device and the bleeding site then fulgurated. Irrigation may be necessary. At the end, the testicular artery, lymphatics, and adventitial tissue should be left intact with the veins transected. Usually at this level, there are one or two large veins with one or two much smaller veins.

Attention is then directed toward the left-hand side. Surprisingly, often in young people there are adhesions between the sigmoid colon and posterior abdominal wall. These can usually be mobilized easily. It is not necessary to perform a complete mobilization because once the vessels are seen and the posterior peritoneum is opened, the adhesions fall away from the operation site.

The only difference on the left-hand side is that with the surgeon remaining standing on the left, the initial peritoneal incision is made LATERAL to the spermatic vessels and the second T incision passes medially from the first incision through the peritoneum over the spermatic vessels (Fig. 22-11A and B).

Upon completion of the procedure, the surgeon reexamines the operation sites, any residual hemostasis is secured, if necessary, residual irrigation fluid is aspirated, and the CO_2 is expelled with removal of the ports and finger examination of the tracts in standard fashion.

Results

Since December 1990, 25 patients have undergone laparoscopic varicocelectomy—21 were bilateral and 4 were unilateral. All patients were being treated for infertility and had either clinical or subclinical varicoceles with a stress pattern on semen analysis. All procedures were performed as outpatients and no patient had to be admitted to the hospital. Average operating time for the bilateral cases was 2 h and 2 min with a range from 1 h and 8 min to 3 h and 38 min. For the unilateral cases it averaged 1 h and 27 min with a range from 55 min to 2 h and 10 min. There were no significant complications; 5 patients, as is not uncommon after any varicocelectomy, had some mild testicular discomfort. The testicular artery was inadvertently transected in 1 patient, and 1 patient developed a secondary hydrocele. This latter occurred early on in the series, at which stage we were ligating the total vascular package, except for the artery. More recently as described, the spermatic veins are selectively transected, leaving lymphatics and testicular artery intact. Pneumoscrotum occurred intraoperatively in several patients; however, by compressing this, especially prior to trocar removal, it settled rapidly without problem. Care should be taken not to compress too vigorously, for the CO_2 will absorb anyway and the compression may be painful postoperatively.

Postoperatively the varicoceles were either not evident at all on physical examination or were significantly reduced in size with no dis-

Chapter 22 Laparoscopic Varicocelectomy

Figure 22-10
A and **B.** Clip applier placing two proximal and two distal clips.

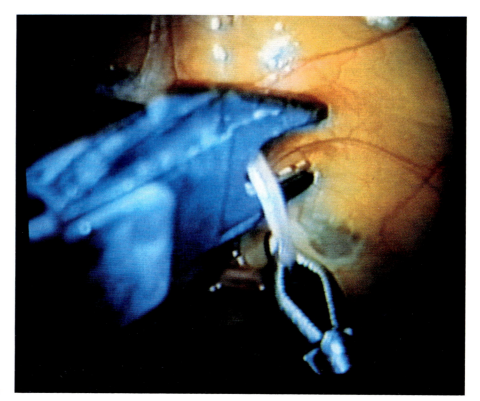

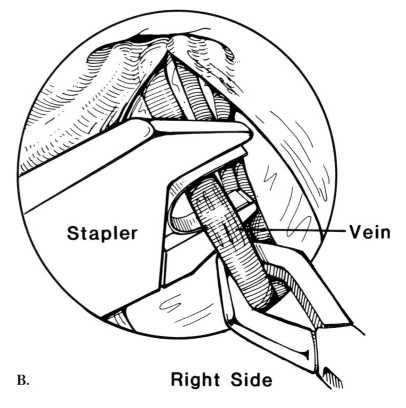

Part Two Laparoscopic Abdominal Surgery

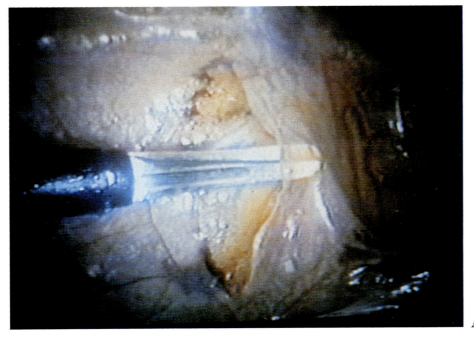

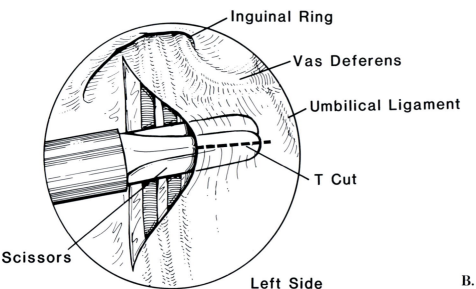

Figure 22-11 A and **B.** Left laparoscopic varicocelectomy. Initial peritonel incision LATERAL to spermatic veins. Second T incision passing medially.

tension Valsalva. All the patients returned to work within 24 to 72 h and required minimal oral analgesics. To date, it is too early to report improvements in semen analysis.

Comment

This is a fairly simple laparoscopic procedure. With care and patience, it would seem to be an excellent way of introducing surgeons into the field of laparoscopic surgery. The technique, as described, has been developed to be performed by a team of surgeon, assistant surgeon, and nurse. With further experience and particularly with the surgeon becoming more adept at using both hands, the procedure could further be modified to be performed by surgeon and nurse assistant only. This procedure, although excellent for a unilateral varicocele, is obviously extremely well-suited to bilateral procedures because no further incision or ports have to be established, and this has become the method of choice in our hands.

References

1. Macomber D, Sanders MM: The spermatozoa count. *N Engl J Med* 200:981, 1929.

2. Cockett ATK, Urry RL, Dougherty KA: The varicocele and semen characteristics. *J Urol* 121:435, 1979.

3. Dubin L, Amelar RD: Varicocelectomy: 986 cases in a twelve-year study. *Urology* 10:446, 1977.

4. Lome LG, Ross L: Varicocelectomy and infertility. *Urology* 9:416, 1977.

5. Narayan P, Amplatz K, Gonzalez R: Varicocele and male subfertility. *Fertil Steril* 36:92, 1981.

6. Amelar RD, Dubin L: *Infertility in the male,* in Kendall R, Karifin L (eds): *Practice of Surgery (Urology).* Philadelphia, Harper and Row, 1984, p. 43.

7. Verrstoppen GR, Steeno OP: Varicocele and the pathogenesis of associated subfertility: A review of the various theories. 1: Varicocelogenesis. *Andrologia* 9:133, 1977.

8. Zorgniotti A, MacLeod J: Studies in temperature, human semen quality, and varicocele. *Fertil Steril* 24:54, 1973.

9. Kaye KW: Modified high varicocelectomy: Outpatient microsurgical procedure. *Urology* 32:13, 1988.

10. Castaneda-Zuniga W, Gonzalez R, Amplatz K: Spermatic vein embolization in the treatment of infertility, in Kaye KW (ed): *Outpatient Urologic Surgery.* Philadelphia, Lea and Febiger, 1985.

11. Sanchez-de Bedajoz E, Diaz-Ramirez F, Marin-Martin J: Tratamiento endoscopico del varicocele. *Arch Esp Urol* 41:15, 1988.

12. Sanchez-de Bedajoz E, Diaz-Ramires F, Vara-Thorbeck C: *J Endourol* 4:371, 1990.

13. Hagood PG et al: Laparoscopic varicocelectomy: Preliminary report on a new technique. *J Urol* 147:73, 1992.

14. Donovan JF, Winfield HN: Laparoscopic varix ligation. *J Urol* 147:77, 1992.

15. Schultz L et al: Laser laparoscopic herniorrhaphy: A clinical trial. Preliminary results. *J Laparoendosc Surg* 1:41, 1990.

23

Laparoscopic Surgery of the Upper Urinary Tract and Retroperitoneum

John C. Hulbert

Urology, a broad specialty encompassing techniques of open surgery, endoscopic surgery, radiologic imaging modalities, and other surgical and nonsurgical disciplines, has recently begun to utilize laparoscopy.[1,2] Its initial use was to facilitate the identification of the impalpable, undescended testes in pediatric urology;[3] more recently it has been applied in adult urology for the removal of pelvic lymph nodes to aid the staging of prostatic and bladder cancer (see Chap. 21) and for the laparoscopic ligation of varicocele.[4] A small number of urologists have pioneered techniques for approaching the upper urinary tract and the retroperitoneum with a laparoscope.[5-7] It is the advantages of such techniques, i.e., the profound improvement in length of hospital stay and the reduction in morbidity and convalescence that have popularized these new techniques. This chapter will review the use of laparoscopy in treating pathology of the upper urinary tract and retroperitoneum.

Informed Consent and Preoperative Preparation

The appropriate informed consent before a new and innovative technique is important. Informed consent should include a discussion with the patient of the innovative nature of these techniques, of their invasive nature, of their benefits and potential complications. Also, the patient must be made aware that there is the possibility of converting to an open operation. The patient should certainly be advised that only a small number of people have performed these techniques and that the possibility of converting to an open operation is higher the fewer the procedures that the surgeon has performed. Preoperative preparation should include the standard history and physical examination and bowel preparation; a light bowel preparation is advisable and is certainly routine. Clearly, a patient who has a history of a coagulation disorder or is a very poor risk for anesthesia presents a contraindication to these techniques, and any patient who has had extensive prior abdominal surgery may be an unlikely candidate for these new techniques.

Positioning of Patient

The difficulties of accessing the upper urinary tract and the retroperitoneum are considerable; unlike the gallbladder or even the pelvic lymph nodes, which are relatively superficial and can be approached usually with a small amount of dissection, the retroperitoneum requires considerable dissection and retraction in order to access adequately. After the induction of anesthesia and the insertion of an endotracheal tube, a nasogastric tube is placed in the stomach and a catheter in the bladder. The patient needs to be positioned in such a way to allow the kidneys, the ureter, and the midline retroperitoneal structures to be accessed; this will require that the patient be positioned on a table that will not only tilt both in a head up and a head down direction but also from side to side; the patient will therefore also need to be secured to the table so that he or she does not roll off.

The patient is turned and placed in a 45° flank position with the flank supported by a sandbag, with the kidney rest slightly raised and the patient secured to the table with straps; the arms are usually placed across the patient on an arm board. The table is tilted to the side initially in such a way as to flatten the patient as much as possible (Fig. 23-1).

The Verres needle is inserted through the umbilicus and a pneumoperitoneum established. Alternatively, a Hasson cannula can be inserted by a direct dissection down to the peritoneum. Once the pneumoperitoneum is established a 10-mm trocar can be placed through the umbilicus and the laparoscope inserted so that a standard laparoscopy can be performed; the table is then flattened so the patient is once again in the 45° flank position, and the degree of tilt can be adjusted as necessary either from side to side or with head up and head down. In order to access the kidney, the ureter, or the midline retroperitoneal structures, the surgeon can utilize very similar supplemental port sites. One is placed immediately lateral to the umbilicus about 4 cm from the midline, and this is usually an 11- or 12-mm port. A second is placed approximately four-finger breadths below the costal margin just lateral to the midline, and this is usually a 5-mm port. A third is placed out in the anterior axillary line, and this is a 5-mm port but may be later changed to a 10-mm port midway through the case.

With the aid of scissors and graspers passed through these ports, the lateral peritoneal attachment of the descending colon, if on the left side, or the ascending colon, if on the right side, are divided from the flexure of the colon all the way down into the pelvis (Fig. 23-2). By further dissection both sharply with scissors and bluntly with a suction irrigator, the colon can then be reflected medially in the plane between Gerota's fascia and the mesentery of the colon (Fig. 23-3). In this way Gerota's fascia may be left intact around the kidney.

After the colon has been mobilized (Fig. 23-4A and B), the ureter should be identified as it crosses the common iliac artery; if the kidney is to be removed, it may be picked up with graspers and dissected in a superior direction; if it is not to be removed, it can be circumscribed

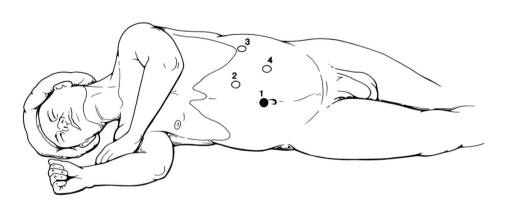

Figure 23-1
Positioning of the patient for the approach to the upper urinary tract or other retroperitoneal structures. The site at which ports may be placed for accessing these structures and regions are indicated. The patient is secured in the 45° flank position.

Figure 23-2
The beginning of the reflection of the descending colon (*a*) by incision of the lateral peritoneum just caudal to the spleen (*b*).

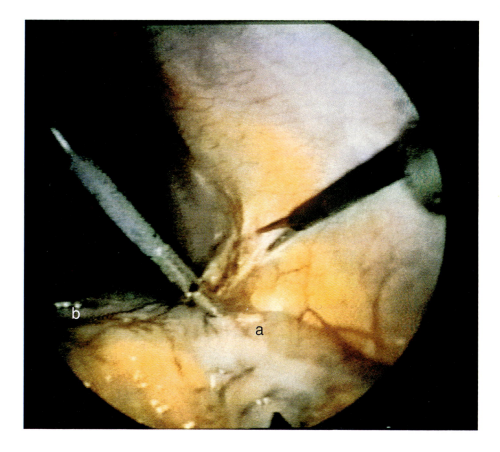

with a ring grasper so that it is not traumatized and gently lifted up and dissected free of its surrounding structures. If the kidney is to be removed, the renal pedicle can then be approached by following the ureter up to the renal hilum; further dissection of the colon medially will reveal the midline retroperitoneal structures, i.e., the aorta, the inferior vena cava, and the right and left renal veins. Once this approach has been appreciated and mastered, it can then be applied in a number of different clinical situations.

Figure 23-3
Positioning of the patient also showing mobilization of the descending colon for the approach to the left kidney or to the retroperitoneal midline structures.

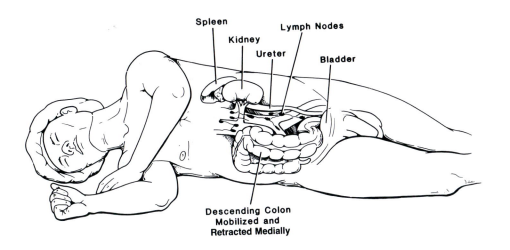

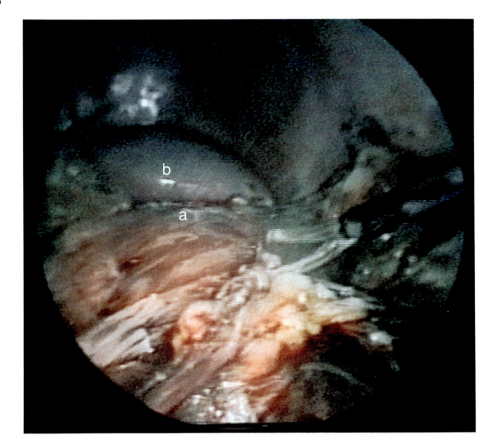

Figure 23-4
A. After reflection of the colon, the kidney (*a*) with Gerota's fascia surrounding can be seen. Note the spleen (*b*) in the superior aspect of this picture.

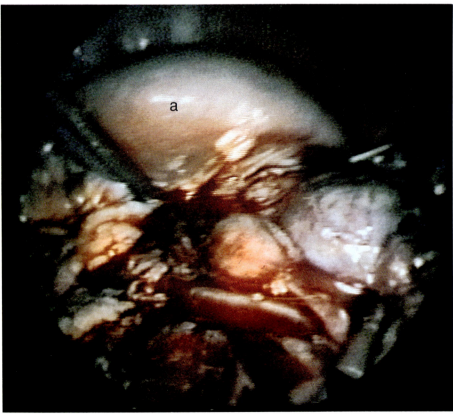

Figure 23-4
B. After opening Gerota's fascia, the surgeon can mobilize the kidney (*a*) more easily. This procedure is applicable to cases that do not involve malignant disease of the kidney.

Removal of the Kidney

With the previously described technique, it is possible to isolate the renal pedicle (Fig. 23-5); in order to control the renal pedicle adequately for removal of the kidney, it may be desirable to embolize the kidney with alcohol immediately prior to the procedure (it is important not to use a coil because this would make it very difficult to clip or staple the renal pedicle). Currently the favored techniques for controlling the renal pedicle are to use a large number of Endoclips or an endoscopic GIA stapler for the renal pedicle that will lay down three lines of staples on either side of the renal pedicle as well as dividing it (Fig. 23-6). Familiarity with the techniques of endoscopic suture ligation, however, will enable a surgeon to tie the renal pedicle as an alternative. Once the kidney's pedicle has been divided and the remaining attachments of the kidney within Gerota's fascia have been dissected, the kidney will lie free in the peritoneal cavity (Fig. 23-7). Note that this type of nephrectomy, simple nephrectomy, does not include removal of the adrenal gland.

The organ itself can then be placed in a small bag (a lap sack) that is inserted through one of the large ports. The end of the bag can then be drawn out through one of the ports so that a

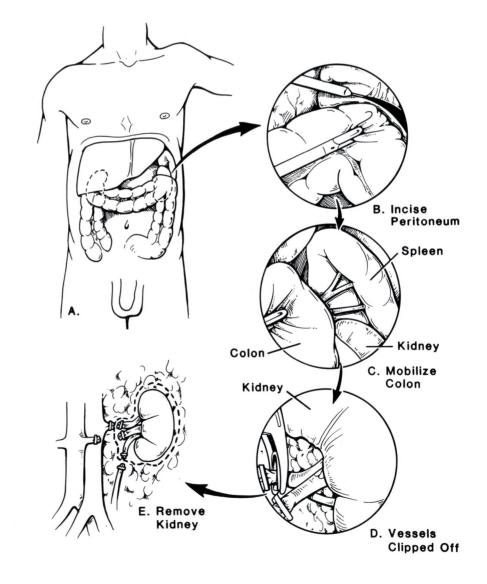

Figure 23-5
A. Initial and basic anatomical approach to the kidney. **B.** Incision of the lateral peritoneal attachments of the colon. **C.** Reflection of the colon to reveal the kidney surrounded by Gerota's fascia with the spleen sitting above it. **D.** Control of the pedicle using vascular clips or, alternatively, vascular staples. **E.** Kidney divided from ureter and pedicle and completely mobilized ready for removal.

Part Two Laparoscopic Abdominal Surgery

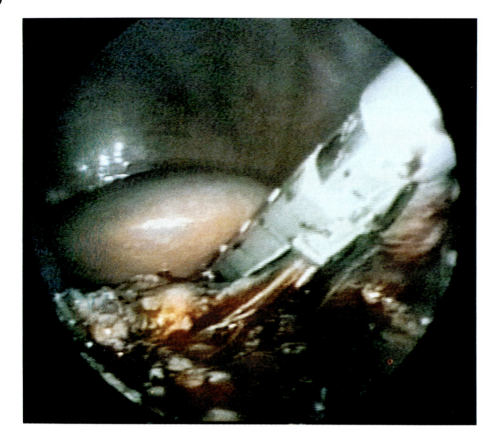

Figure 23-6
Control of the renal pedicle, using a vascular stapling device.

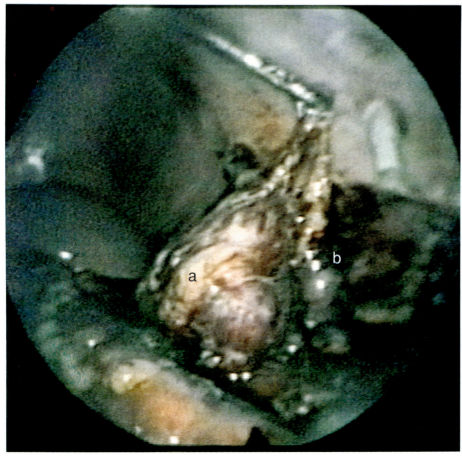

Figure 23-7
The completely mobilized kidney (*a*) free of the ureter and of its blood supply within the abdominal cavity. The divided renal pedicle (*b*) is seen.

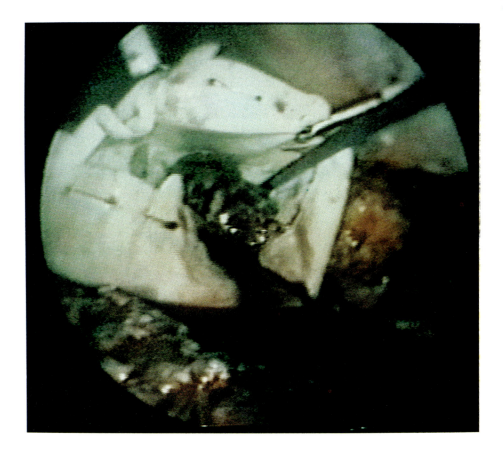

Figure 23-8
The detached organ is placed inside a lap sack prior to its morcellation and removal.

morcellating device that is either hand-controlled or mechanical can be passed through the neck of the sack and the organ fragmented. In other words, the kidney is fragmented and then removed from inside the bag through the laparoscopy port (Fig. 23-8).

The current indications for this technique are for benign disease of the kidney requiring nephrectomy; these are relatively few but important, and it is a very useful technique for removing small atrophic kidneys in patients with renal hypertension as a result of unilateral renal disease or in patients with small, scarred pyelonephritic kidneys with either flank pain or recurrent infection (provided that the contralateral kidney is normal). At the present time, this technique is not being advocated for patients with carcinoma of the kidney because the criteria that need to be met when we perform open surgery for renal cancer have yet to be completely and successfully fulfilled by laparoscopic surgery. The possibility of spillage of malignant cells exists, and we will need to demonstrate that the basic principles of open surgery for malignant disease of the kidney are being met. The limited experience of this technique has already indicated a reduction in the hospital stay to 2 or 3 days and a convalescence of 2 to 3 weeks. The standard hospital stay for open surgical nephrectomy is 1 to 2 weeks with a convalescence of up to 1 year. In time, as the technique is refined, selected patients with malignant diseases of the kidney may become candidates, and this technique may become more widely accepted as experience grows.

Renal Cystic Disease

Cystic disease of the kidney is common, but the vast majority of patients with renal cysts require no treatment if they have no symptoms. Some patients with cystic disease, however, particularly patients with polycystic kidney disease, develop pain. Our techniques up until now have included percutaneous aspiration with attempts at sclerosis of these cysts, techniques that are associated with a high recurrence rate, and for those who fail these techniques, open surgery, which is associated with a considerable morbidity and a protracted convalescence. Polycystic kidney patients with flank pain are a particular problem as it is hard to target the affected cyst accurately by percutaneous means; in addition, to perform bilateral cyst decortication (Rovsing's operation) through a long incision—a chevron incision—is a very major procedure with considerable morbidity and a long convalescence. Laparoscopy may be used to approach the cystic kidney and has been performed in selected patients successfully; the advantage of the percutaneous technique is that much of the cystic wall can be excised and therefore the possibility of recurrence is reduced (Fig. 23-9). Caution, however, must be used in assuring that patients do not have a malignancy in the wall of the cyst; this can be minimized by prior aspiration of the cyst percutaneously and analysis of the cyst fluid for malignant cells. Large anteriorly located renal

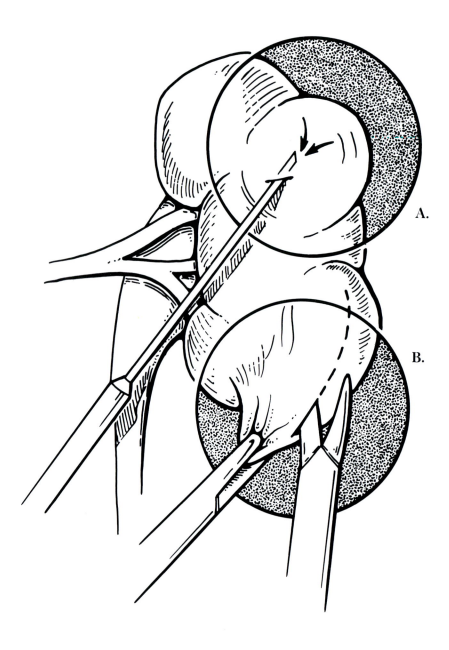

Figure 23-9
A. Drainage of renal cysts should precede decortication to identify possible malignancy by the surgeon's performing immediate cytology on the aspirate. **B.** Renal cystic decortication (i.e., the excising of that part of the cyst that extends outside the renal substance). Use of the argon beam coagulator here will help control minor bleeding from the edge of the cyst wall.

cysts are most suitable for this technique, although it has been possible to approach cysts on the posterior aspect of the kidney by turning the kidney medially to access them more easily. This technique may have a role in the management of selected patients with symptomatic cystic disease of the kidney, although prior attempts at percutaneous drainage should have been performed before considering laparoscopic decortication. Further experience and long-term results need to be evaluated before determining just how extensive the role of this technique will be in the future.

Ureterolysis

Retroperitoneal fibrosis is rare; however, current techniques for the surgical management of retroperitoneal fibrosis require the complete mobilization and lateralization of the ureter—i.e., ureterolysis. The same technique can and has been performed through a laparoscope. The process of cicatrization that encases the ureter may result in difficulty in mobilization. Indeed, some cases of supposed retroperitoneal fibrosis may have malignant encasement of the ureter. Laparoscopy can therefore perform a diagnostic purpose here in determining the etiology of the ureteral obstruction if a computed tomography (CT) scan or other imaging technique has failed to indicate the presence of malignancy. The lateralization of the ureter that is important in preventing recurrence may also be performed through a laparoscope aided by some recent developments in stapling techniques allowing stapling of tissues one to another. Although it is key to staple periureteral tissue to the lateral abdominal wall, one must ensure that the ureter itself is not being damaged (Fig. 23-10). Al-

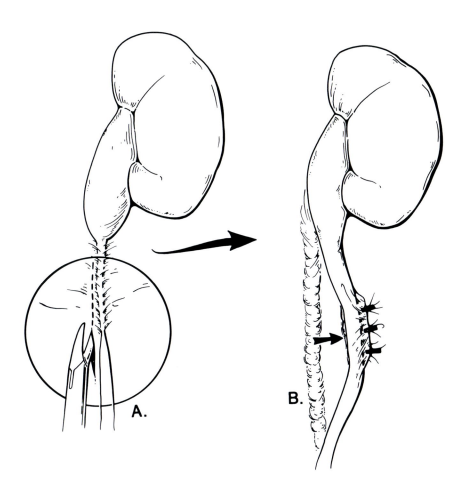

Figure 23-10
The technique of laparoscopic ureterolysis. **A.** The affected segment of the ureter is mobilized, using sharp and blunt dissection. **B.** The ureter is lateralized with Endohernia clips, with the staples placed between the periureteral tissue and the retroperitoneal wall.

though its use in the management of retroperitoneal fibrosis is currently controversial, selected patients may benefit from this approach. If the approach proves to be unsuccessful, one can then convert to an open operation immediately.

Other Applications in the Upper Urinary Tract

It is feasible to perform a number of other techniques on the upper urinary tract. Selected patients with large calculi in the upper ureter may not be entirely suitable for shock wave lithotripsy, percutaneous surgery, or ureteroscopic surgery. In reality, this condition is seen in a small number of patients and is usually limited to patients with very large stones in the upper or mid-ureter. These patients may ordinarily be considered for open ureterolithotomy even in these days, but they could have their stones removed laparoscopically because it is not difficult to open the ureter to remove a stone and then to approximate the edges gently with a ureteral stent in place to allow adequate healing. Reports exist of this procedure having been performed, although none has yet been published.

Reimplantation of the ureter is under consideration as is ureteroureterostomy. Both have been performed in the laboratory abated by techniques of laser welding with the KPT laser. Ureteroenteric anastomosis for urinary diversion and cutaneous ureterostomy may be performed, and anecdotal reports exist of these having been attempted.

Laparoscopy of Midline Retroperitoneal Structures

It has been demonstrated that the kidney in the upper urinary tract can be successfully approached with the laparoscope. With a small amount of further dissection, the midline retroperitoneal structures can be revealed, i.e., the aorta and the inferior vena cava. Retroperitoneal lymphadenectomy for testes cancer

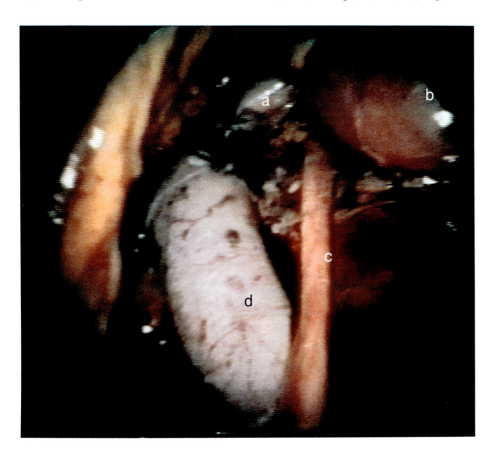

Figure 23-11
View of the retroperitoneal structures after laparoscopic retroperitoneal lymph node dissection. Note the anomalous left-sided vena cava (*a*), lower pole of the left kidney (*b*), with Gerota's fascia removed, and the exposed left ureter (*c*) and the left renal vein (*d*).

is a well-recognized treatment for both staging and for therapeutic purposes. This has now been performed through a laparoscope successfully, although it is not advocated as a replacement for the standard open technique of retroperitoneal lymphadenectomy. It should be regarded rather as an extended lymph node sampling in patients who would otherwise have undergone surveillance for clinical Stage A testes cancer. Surveillance has recently been reviewed more critically because of reports of bulky retroperitoneal recurrence years after the initiation of the surveillance protocol. Surveillance alone overlooks patients who have clinical Stage A disease and actually have pathological Stage B-I or early B-II disease, with macrometastases or small micrometastases in the retroperitoneal nodes.[8] Laparoscopy has been successfully performed to access and remove these targeted nodes for a left-sided testes tumor. This requires that the left aortic, interaorto-caval, and the preaortic nodes should be removed. For a right-sided testes tumor, the right caval, precaval, and the interaorto-caval nodes as far as the bifurcation of the aorta need to be removed (Fig. 23-11). It is to be hoped that this technique may gain acceptance for increasing the accuracy of staging of clinical Stage A testes cancer and therefore optimizing the treatment of this disease.

In conclusion, laparoscopic techniques are being extended to the upper urinary tract and the retroperitoneum and are changing our thinking with regard to the management of certain diseases. The indications for the use of these techniques in the upper urinary tract and retroperitoneum will increase and in the future will include such techniques as partial nephrectomy, closed renal biopsy, ureteroanastomoses, pyeloplasty, adrenalectomy, and even radical nephrectomy. These techniques will become feasible as instrumentation and skill with these techniques develop.

References

1. Gordon AG, Magos AL: The development of laparoscopic surgery. *Clin Obstet Gynecol* 3(3):429–446, 1989.

2. Spaw AT, Reddick EJ, Olsen DO: Laparoscopic laser cholecystectomy; analysis of 500 procedures. *Surg Lap Endosc* 1:2–7, 1991.

3. Weiss RM, Seashore JH: Laparoscopy in the management of the nonpalpable testis. *J Urol* 138(2):382–384, 1987.

4. Winfield HN et al: Urological laparoscopic surgery. *J Urol* 146:941–948, 1992.

5. Clayman RV et al: Laparoscopic nephrectomy: Initial case report. *J Urol* 146:278–282, 1991.

6. Hulbert JC, Shepard TG, Evans RM: Laparoscopic surgery for renal cystic disease. *J Urol* 147:433A, 1992.

7. Hulbert JC, Fraley EE: Laparoscopic retroperitoneal lymphadenectomy: New approach to pathological staging of clinical Stage I germ cell tumors of the testes. *J Endourol* 6, 1992, in press.

8. Pizzocaro G et al: Difficulties of a surveillant study omitting retroperitoneal lymphadenectomy in clinical Stage I nonseminomatous germ cell tumors of the testes. *J Urol* 138:1393–1396, 1987.

24

Laparoscopic Bowel Resection

Joseph J. Pietrafitta

Increased technical ability has allowed the general surgeon to begin to perform more complicated surgical procedures in a safe and an effective manner. Resection of the bowel, both small and large, challenges the surgeon from a technical as well as an intellectual standpoint. Development of endoscopic staplers has to a large extent made these operations feasible. Although bowel resections are currently being performed on a limited basis, the future expansion of these techniques appears to be inevitable.[1-7]

A number of steps are involved in resection of the bowel. They include (1) trocar placement, identification of resection margins, (3) suspension of the bowel, (4) transection and securing of the mesentery, (5) transection of the bowel, (6) removal of the specimen, and (7) reanastomosis. Each of these aspects has its own inherent difficulties, with a number of technical innovations that have made laparoscopic bowel resection possible.

I will review, in a step-by-step fashion, the major procedures, including small bowel resection, loop and end colostomy, mucous fistula formulation, colostomy closure, right colectomy, and finally sigmoid and low anterior resection.

Trocar Placement

A very important aspect of bowel work is trocar placement. In general, an initial view of the abdomen is obtained through a standard supraumbilical puncture with a 10-mm trocar for telescope insertion. After an initial survey is accomplished, additional trocars must be placed. Three or four additional trocars will usually be required. Placement of the second and third trocars is usually opposite the loop that is to be resected. Both should be 12 mm in size to allow introduction of the endoscopic linear stapler. For example, if the right colon is to be removed, these two trocars (numbers 2 and 3) should be placed on the left side of the abdomen, one in the left upper and the other in the left lower quadrant. The fourth trocar is then placed in the upper or lower quadrant on the right side when additional traction is necessary. If complete access to all quadrants of the abdomen is desired then a total of four trocars, all 12 mm

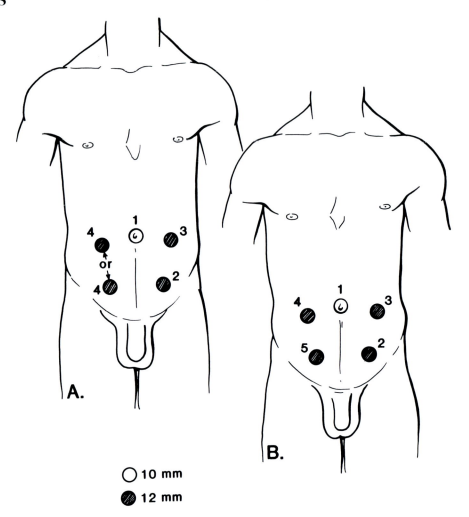

Figure 24-1
A. Trocar placement for right colectomy, indicating order of placement: no. 1—10 mm at the umbilicus, no. 2—12 mm in the left lower quadrant, no. 3—12 mm in the left upper quadrant, no. 4—usually necessary right upper or lower quadrant. **B.** An optional fifth trocar can be placed in the other right quadrant not occupied by no. 4.

in size, are placed, one in each quadrant (Fig. 24-1). Adequate trocar separation must be emphasized. Trocars that are not separated by at least 3 in. behave as a single trocar from the standpoint of bimanual manipulation.

Identification of Resection Margins

In open abdominal surgery, individual lesions can be easily palpated. In laparoscopic colon work, the surgeon must rely on preoperative assessment and to some degree intraoperative visual assessment of anatomical landmarks to assure inclusion of the specific lesion in the resected specimen.

The most useful preoperative aid, namely colonoscopy, may be extremely helpful. In the patient who is undergoing laparoscopic closure of a colostomy and mucous fistula, it is useful to minimize the length of the distal segment in order to allow easy introduction of the circular stapler transanally. With preoperative colonoscopy, a determination might be made that partial resection of the distal segment of bowel is warranted. Techniques of preoperative assessment may become even more important when more limited resections are performed for isolated lesions, especially of a benign nature. In the patient undergoing a laparoscopic colon resection, landmarks are often obscured by omentum, mesenteric fat, and previous abdominal surgery. A concerted effort is needed to identify specifically the segment of bowel to be removed. Once this has been done, the resection is begun.

Suspension of the Bowel

In order to mobilize the colon, it is necessary to place the mesentery on stretch. This is performed by attaching the colon to the abdominal wall just inside the proximal as well as the distal resection margins. This technique is most commonly used with resections of the transverse, descending, and sigmoid colons. This technique is less useful with resections of the right colon.

Prior to attempting to suspend the bowel, however, all lateral attachments of the colon (right and left) must first be taken. The colon is placed on traction toward the midline, using bowel (Babcock) graspers. The peritoneal attachments are cut. This freeing up of the colon will allow the bowel enough mobility to be suspended to the abdominal wall.

There are two techniques that are available. The first is performed using heavy suture (no. 0 or greater). The suture is passed through the abdominal wall into the peritoneal cavity. It is grasped intraperitoneally and passed under the bowel through the mesentery and back up through the abdominal wall. The suture is tightened, drawing the bowel up to the abdominal wall. It is tied or clamped externally, securing the bowel in position. Usually two sutures are placed, one at each resection margin (Fig. 24-2).

The alternate method is to use a device called a *bowel suspender*. This device is 10 mm in diameter, is made of a flexible plastic material, has a preformed circular shape, comes in two sizes (circle diameter of 30 or 40 mm, respectively), has interlocking ends, allows a single suture to be attached to one end for attachment to the abdominal wall, and can be introduced down a trocar with a pusher. The entire device is disposable (Fig. 24-3).

Once the bowel is suspended with tension placed on the mesentery, transection of the mesentery becomes much simpler. There is no longer any need to tie up trocars and instruments holding up the bowel in order to work on it (Fig. 24-4).

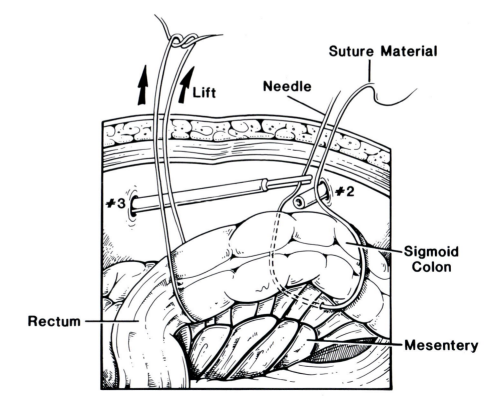

Figure 24-2
Sigmoid colon suspended up to the abdominal wall, using two heavy sutures placing tension on the mesentery.

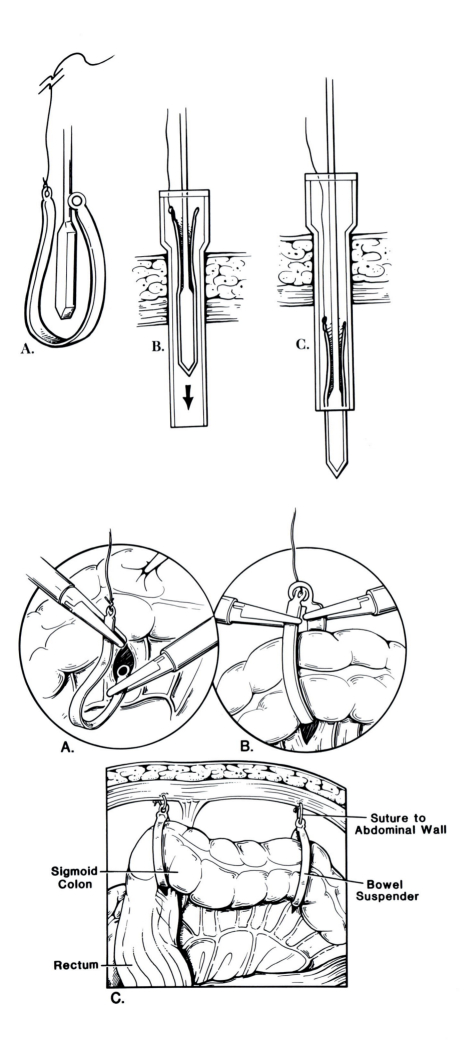

Figure 24-3
A. Bowel suspender with pusher. **B** and **C.** The suspender is inserted through the cannula and placed around the intestine under video control.

Figure 24-4
Laparoscopic view showing: **A** and **B.** the device being placed around the bowel, and **C.** the bowel suspended to the abdominal wall.

Transection and Securing of the Mesentery

Transection of the mesentery can be a formidable task in some instances. In a patient who is thin and who has never had any previous abdominal surgery or inflammatory conditions, mesenteric transection is not usually very difficult. Many patients, however, have had previous surgery or have had previous inflammatory conditions that make the dissection difficult. It is the prudent surgeon who knows when this portion of the operation is no longer feasible and must be performed open.

There are several methods of handling the mesentery in terms of controlling blood vessels and cutting tissue. The vessels can be skeletonized, secured, and cut or the mesentery can be treated with mass ligation. Bipolar cautery and laparoscopic linear vascular stapling devices (staple height of 3.0 mm) are the only two tools for mass ligation.

In order to skeletonize the blood vessels, additional maneuvers are usually necessary, namely *transillumination*. A second telescope is placed behind the colon to be transilluminated. This is for light delivery only and not for viewing. The light intensity of the viewing telescope is decreased. The blood vessels can then be viewed transilluminated from behind (Fig. 24-5).

Once the vessels are identified and isolated, control of smaller blood vessels can be accomplished with bipolar cautery, monopolar cautery, endoscopic clips, and vascular linear staplers. Larger blood vessels require suture ligation, the application of clips, or the use of the vascular linear staplers (Fig. 24-6).

Cutting of tissue can be performed with a variety of instruments and devices, including regular scissors, cautery scissors, cautery hook or similar instruments of different configurations (needle point, spatula, etc.), contact laser fibers, and linear staplers. The best coagulation is obtained with cautery devices, and the cleanest most precise cutting is obtained with laser devices.

Mention should be made at this time about extended mobilization beyond the suspended portion of the bowel by using extracorporeal traction. The colon can be exteriorized either

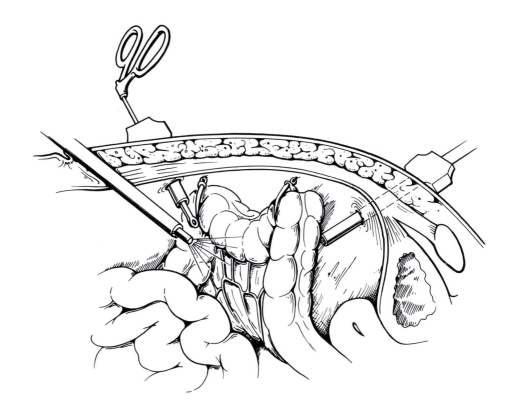

Figure 24-5
Transillumination of the sigmoid colon by placing the laparoscope in the 12-mm trocar in the left lower quadrant and using a fiber optic light source (another laparoscope) to illuminate through the umbilical port.

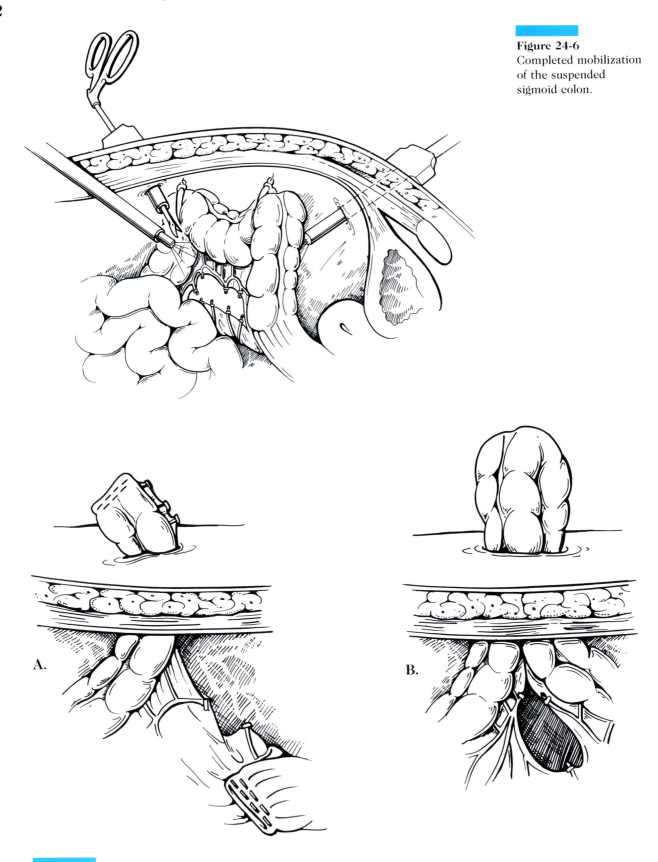

Figure 24-6
Completed mobilization of the suspended sigmoid colon.

Figure 24-7
A. External view of exteriorized bowel with transected end. **B.** External view of exteriorized bowel loop prior to transection.

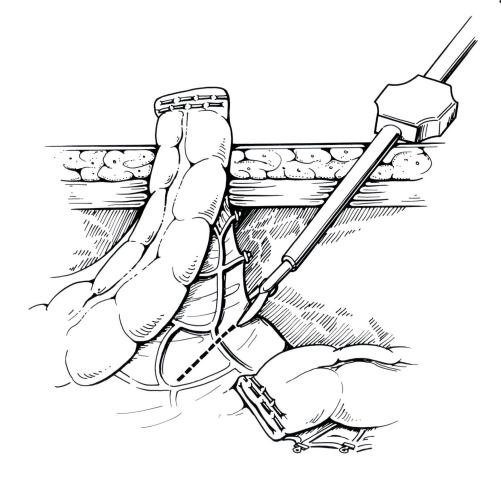

Figure 24-8
Internal view of mesentery after bowel has been exteriorized. Traction can be applied so that continued dissection can be done on the mesentery.

as a single transected end or an untransected loop through either an enlarged trocar hole or a separate incision. If the incision is fashioned so that the bowel occludes the opening when withdrawn, pneumoperitoneum can be maintained. In this way, external traction can be applied to the mesentery while maintaining pneumoperitoneum and laparoscopic view and continuing to work on the mesentery laparoscopically (Figs. 24-7 and 24-8).

Transection of the Bowel

Once the bowel is adequately mobilized and the mesentery is transected, the colon must be transected. This is accomplished with the linear cutter. This device is currently available in a 3-cm length applying either two triple staple rows or two double staple rows depending on which device is used. A 6-cm long stapler will ultimately become available. It should be mentioned that a 3-cm stapler will fit down a 12-mm trocar. The 6-cm staplers will require a 17- or 18-mm trocar (Fig. 24-9C). It may be preferable to use two sequential applications of a 3-cm stapler rather than using a 6-cm stapler in order to minimize the size of the trocar that is used. Given the choice of a 3.0-mm or a 3.5-mm staple height, you would invariably choose the 3.5-mm staple to transect the colon. There are tissue (colon) thickness measuring devices that are available to help in choosing the appropriate staple height. A 3.0-cm stapler will completely transect a segment of colon that is 2.0 cm in diameter. Most all segments of both large and small bowel for that matter are greater than 2.0 cm in diameter.

A decision regarding which resection margins should be transected intraabdominally will be determined based upon the type of resection that is being performed. In a low anterior resection, sigmoid resection, formal left colectomy, or subtotal colectomy, the colon should be transected only at the distal resection margin, forming a Hartmann's pouch (Fig. 24-9). In right-sided work, both resection margins are transected if an intracorporeal side-to-side anastomosis is to be fashioned (Fig. 24-10). If an extracorporeal anastomosis is to be performed, the entire loop is exteriorized, amputated externally, and an extracorporeal anastomosis is fashioned.

Removal of the Specimen

With left colon work, the proximal colon should be withdrawn through an enlarged trocar site or a separate incision in the left lower quadrant after intraabdominal transection of the bowel (Fig. 24-11). The colon is then amputated.

An alternate method is to exteriorize the en-

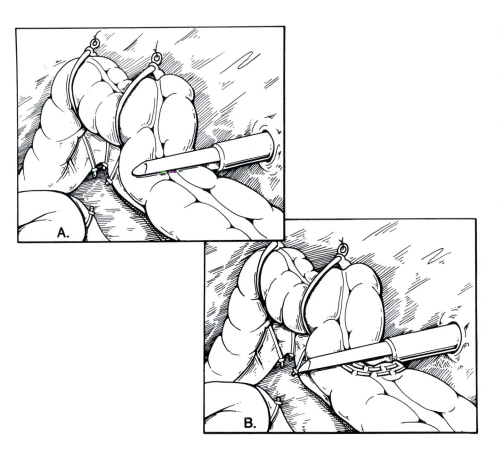

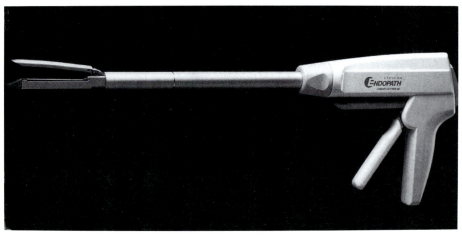

Figure 24-9
A. Because of the relatively small size of the stapling device, one firing may result in a partial transection of the suspended sigmoid colon segment. **B.** A complete transection of the suspended colon segment is accomplished by firing the stapler a second time, thus forming a Hartmann's pouch. **C.** The 6-cm stapler requires a 17- or 18-mm trocar for insertion.

Chapter 24 Laparoscopic Bowel Resection

Figure 24-9
D. 3-cm stapler applied to the colon, which is transected **(E)** after firing.

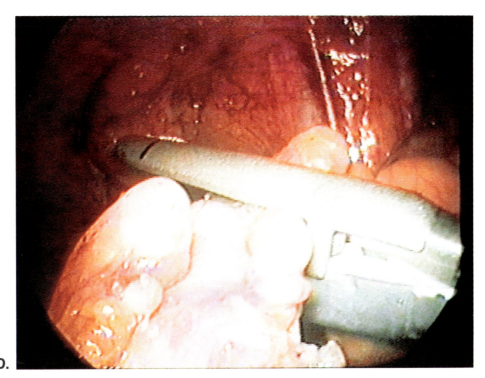

D.

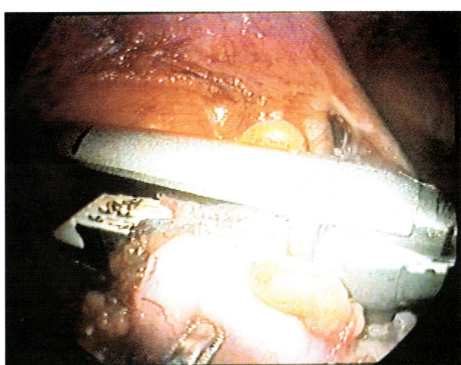

E.

tire segment, remove the specimen, and perform an extracorporeal anastomosis (Fig. 24-12). Because reanastomosis on the left side, using circular staplers, is relatively simple, the method of intracorporeal anastomosis using a circular stapler is preferred.

On the right side, there are similarly two methods of specimen removal and reanastomosis. In one method, the entire segment can be exteriorized, the specimen removed, and an extracorporeal anastomosis performed (Fig. 24-13). In the other method, both ends can be

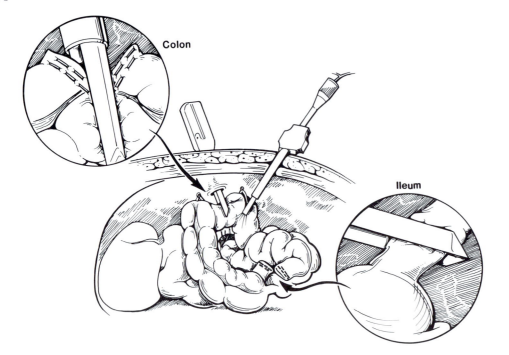

Figure 24-10
Complete transection of the distal ileum and the right transverse colon prior to removal of the right colon.

transected intraabdominally and the specimen removed with a totally intracorporeal anastomosis performed (Fig. 24-14).

A final point should be made concerning specimen removal. In order to resect more bowel, the pneumoperitoneum should be released prior to amputation of the specimen. In that way a longer segment can be removed (Fig. 24-15).

Reanastomosis

There are three major techniques of reanastomosis that are available to the surgeon who is performing laparoscopic colon resections. The type that is chosen depends on which portion of the colon is being removed and the ability of the surgeon to perform intracorporeal anastomoses.

1. Intracorporeal End-to-End Anastomoses

When any portion of the left colon is removed (low anterior resection, sigmoid resection, formal left colectomy, or subtotal colectomy) and an anastomosis is to be performed within 25 to 35 cm of the anus, an intracorporeal circular stapled anastomosis should be performed. As

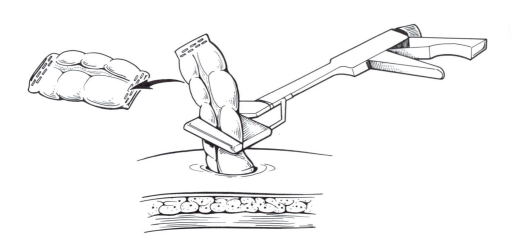

Figure 24-11
The proximal colon can be exteriorized during a sigmoid resection, allowing the second staple transection to be performed extracorporeally.

Chapter 24 Laparoscopic Bowel Resection

Figure 24-12
The sigmoid colon can be exteriorized as a loop and a totally extracorporeal resection and reanastomosis performed.

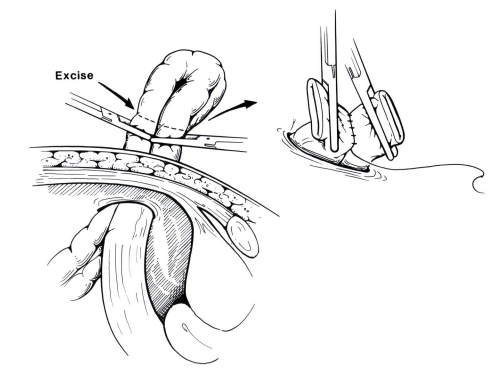

has been previously shown, the proximal end of the bowel has been brought out through the abdominal wall. The specimen has been amputated. At this point, a purse-string suture is placed in the proximal cut end of the bowel.

The anvil of the circular stapler is then introduced into the bowel and the purse-string suture is tied (Fig. 24-16A).

The entire colon is then replaced within the abdominal cavity. The enlarged trocar hole or

Figure 24-13
Exteriorized right colon and distal ileum are brought out through an enlarged trocar site on the right side of the abdomen. Then an extracorporeal resection and reanastomosis can be done.

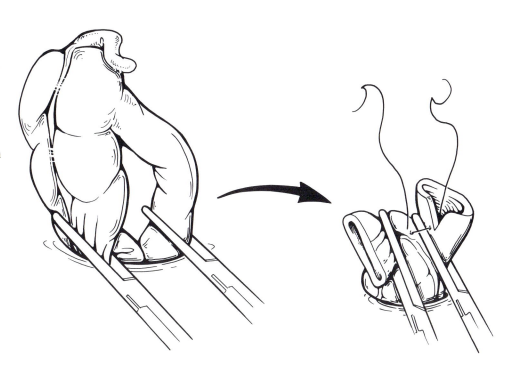

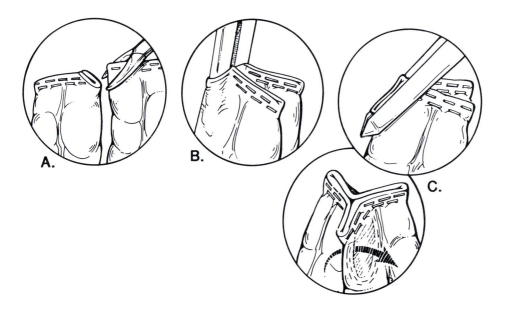

Figure 24-14
A totally intracorporeal anastomosis is done by (**A**) aligning the transected ends of colon side by side and cutting off a corner of the stapled edge. **B.** Then the stapling device can be inserted and fired. **C.** The colotomy is closed with another staple line creating a stapled anastomosis.

incision made to remove the specimen is then closed (Fig. 24-16B).

At this point, the circular stapler is introduced per anus. Its introduction can be viewed laparoscopically. When the stapler head can be seen approximating the closed end of the distal colon, the stapler is opened and the trocar is used to puncture through the bowel wall. The plastic trocar is removed using a special extraction device. The same device is used to insert the anvil into the stapler shaft (Fig. 24-17).

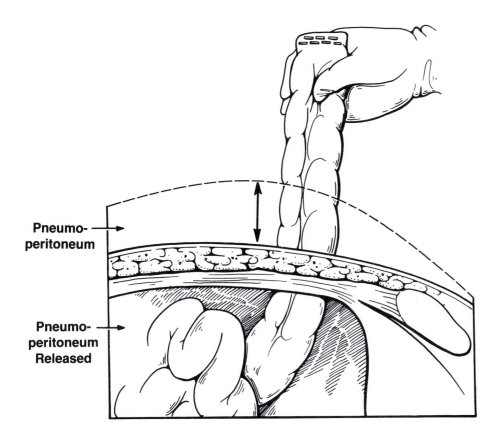

Figure 24-15
The length of exteriorized sigmoid is different with the pneumoperitoneum maintained compared with the pneumoperitoneum decompressed.

Figure 24-16
A. Proximal bowel with purse-string suture and anvil in place. **B.** Closed opening in abdominal wall with the colon back inside abdominal cavity with attached anvil.

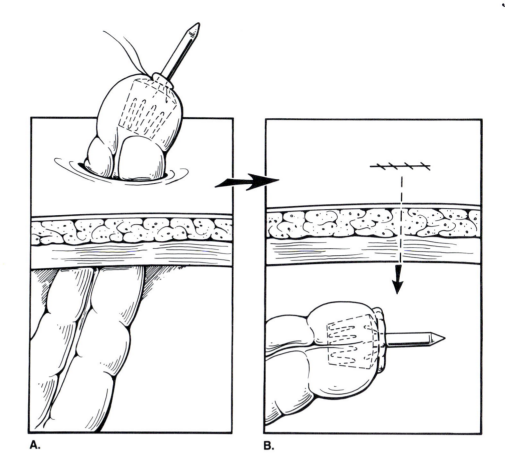

Figure 24-17
A. The stapler is passed through the anus and rectum. When the head is seen at the distal staple line, the trocar is passed through the bowel wall and removed, using a special extraction tool. **B.** The same tool used to introduce the anvil into the stapler shaft. **C.** The stapler is then closed and fired, completing the anastomosis. **D.** The stapler can then be removed.

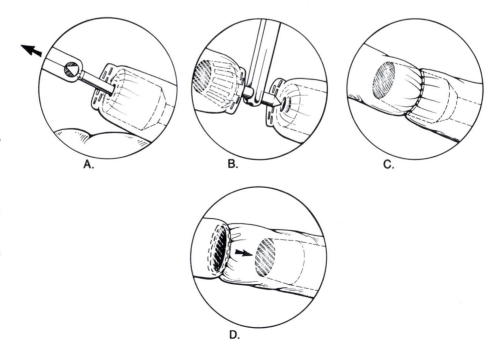

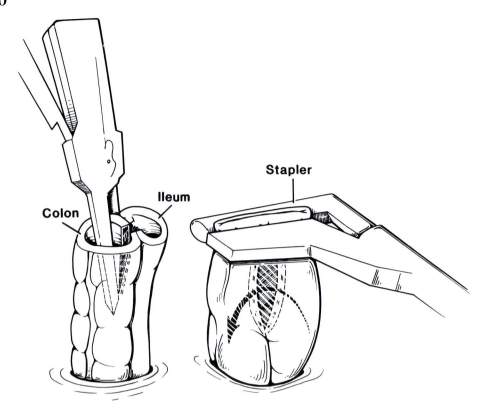

Figure 24-18
Extracorporeal anastomosis in a right colectomy.

2. Extracorporeal End-to-End or Side-to-Side Anastomosis

An alternate method is performance of an extracorporeal anastomosis with both ends exteriorized. The anastomosis can be hand sewn end to end or stapled side to side. This technique can occasionally be used in sigmoid resections but is not possible with low resections. This technique can also be used to perform an anastomosis on the right side in right colectomy (Fig. 24-18).

3. Intracorporeal Side-to-Side Stapled Anastomosis

In a right colectomy, a circular stapler cannot be used to perform an intracorporeal anastomosis. In this case, either an extracorporeal hand sewn end-to-end or stapled side-to-side anastomosis is performed; otherwise, a totally intracorporeal stapled anastomosis must be done. If a totally intracorporeal anastomosis is to be performed, it must be done in a side-to-side functional end-to-end fashion using linear staplers.

The right colon is removed by transecting both the ileum and right transverse colon intracorporeally. The specimen is then removed. The two ends are approximated side to side and held in approximation using a Babcock clamp on the antimesenteric border. The corners of both bowel limbs are cut off. The linear stapler is then used to fashion a side-to-side anastomosis. If the 3-cm linear cutter is used, two applications are necessary in order to prevent an anastomotic stricture.

Other Procedures

End Colostomy

Laparoscopic techniques can be used to fashion an end colostomy. Trocar placement in this procedure is identical to trocar placement for a sigmoid or a low anterior resection (Fig. 24-19).

The bowel is first suspended to the anterior abdominal wall. The mesentery is split toward its root. The bowel is transected distally leaving the distal segment as a Hartmann's pouch. The proximal colon is then grasped using a Babcock through the 10-mm trocar on the left side. The

Chapter 24 Laparoscopic Bowel Resection

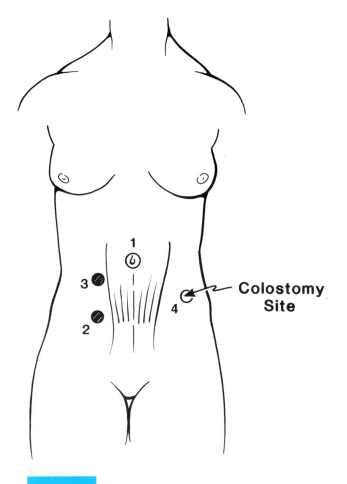

Figure 24-19
A total of 4 trocars are placed: no. 1—10 mm at the umbilicus, no. 2—12 mm in the right lower quadrant, no. 3—10 mm-trocar on the right, lateral to the rectus and just below the level of the umbilicus, no. 4—10-mm trocar at the site where the colostomy will be placed.

trocar is removed and the trocar site is enlarged, allowing the end of the colon to be withdrawn. The colostomy is matured to the skin (Fig. 24-20).

Securing the colon to the abdominal wall to prevent retraction can be performed through the skin incision with the colon being sutured to the fascia, using a single suture in each of the four quadrants of the colon (Fig. 24-21). If the mesenteric mobilization is short, closure to the abdominal wall intraperitoneally is probably not necessary. The mesentery can, however, be sutured to the lateral abdominal wall if desired.

Mucous Fistula

It is a simple matter to perform a mucous fistula rather than leave a Hartmann's pouch. In this case, the surgeon has to be sure that when he or she transects the colon, enough distal length is left to bring the distal segment to the anterior abdominal wall. An additional trocar is placed at the site of the mucous fistula. This trocar should be 10 mm in size. The distal colon is grasped with a Babcock clamp placed through the trocar. The bowel is brought up to the abdominal wall. The trocar is removed. The trocar site is enlarged. The distal colon is withdrawn and matured to the skin (Fig. 24-22).

Various locations can be chosen for mucous fistula placement. In general, they may be placed either in the left lower quadrant of the abdominal wall or in the midline. The left lower quadrant location is preferable. This location makes subsequent mobilization of the mucous fistula for closure somewhat easier because the distal colon does not have to be dissected off the bladder.

Colostomy Closure

Colostomy closure can readily be performed laparoscopically. It is actually simpler to close a colostomy and mucous fistula rather than to close a colostomy and Hartmann's pouch. Because the distal colon in a mucous fistula is already suspended, mobilization becomes a simple matter. In this procedure, three trocars are placed, one at the umbilicus for the telescope and two on the right side for the introduction of instruments (Fig. 24-23).

The first step is to mobilize the distal segment and transect it low in the pelvis. The mucous fistula with its attached colon is left hanging from the abdominal wall (Fig. 24-24). The mesentery of the proximal colon is mobilized. The proximal colon is also mobilized from the peritoneum and fascia intraperitoneally. Once this is completed, the colostomy is excised at the skin level and the colon is brought out as in a primary laparoscopic resection (Fig. 24-25). The purse-string suture is placed, the anvil inserted, and the colon replaced back within the peritoneal cavity.

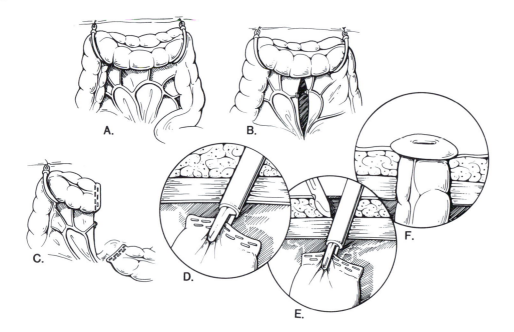

Figure 24-20
A. Bowel suspended to the abdominal wall. **B.** Mesentery split toward its root. **C.** Distal bowel transected leaving a Hartmann's pouch distally. **D.** Proximal colon grasped and brought to the abdominal wall. **E.** Cut down at trocar site to exteriorize the proximal colon. **F.** Colostomy matured. **G.** Transected sigmoid colon retracted to the anterior abdominal wall.

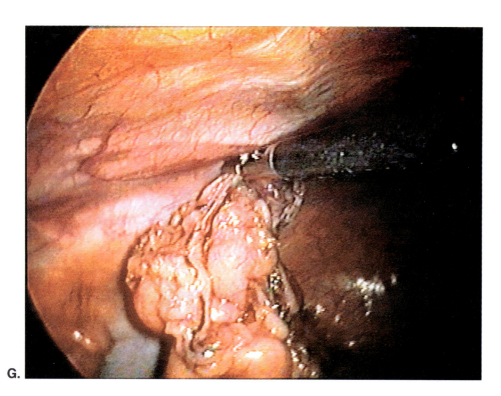

G.

Figure 24-21
Suture placement to secure the colon to the anterior abdominal wall to prevent retraction.

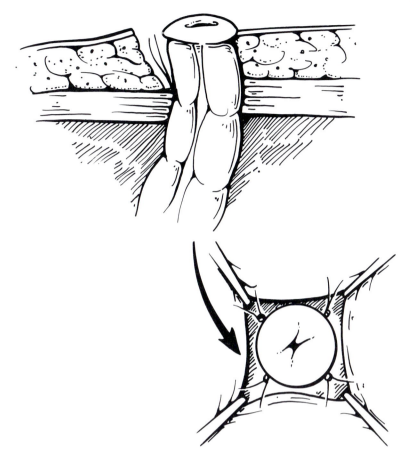

Figure 24-22
A. Additional trocar introduced at the proposed mucous fistula site. **B.** Distal colon grasped and brought up to the abdominal wall. Cut down at trocar site to exteriorize the proximal colon. **C.** Mucous fistula matured.

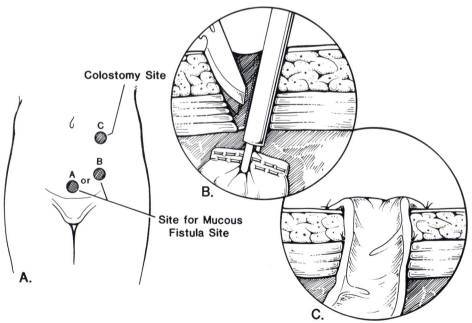

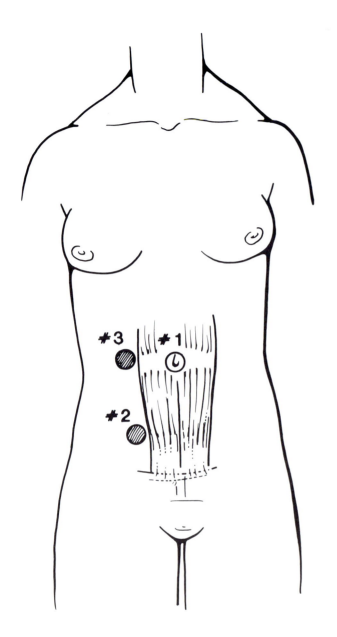

Figure 24-23
Three trocars are placed. A 10-mm trocar at the umbilicus for the telescope. A 12-mm trocar in the right lower quadrant for introduction of the linear stapler. A 10-mm trocar on the right side of the abdomen at the level of the umbilicus lateral to the rectus muscle.

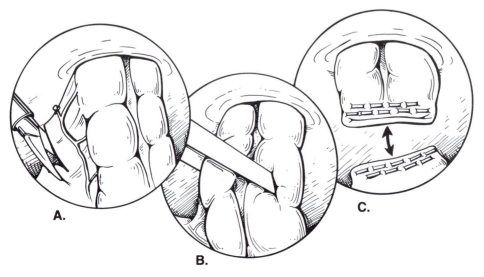

Figure 24-24
A. Mucous fistula is mobilized and **(B)** transected, being converted to a Hartmann's pouch **(C)**.

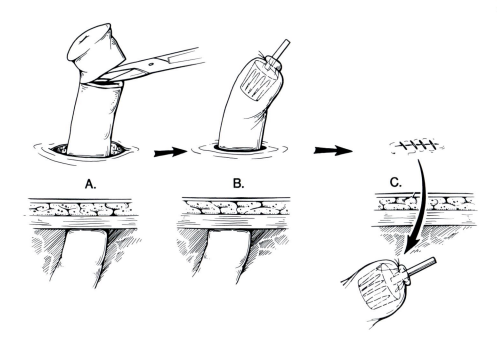

Figure 24-25
A. The colostomy is excised at the skin level and removed by transecting the proximal colon. **B.** A purse-string and anvil are placed. **C.** The proximal colon is placed back within the peritoneal cavity for eventual anastomosis with the end-to-end stapler. Once the proximal colon is placed back within the peritoneal cavity, the anastomosis is performed using the end-to-end stapler.

References

1. Cooperman AM et al: Laparoscopic colon resection: A case report. *J Laparoendosc Surg* 1(4):221–224, 1991.

2. Lange V et al: Laparoscopic creation of a loop colostomy. *J Laparoendosc Surg* 1(5):307–312, 1991.

3. Redwine DB, Sharpe DR: Laparoscopic segmental resection of the sigmoid colon for endometriosis. *J Laparoendosc Surg* 1(4):217–220, 1991.

4. Reich H, McGlynn F, Budin R: Laparoscopic repair of full-thickness bowel injury. *J Laparoendosc Surg* 1(2):119–122, 1991.

5. Saclarides TJ et al: Laparoscopic removal of a large colonic lipoma. Report of a case. *Dis Colon Rectum* 34(11):1027–1029, 1991.

6. Schlinkert RT. Laparoscopic-assisted right hemicolectomy. *Dis Colon Rectum* 34(11):1030–1031, 1991.

7. Ballantyne G et al: Laparoscopic colectomies. *Laparosc Focus* 1(3):1–12, 1992.

25

Laparoscopic Surgery in Children and Infants

Hock L. Tan

The possibility of performing surgery with minimal iatrogenic trauma has the same validity for children as it has for adult general surgery. However, until recently, most reports of successful pediatric laparoscopic surgery have been for older children, and laparoscopy for smaller infants and babies has been confined to diagnostic procedures. The reason for the delay is the lack of suitable instrumentation.

The author has been developing laparoscopic instrumentation for use in infants and older babies, which has extended the usefulness of laparoscopy in these patients.

Laparoscopic Equipment

The standard laparoscopic equipment for adult procedures is unsuitable for use in young children. The length of the adult telescope and the diameter of its cannula make it unwieldy for babies. For example, it makes no sense to make several 10-mm incisions for large cannulas when many pediatric procedures are performed through incisions that are often not much more than 2 to 3 cm long. The bevels of the larger trocars are also too long, and the tip reaches the posterior abdominal wall in small babies when the trocars are established and severely restricts access to any anterior structures. We have designed a telescope and a complete set of instruments for use through 4-mm cannulas that overcome these technical problems.

Current staplers and clip applicators, however, still require a large instrument port, and this limits our present capacity to use these devices in the very young. We are developing new staplers and clip applicators suitable for smaller ports, and this will eventually enhance our ability. In older children it is possible to introduce clips and staplers through the umbilical port with minimal iatrogenic and cosmetic trauma. In general, the adult laparoscopic set can be used effectively in older children (from around the age of 8 onward). However, when dealing with children younger than 8 years old, there are several essential differences in the laparoscopic technique that are related to differences in anatomy or size. These will be discussed.

Anatomic Considerations

The umbilicus is very busy in a neonate (Fig. 25-1). The two umbilical arteries (lateral umbilical ligaments) and the umbilical vein (ligamentum teres) are not obliterated for several weeks. Care must be taken to avoid opening these structures because there is a potential risk of gas embolism if a Verres needle is inadvertently inserted into these structures and CO_2 insufflated unknowingly.

The falciform ligament and the umbilical vein remnant (ligamentum teres) are very prominent structures in infants and children (Fig. 25-2). A Verres needle introduced into the upper abdomen will easily dissect between the two loosely attached folds of peritoneum forming the falciform ligament, and we can easily be misled into thinking that the Verres needle is in the abdomen and insufflate the falciform ligament instead.

The neonatal bladder is an intraabdominal organ, and the urachal remnant is attached to the umbilicus. It would be easy to puncture the urachus and perforate the bladder with a Verres needle. It is therefore mandatory to ensure that the bladder is completely empty immediately prior to surgery.

Unlike in the adult, in children the different layers of the abdomen are very loosely attached

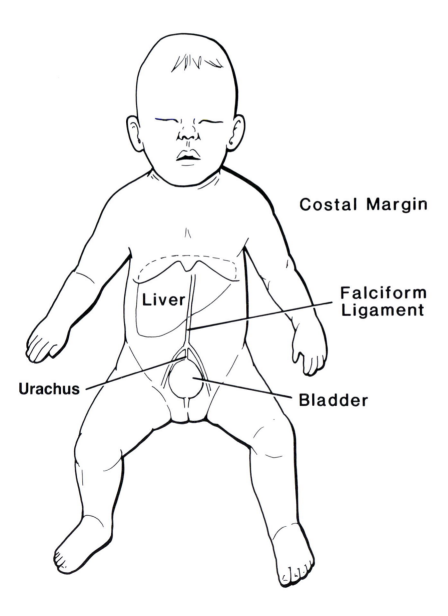

Figure 25-1
Anatomic relationships of the bladder, urachus, umbilical arteries, ligamentum teres, falciform ligament, and liver to the umbilicus in the neonate.

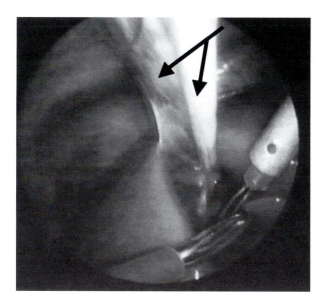

Figure 25-2
The prominent umbilical vein (ligamentum teres) and falciform ligament in the neonate (arrow).

to each other, and lifting the abdomen to establish a trocar simply allows the abdominal muscle to separate from the skin and subcutaneous tissues, making trocar placements more difficult. The peritoneum is also the toughest layer of the abdomen to puncture in an infant and is very loosely attached to the anterior abdominal wall, particularly in the region between the symphysis pubis and the umbilicus. The peritoneum has an inherent tendency to tent away from an advancing needle or trocar. Because of these properties, it can be very difficult to feel if a Verres needle has actually punctured the peritoneum in a child inasmuch as the peritoneum will dissect away from the abdominal wall with the advancing Verres needle (Fig. 25-3). The saline drop test is equally unreliable because of this laxity of peritoneal attachment.

Similarly, monitoring the insufflation pressure is not helpful in determining if gas is being insufflated into the correct cavity. The author has seen CO_2 dissecting all the way around into the posterior parietal peritoneum from an anterior puncture in his initial experience with laparoscopic surgery. The neonatal and infant liver overhangs the costal margin, and its lower margin reaches the umbilicus in neonates. There is a risk of injury to the liver if blind punctures are made in the upper abdomen in very young infants. Even under direct internal endoscopic control, the tip of the cannulas can be perilously close to the anterior surface of the liver (Fig. 25-4). The inferior vena cava and

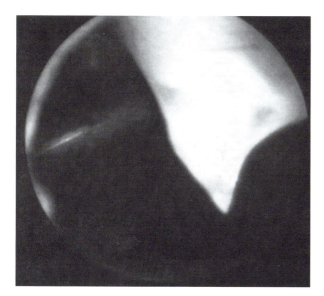

Figure 25-3
The peritoneum is a very sturdy tissue in the neonate, and it will tent away from the muscle and fascia when needles or trocars are inserted.

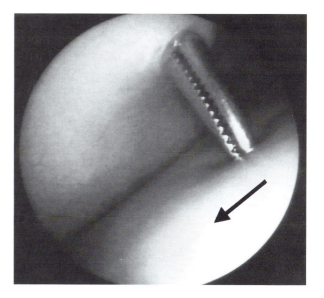

Figure 25-4
The anterior surface of the liver (arrow) is perilously close to the abdominal wall despite a pneumoperitoneum of 10-mmHg pressure.

aorta are barely 1 cm away from the anterior abdominal wall.

Because of the differences highlighted, we do not believe using a Verres needle to create the pneumoperitoneum is safe in small babies and infants.

Establishing the Pneumoperitoneum

To establish the pneumoperitoneum, we recommend the Hasson method. We make a small incision in the circular periumbilical skin crease. In small babies, a supraumbilical approach is easier because there is only one structure (the umbilical vein) to deal with, as opposed to the two umbilical arteries and urachus if one chooses an infraumbilical approach. This difference is much less apparent in older children.

The linea alba is identified, and a small transverse incision is made through the linea alba. We then identify either the umbilical vein (when using a supraumbilical approach) or the urachal remnant and lateral umbilical ligament (when using the infraumbilical approach) and pick up these structures with a hemostat. The peritoneum can then be easily opened on either side of one of these structures with a pair of iris scissors, and the instrument port introduced directly into the abdominal cavity, and insufflation begun. Use maximum pressures of 7 to 10 mmHg in neonates, 12 mmHg in older children.

A purse-string suture or vertical inverting mattress sutures should be placed on either side of the cannula to minimize gas leak and to help stabilize the 4-mm port. Miniature Hasson type cannulas are currently being developed that will reduce gas leaks.

Cannula Placement

Even at maximum insufflation, there is very little room in a baby to perform laparoscopic procedures such as intracorporeal knot tying, and the proximity of adjoining viscera makes the use of diathermy more hazardous. However, the baby's small size also means that the surgeon has very easy visual access to every abdominal viscera apart from the retroperitoneal structures.

Because the surgeon has to work in a small area, the instrument cannulas often have to be very close to each other, and we have to be careful that instrument clashes do not occur. In choosing trocar sites, it is better to establish the instrument ports further away from the operative field and not directly above the operative field because this allows more room for manipulation of the instruments. Having the instrument port too close to the area you wish to operate on will severely impede your ability to retract or manipulate viscera when required. In choosing trocar placement, always place the instrument trocars ahead of the endoscope to facilitate identification of "lost" instruments.

We have found the easiest and least traumatic way of establishing the instrument ports is to make a full thickness incision through the entire thickness of the anterior abdominal wall, including the peritoneum, with a no. 11 scalpel blade. The middle finger should rest on the blade as a guard to prevent the blade from penetrating too far into the abdominal wall and damaging the underlying viscera. The tip of the no. 11 scalpel blade should always be in full endoscopic view because the tip of the blade is close to the underlying abdominal viscera and can do damage by an injudicious stab. Once the peritoneum has been punctured by the no. 11 scalpel blade, the incision in the peritoneum should be enlarged to about 5-mm length to facilitate the next step.

A pair of straight mosquito hemostat forceps is inserted through the incision, the tip advanced through the peritoneal incision, and a tract created by spreading the hemostats. The instrument cannulas can then be inserted through the tract effortlessly, although it is still necessary to use a "screwing" action to advance the cannula through the layers of the anterior abdominal wall. The peritoneum in the suprapubic area is particularly difficult to penetrate in infants because of the loose attachment of the peritoneum to the undersurface of the abdominal wall (inasmuch as it has to accommodate the infantile bladder as it distends).

Most pediatric procedures can be performed using 4-mm or 5.5-mm cannulas, but it is sometimes necessary to use a larger (10-mm) port to extract viscera, such as appendixes or gallbladders, or if stapling is required. The best position for the placement of large trocars is through the linea alba via a small periumbilical incision. It is easy to extend this incision circumferentially to accommodate the 10-mm cannula with minimal cosmetic or iatrogenic trauma.

Pyloromyotomy (Ramstedt's Operation)

Pyloromyotomy is an operation that lends itself to laparoscopic surgery and requires only one 4-mm telescopic port and two 4-mm instrument ports. The patient is positioned at the foot of the operating table. The 4-mm telescope trocar is established in the manner already described earlier in this chapter. The surgeon initially stands on the patient's right while this first trocar is being established. The surgeon should then reposition himself or herself to sit at the end of the table, facing the patient's feet. The assistant surgeon should stand on the surgeon's right, and the scrub nurse on the surgeon's left. The anesthesiologist is at the front of the table on the surgeon's right. The operating table is tilted head up to allow the abdominal viscera to fall away from the operative field. The video monitor is positioned at the front of the operating table. This arrangement allows everyone involved in the operation to have an excellent view of the entire endoscopic proceeding on the one monitor (Fig. 25-5).

An insufflation pressure of 7 mmHg is adequate, although it can be increased to 10 mmHg if necessary. Two instrument ports are established in each upper quadrant of the abdomen under direct video-endoscopic control. Once again, special care has to be taken when inserting these ports because the liver is only about 1 cm away from the anterior abdominal wall. The ports should be placed midway be-

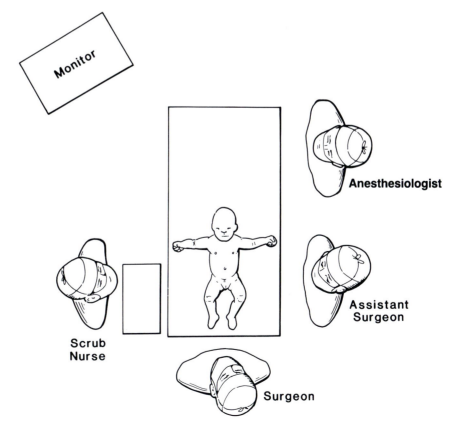

Figure 25-5
The operating room setup for performing laparoscopic pyloromyotomy in the infant.

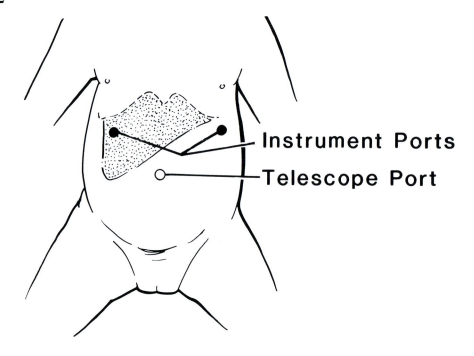

Figure 25-6
The placement of instrument and telescope ports for pyloromyotomy in the infant.

tween the umbilicus and the costal margin, lateral to the nipple line (Fig. 25-6).

The gastric antrum and pylorus are identified by retracting the free edge of the liver upward and away from the stomach with the right upper quadrant grasper. The transverse colon can occasionally obscure the view, but it can be swept inferiorly away from the operation field.

While the liver is retracted with the left upper quadrant port, the duodenum just distal to the vein of Mayo should be firmly grasped by the atraumatic graspers in the right upper quadrant port. Do not attempt to hold the pyloric tumor because the forceps will slip off the firm tumor, and it will be difficult if not impossible to incise the tumor owing to instrument clash.

The duodenum and pylorus are retracted inferiorly away from the liver edge. If the liver edge is still obscuring the vision, it can be swept upward and tucked under the pylorus momentarily with the left upper quadrant grabber. The extent of the tumor can be identified quite readily by "palpating" it with the left-sided atraumatic graspers. The normal antrum is easily indented, and there is an abrupt junction identifiable between it and the firm pyloric tumor.

The endotome is introduced through the left upper quadrant port; the blade advanced out of its sheath in its entirety. The seromyotomy should be started at the duodenal end. The incision is extended toward the antrum about 3 to 4 mm beyond the extent of the tumor (Fig. 25-7). Countertraction should be applied with the atraumatic graspers holding on to the duodenum. It is not possible to cut in the opposite

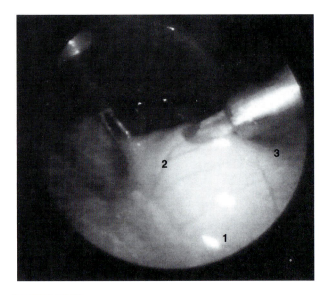

Figure 25-7
The initial incision in the pyloric tumor is made with an endotome. Note the vein of Mayo.
1 = Duodenum. 2 = Vein of Mayo. 3 = Antrum.

direction because the countertraction is important. The initial incision has to be deep or else it will be difficult to introduce the spreader.

The endotome is exchanged for the pyloric spreader, which is thrust through the incision until slight resistance from the intact mucosa is felt. It is important to ensure that the spreader is through the entire thickness of the tumor because the tumor will be otherwise difficult to split, and the edges will tear. The tumor is spread widely, beginning at the duodenal end. It is necessary to move the forceps further up the antral end to spread the most proximal fibers of the pyloric tumor. The mucosa should be inspected when the jaws of the spreader are wide apart. This is the best time to inspect it closely before the edges of the tumor bleed (Fig. 25-8). Sufficient air should be insufflated by the anesthesiologist via a nasogastric tube on completion of the pyloromyotomy to exclude an inadvertent perforation. The mucosa will be seen to bulge.

The abdomen is desufflated and the mini-incisions closed by repairing the linea alba with one or two absorbable sutures and subcuticular skin closure. The patient can be fed the same day and discharged once feeding is established, usually on the following day. In our preliminary series, we have the impression that children do not vomit much following laparoscopic pyloromyotomy. This may be due to the minimal handling of the stomach. The entire operation is performed in situ as opposed to the open operation where considerable traction on the stomach is required to deliver the tumor.

Laparoscopy for Undescended Testes

Undescended testes is one of the most common conditions requiring surgical correction in the pediatric age group. However, in most children the testis is easily palpable in the superficial inguinal pouch and there is no indication for laparoscopy in these patients because orchidopexy is straightforward in these cases.

Laparoscopy is therefore indicated only in the patient with impalpable testis. The evidence is mounting that orchidopexy should be performed earlier to preserve spermatogenesis. We therefore recommend diagnostic laparoscopy at 12 months of age if the testes are still impalpable at that age. It is unrealistic to expect any further testicular descent beyond this age even in the extremely premature infant.

Diagnostic laparoscopy will establish if the testis is intraabdominal and offers the surgeon the option of ligating the testicular vessels to allow for collateral circulation to develop via the vessels to the vas. This enables the testis to be brought down on the vessel to the vas at some future date. The testicular vessels can be easily ligated without interfering with the operative field at subsequent open surgery.

Consent should be obtained for orchidectomy, open exploration, or ligation of the testicular vessels. The surgeon should stand on the contralateral side. We have found a 4-mm telescope more than adequate for diagnostic and therapeutic purposes. The video monitor should be positioned directly in front of the surgeon. The patient is tilted head down and rolled toward the surgeon to allow the viscera

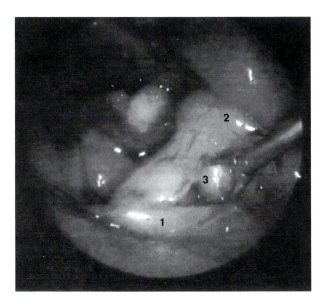

Figure 25-8
The spreader is shifted more proximally to complete pyloromyotomy at the antral end. Note that the mucosa is best inspected at this time.
1 = Duodenum. 2 = Antrum. 3 = Mucosa pouting through the myotomy.

to fall away from the operation site. A diagnostic laparoscopy should be performed before establishing the instrument trocars. The internal inguinal ring should be inspected first. Its internal landmark is easily identified by following the external iliac vessels to their junction with the inferior epigastric vessels. If the vas deferens and testicular vessels are seen entering the internal inguinal ring, and if an indirect hernia is present, then the testis is intracanalicular (within a complete inguinal hernial sac). In this instance, you should proceed to an open orchidopexy, and the testes generally can be brought down satisfactorily without prior ligation of the testicular vessels.

If both the vas and testicular vessels enter the internal inguinal ring, the testis is either absent or it will be small and dysplastic. You should proceed to an open operation to explore the inguinal canal and perform an orchidectomy under the same anesthetic. If the vas or testicular vessels are not readily identifiable at the internal ring, then two 4-mm instrument ports should be inserted, one in the ipsilateral iliac fossa and the other in the ipsilateral upper quadrant of the abdomen.

It is probably easiest to look for the vas deferens first. It can usually be seen best where it crosses the lateral umbilical ligaments (umbilical arteries). The vas can then be followed laterally to either its testis or to its blind ending. If a small dysplastic testis is found, an orchidectomy can be performed using two Endoloops to ligate the vessels in continuity before excision of the testis. These dysplastic testes are usually very small and can be removed through the umbilicus without changing to a larger trocar.

If a sizable testes is located, the testicular vessels can be ligated. This can be performed without having to change to a larger instrument port. The peritoneum overlying the testicular vessels is divided by sharp Endoshears dissection. This allows the testicular artery to be picked up and two endoknots (with the needle removed) placed around it. An extracorporeal knot completes the procedure. The collateral supply will develop and orchidopexy performed later by bringing the testis down on the blood supply to the vas.

Laparoscopy for Pediatric Malignancies

Most pediatric malignancies are sarcomas. The management of pediatric malignancies has undergone significant changes in recent years. Chemotherapy in combination with local radiotherapy and limited excision preserves function without compromising the cure rate. This is now the favored treatment modality for many pediatric malignancies.

Laparoscopy is helpful in the staging of childhood tumors because the view through the endoscope is even better than that in an open operation. The only area inaccessible is the retroperitoneum. Many pediatric patients with malignancies have poor wound healing and suffer wound dehiscence or ventral hernias following open laparotomy owing to the chemotherapy regime. Laparoscopy eliminates the risk of dehiscence and ventral hernia.

Transperineal high dose radiotherapy with iridium wire has been employed in pelvic malignancies, but a major morbidity associated with this is ablation of ovarian function. This can be prevented by oophoropexy, which reduces the radiation dose to the ovary.

Oophoropexy

Oophoropexy can be a complex organizational problem, and it is essential to coordinate the services of the radiotherapist, the orthopedic surgeon, and the radiologist, as well as the pediatric surgeon, prior to surgery. The aim is to perform a staging laparoscopy, oophoropexy, and transperineal insertion of hollow needles for iridium needle brachytherapy. The patient will have to be immobilized in a hip spica, to prevent accidental dislodgment of the hollow needles, and, under the same anesthetic, moved to radiology to check the position of the needles with a computed tomography (CT) scan for calculation of the radiation dose.

The patient is positioned at the foot of the table in the Lloyd Davies position and the bladder catheterized with a silastic urethral Foley catheter. The patient is tilted head down and

Figure 25-9
The patient position and operating room setup for oophoropexy before radiation treatment of the pelvis.

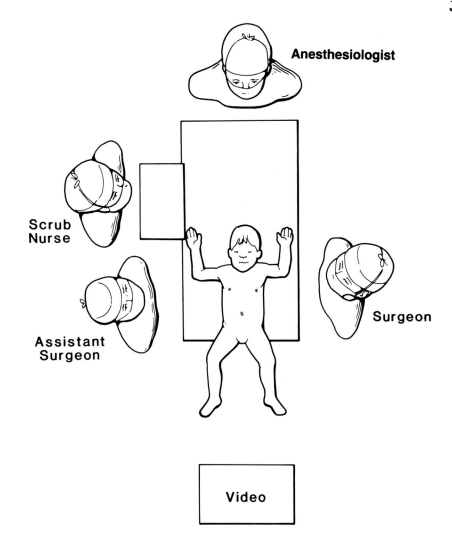

rolled toward the surgeon, to allow the viscera to be retracted away from the pelvis. The surgeon stands on the contralateral side of the ovary being fixed, and the video monitor is positioned between the patient's legs. The assistant stands on the ipsilateral side. The scrub nurse stands next to the assistant surgeon (Fig. 25-9).

The 4-mm telescope port is introduced through the umbilicus, using the technique previously described. Two more ports are established, one in each iliac fossa under direct internal video endoscopic control. Care is taken to avoid placing the trocars through the inferior epigastric vessels (which are prominent in this position). Atraumatic graspers are introduced into each instrument port, and a pelviscopy is performed. The atraumatic graspers can be used to manipulate the uterus, adnexa, and all intrapelvic viscera to allow careful inspection of the pelvic viscera and wall and any suspicious tissue or node biopsied. The ovary is easily identified as a small golden yellow organ by following the fallopian tube laterally. It should be grasped by the atraumatic forceps in the left-sided instrument port and retracted away from the pelvic brim into the abdomen proper (Fig. 25-10).

A laparoscopic suture is introduced through the right iliac fossa port and mounted on a 3-mm needle holder. The ovary is then grasped with the grasper, and one stitch is placed through the body of the ovary (Fig. 25-11). Sufficient length of suture is then drawn through the ovary to allow the end of the needle to be delivered extracorporeally. The peritoneum of the ipsilateral lateral abdominal wall 2 cm above

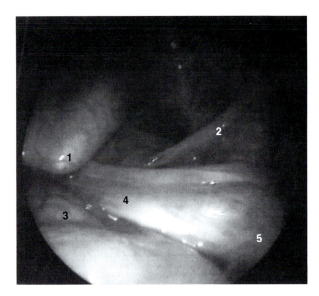

Figure 25-10
The ovary is grasped and pulled over the pelvic brim in order to fix it to the lateral abdominal wall.
1 = Preperitoneal radioactive implant. 2 = Pelvic brim. 3 = Rectum. 4 = Fallopian tube. 5 = Ovary.

the pelvic brim is picked up with the grasper and stitched with the same suture. An extracorporeal knot completes the fixation of the ovary to the lateral abdominal wall.

The umbilical telescope port is removed after both ovaries have been fixed, and the umbilical incision extended to allow the introduction of a 10-mm cannula. The telescope is reintroduced into either of the two instrument ports, a clip applicator is introduced through the 10-mm umbilical port, and a titanium clip applied onto the body of each ovary under direct visual control. This will allow the radiotherapist to calculate the dose to the ovary because the radio-opaque marker is visible on a plain x-ray. The hollow radiation needles are inserted under direct laparoscopic control, and the child's legs immobilized in a hip spica on completion of the procedure. The cosmetic advantage of this technique is apparent in Fig. 25-12.

Discussion

Although pediatric laparoscopic surgery is still in its infancy, the development of equipment suitable for smaller instrument ports will in-

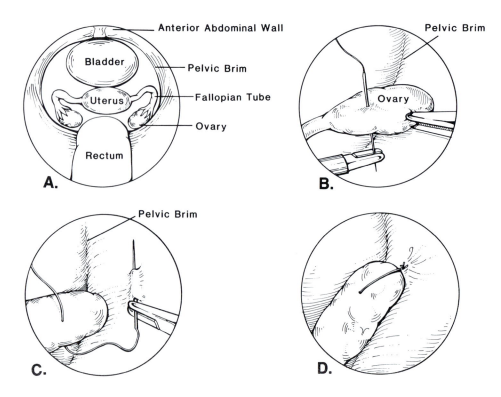

Figure 25-11
A. Normal pelvic anatomy. **B.** A laparoscopic suture is passed through the ovary and then **(C.)** through the lateral abdominal wall above the pelvic brim. **D.** An extracorporeal knot completes the fixation.

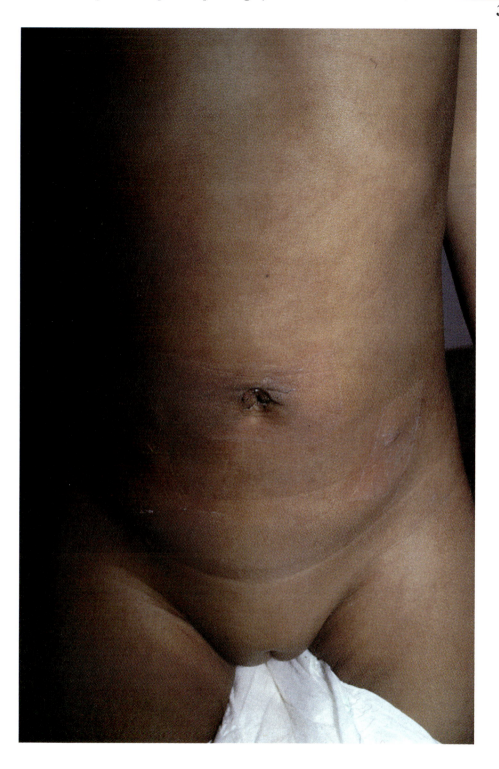

Figure 25-12
There is minimal cosmetic deformity seen with this technique.

evitably see laparoscopy being adopted by more pediatric surgeons as they develop skills in laparoscopy. There are a few important factors to consider when it comes to the performing of safe pediatric laparoscopy.

The fact that laparoscopic surgery is minimally invasive does not mean it is minor surgery. There is potential to cause great harm if improper techniques are employed, especially in small infants and babies simply because there is less room for error. Bleeding has more serious implications, not only because of the smaller blood volume but also because blood will absorb much of the reflected light, and this can compromise the illumination very quickly, especially when small endoscopes are used. The relative toughness of the infant peritoneum, the ease with which it strips off the anterior abdominal wall, and the proximity of underlying viscera make it potentially hazardous to use the Verres needle technique for establishing a pneumoperitoneum.

In spite of these relative drawbacks, the fact that laparoscopic surgery offers a means of performing surgical procedures with minimal iatrogenic trauma remains a very attractive proposition. This attraction will popularize laparoscopy in children in the future.

Bibliography

Alain JL et al: Extramucosal pyloromyotomy by laparoscopy. *J Pediatr Surg* 26:1191–1192, 1991.

Donaldson S, Kaplan H: Complications of treatment of Hodgkin's disease in children. *Cancer Treat Reports* 66(4):977–989, 1992.

Flamant F et al: Long-term sequelae of conservative treatment by surgery, brachytherapy and chemotherapy for vulval and vaginal rhabdomyosarcoma in children. *J Clin Oncol* 8(11):1847–1853, 1990.

Gans SL, Austin E: The techniques of laparoscopy, in Gans SL (ed): *Pediatric Endoscopy*. Orlando, FL, Grune & Stratton, 1983.

Gans SL, Berci G: Advances in endoscopy of infants and children. *J Pediatr Surg* 6:199–233, 1971.

Gans SL, Berci G: Peritoneoscopy in infants and children. *J Pediatr Surg* 8:399–405, 1973.

Hay SD et al: Sarcomas of the vagina and uterus: The intergroup rhabdomyosarcoma study. *J Paediatr Surg* 36:718–724, 1985.

Loughlin K et al: Genitourinary rhabdomyosarcoma in children. *Cancer* 63:1600–1606, 1989.

Newman KD et al: Laparoscopic cholecystectomy in pediatric patients. *J Pediatr Surg* 26:1184–1185, 1991.

Piouvost M et al: Transposition ovarienne percoelioscopique avant curietherapie dans les cancers du col uterin stade 1A et 1B. *J Gynecol Obstet Biol Reprod (Paris)* 30:361–365, 1991.

Rodgers BM et al: Laparoscopy in the diagnosis and treatment of malfunctioning ventriculoperitoneal shunt, in Gans SL (ed): *Pediatric Endoscopy*. Orlando, FL, Grune & Stratton, 1991.

Sackier JM: Editorial. *J Pediatr Surg* 26:1145–1147, 1991.

Spicer RD: Infantile hypertrophic pyloric stenosis: A review. *Br J Surg* 69:128–135, 1982.

Stauffer UG: Laparoscopy in hepatology and biliary diseases, in Gans SL (ed): *Pediatric Endoscopy*. Orlando, FL, Grune & Stratton, 1983.

Stillman R et al: Ovarian failure in long term survivors of childhood malignancy. *Am J Obstet Gynecol* 139(1):62–66, 1981.

Tan HL, Najmaldin A: Laparoscopic pyloromyotomy for infantile pyloric stenosis (in press). *J Pediatr Surg* (international).

Valla JS et al: Laparoscopic appendicectomy in children: Report of 465 cases. *Surg Laparosc Endosc* 1:166–172, 1991.

Waldschmidt J, Schier F: Laparoscopical surgery in neonates and infants. *Eur J Pediatr Surg* 1:145–150, 1991.

Wickham JEA: Editorial. *Minimally Invasive Ther* 1:1–5, 1991.

Zeidan B et al: Recent results of treatment of infantile pyloric stenosis. *Arch Dis Child* 63:1060–1064, 1988.

26

Reimbursement for Laparoscopic Procedures

Shelley R. Coupanger

Reimbursement for the laparoscopic procedures is a new issue for the physician and the insurance carriers.[1] Because of the advanced skill and technical components needed, this type of procedure may be reimbursed at a different rate than reimbursement for the standard procedure.

In order to obtain a fair reimbursement, it is necessary to educate the insurance carriers. Laparoscopic procedures should be presented to the carriers as operations different from incisional surgery of the same nature. Use an unlisted code for that area of the body. For example, a laparoscopic hernia repair would be coded 49999 instead of 49505. Then a fair surgical fee needs to be determined by the surgeon.

Once the coding and fee are determined, it is necessary to work with the insurance carrier to establish a fair reimbursement. The two key components of this are a predetermination package and the appeal process.

First the predetermination letter and package are sent to the insurance carriers before the procedure is scheduled. The predetermination letter states the patient's preoperative diagnosis, what type of surgery is planned, the procedure code, and what the charges will be. The insurance carrier can then determine if this is a covered service. The package contains a letter describing in layman terms the procedure in its most detailed form and any additional information pertaining to the laparoscopic procedure. This would include articles from major medical publications, letters, and/or studies done by other physicians.

This early information provides the insurance carriers and their policy review committees with the time and opportunity to understand the advantages of the laparoscopic procedure and to form their coverage policy. In this initial stage, the only information requested is their coverage policy and not the amount of reimbursement. The main objective is to establish with the insurance carriers that the laparoscopic procedure is an accepted and different procedure from the incisional counterpart. Also, after reviewing the predetermination package, the carrier may make a decision regarding the amount of the reimbursement. In these cases, payment is received in a timely fashion. In other cases, the amount of reimbursement can be negotiated or appealed at a later date.

Using this method will help to identify insurance carriers that will cover the laparoscopic procedure and those that will not. If the insurance carriers deny the procedure, the reason needs to be determined. The majority may state that they consider the procedure to be experimental. In these settings, direct face-to-face meetings with the insurance medical directors and/or their policy committees to review the procedure specifically can be very successful. Many denials are due simply to a misunderstanding concerning what is being done specifically.

If the insurance company refuses coverage, there are three further options. One is for the patient to take the matter directly to the carrier to see if the carrier can effect a change in the policy. This often can be very successful because the patients are the ones who pay the premiums and not the physicians. The other options are for the patient to pay for the procedure out of pocket or consent to the incisional procedure.

This approach to billing and coding for laparoscopic procedures still results in a number of underpayments. These should be dealt with on a case-by-case basis; however, the appeal process is the most direct approach. This is the final step in receiving fair reimbursement.

If there is a significant underpayment for a laparoscopic procedure, the carrier should be sent an appeal package. The appeal package should contain a letter stating that the carrier has underpaid for the procedure and explaining why the reimbursement should be at a higher level. Also include in the appeal package a "usual, reasonable, and customary" letter that requests the data the company is using to establish its payment amount. Examples of what other carriers are paying for the same procedure should be included. We attach copies of the explanation of benefits as further proof. Lastly, we supply the companies with the operative note, articles, or any other supportive documentation that relates to the procedure.

These approaches may be time consuming, but they are direct and truthful. The insurance carriers have generally appreciated the forthright nature of the discussions, and over time a relationship of trust is created.

References

1. Coupanger SR, Schultz LS: Laser laparoscopic cholecystectomy reimbursement issues: Current Status. *Lasers Surg Med* (supplement 3), 1991.

Index

Note: Page numbers in *italics* indicate figures; page numbers followed by *t* indicate tables.

Abdominal attachments, pediatric laparoscopic surgery and, 328–330, *329*
Abdominal wall pain, postoperative, cholecystectomy and, 132
Abdominal wall problems, as complication of cholecystectomy, 228–229, *231*, 232
Abscesses, 92
　as complication of cholecystectomy, 226–227, *231*
　hepatic, 95
　ruptured appendicitis with, 113–115, *114*, *115*
Adhesions, *162*, 162–163
　cholecystectomy and, 131
　cholecystocholangiography and, 142
　as contraindication to laparoscopy, 76–77
　lysis of, 97, 99, 100, *100*, 100t
　procedure failure and, 78
Alternating current (AC), 50–51
Anesthesia, 69–72
　anesthetic techniques and, 69–70
　cardiovascular effects of, 70–71
　gastrointestinal effects of, 72
　pain control and, 72
　pulmonary effects of, 71
Antiemetics, inguinal herniorrhaphy and, 261
Antireflux surgery, 245–253, *246–252*
Appeal package, 340
Appendectomy, 103–116, *104–111*
　advantages of laparoscopy for, 115–116, 116t
　retrocecal appendicitis and, *112*, 112–113, *113*
　ruptured appendicitis with abscess and, 113–115, *114*, *115*
Appendix:
　preventing rupture of, 106–107, *107*
　removal from abdominal cavity, 110, *110–111*, 112
　transection of, 107, *108*, 109
Argon beam cautery, intraoperative bleeding and, 151
Argon beam coagulator (ABC), 53
Argon laser, 43, 45, 47

Bile duct transection, as complication of cholecystectomy, 218–221, *220–222*, *224–227*, 226t

Bile leaks, as complication of cholecystectomy, 221–223, *228–230*
Bilomas, as complication of cholecystectomy, 221–223, *228–230*
Biopsies:
　of hepatic tumors, 94–95
　intraabdominal, technique for, 95, *96–98*
　of tumors, 94–95
Bipolar cautery, 19, *20*, *21*, 22–23, 50, *50*
　intraoperative bleeding and, 150
Bipolar electrogenerators, 77
Bipolar graspers, 54–55
Bladder:
　cancer of, pelvic lymphadenectomy and (*see* Pelvic lymphadenectomy)
　injuries to, 80
　observation of, 92
　pediatric laparoscopic surgery and, 328, *329*
Bleeding, 79, *79*
　intraoperative, management of, 149–151, *150–157*, 154–155
"Bovie" units, 48
Bowel injuries, 79–80
Bowel obstruction, following laparoscopy, 80
Bowel resection, 307–325
　identification of margins for, 308–309
　reanastomosis and, 316–320
　　extracorporeal end-to-end of side-to-side anastomosis and, 320, *320*
　　intracorporeal end-to-end anastomoses and, 316–318, *319*
　　intracorporeal side-to-side stapled anastomosis and, 320
　specimen removal and, 314–316, *316–318*
　suspension of bowel and, 309, *309*, *310*
　transection and securing of mesentery and, 311, *311–313*, 313
　transection of bowel and, 313–314, *314–316*
　trocar placement for, 307–308, *308*
Bowel suspender, 309, *310*
Brightness control, 36
Bupivacaine, postoperative pain control and, 72
Burn injuries, as complication of cholecystectomy, 223

341

Index

Camera(s), 35
  single-chip, 34
Camera control unit (CCU), 35
Cancer:
  of bladder, pelvic lymphadenectomy and (see Pelvic lymphadenectomy)
  pediatric, laparoscopy for, 334
  of prostate, pelvic lymphadenectomy and (see Pelvic lymphadenectomy)
  testicular, retroperitoneal lymphadenectomy for, *304*, 304–305
  uterine transmural, 92
Cannulas, 11, *12–16*
  disposable, 11, *13*
  for pediatric laparoscopic surgery, 327
  placement of, for pediatric laparoscopic surgery, 330–331
  redirection of, in obese patient, *161*, 161–162
Carbon dioxide embolism, anesthesia and, 70
Carbon dioxide insufflator, *10*, 10–11
Carbon dioxide (CO_2) laser, 43, 45
  power density of, 45, *46*
Cardiac decompensation, as contraindication to laparoscopy, 76
Cardiovascular effects, of anesthesia, 70–71
Cart, setting up, 36–37, *37*, *38*
Cautery:
  argon beam, 53
    intraoperative bleeding and, 151
  biopsies using, 95, *98*
  bipolar, 19, *20*, *21*, 22–23, 50, *50*
    intraoperative bleeding and, 150
  electric(see Electrocautery)
  electrosurgery differentiated from, *48*, 48–49
  monopolar, 19, 50, *50*
  unipolar, intraoperative bleeding and, 150
Cautery units, 42
Charge couple device (CCD), 35
Chenodeoxycholic acid (CDCA), 205–206
Children (see Pediatric surgery)
Cholangiography, 137–146
  in acute cholecystitis, 157
  cholecystocholangiography and, 137–140, *138–142*, 142
  completion, 181, *182*
  cystic duct, 143, *143–147*, 145–146, 147t
  intraoperative, 170–171, *171*
  transcystic duct common bile duct access and, 190–192, *192*
Cholecystectomy, 2–3, 119–135, *120–122*
  complications of, 134, 217–232, 218t, 219t
    abdominal wall problems as, 228–229, *231*, *232*
    abscess formation as, 226–227, *231*
  bile duct transection as, 218–221, *220–222*, *224–227*, 226t
  bile leaks and bilomas as, 221–223, *228–230*
  intestinal injuries as, 223, *230*
  retained common bile duct stones as, 227–228
  splenic or renal injuries as, 223
  vascular injuries as, 223
  drains and, 130
  future of, 134–135, *135*
  indications for, 130–132, 133t
  initial clinical cases using, 121–123
  laparolithic, laser, 134, *135*
  operative technique for, 123–130, *123–133*
  results with, 132–134, 133t, 134t
Cholecystitis:
  acute, management of, 155–157, 156t, *158–160*, 159
  cholecystectomy and, 131
Cholecystocholangiography, 137–140, *138–142*, 142
  cholecystectomy and, 124, *125*
  inability to perform, 142
  transcystic duct common bile duct access and, 193, 199
Cholecystography, oral, asymptomatic stones and, 204–205
Choledochoscopy, transcystic, 173, *175–177*, 185–186
Choledochotomy, direct, *183–186*, 183–187
Cholelithiasis:
  cholecystectomy and, 130–131
  nonsurgical, 203–214
    asymptomatic stones and, 203–205
    contact dissolution and, 211–212, *212*
    gallstone lithotripsy and, 206–211, *208*, *210*
    oral dissolution and, *205*, 205–206, *207*
    percutaneous gallbladder ablation and, 213–214
    stone recurrence and, 212–213, *213*
Circulatory impairment, anesthesia and, 70
Clip applicators, for pediatric laparoscopic surgery, 327
"Coag" mode, *52*, 52–53
Coagulation methods, 19, *20*, *21*, 22–23
Codeine, following inguinal herniorrhaphy, 268
Coding, for reimbursement, 339
Coherence, of laser light, 44
Collimation, of laser light, 44
Colon resection (see Bowel resection)
Color:
  of lasers, 36, 44, *45*
  video systems and, 33–34
Color balance, troubleshooting and, 39

Colostomy:
    closure of, 321, *324*, 325, *325*
    end, 320–321, *321–323*
Common bile duct access, transcystic duct, 189–190, *190–198*, 192–193, 199–201, *200*
Common bile duct exploration, 169–187
    direct, *183–186*, 183–187
    through cystic duct, 170–171, *171–182*, 173, 175–179, 181, 183
Common bile duct stones (*see* Stones)
Complications, 75–82, 76*t*
    bleeding as, 79, *79*
    of cholecystectomy (*see* Cholecystectomy, complications of)
    contraindications to laparoscopy and, 76*t*, 76–77, 77*t*
    equipment failure and, 77–78, *78*
    gastrointestinal, 79–80
    genitourinary, 80
    infection as, 80–81
    of inguinal herniorrhaphy, 267–268, 268*t*
    physiology of laparoscopy and, 76
    postoperative, 81
    procedure failure and, 78
Conduction heat transfer, 42
Consent (*see* Informed consent)
Contact dissolution, *203*, 211–212
"Contact" laser fibers, 42
Contrast control, 36
Convection heat transfer, 42
Convergence, depth perception and, 85
Credentialing, 57–58, 58*t*
Culdoscopy, 7
Current, 51
    "cut" and "coag" modes and, 52, *52*
"Cut" mode, *52*, 52–53
Cyst(s):
    hepatic, 94, *94*
    ovarian, 93
    renal, 301–303, *302*
Cystic artery, intraoperative bleeding and, 151, *152–153*, 154
Cystic duct:
    closure of, 181, *182*
    dissection for, for cholecystectomy, 126–127, *126–128*
    occlusion of, 213
Cystic duct cholangiography, 143, *143–147*, 145–146, 147*t*
Cystic hematoma, 92–93
Cystitis, as complication of laparoscopy, 81

Depth perception, loss of, 85–86
Desiccation, 53–55

Diagnostic laparoscopy, 91–92, 95, 97
Diaphragmatic hernias, congenital, 93–94
Diethyl ether, stone dissolution and, 211
Direct current (DC), 51
Disposable equipment:
    cost of, 62
    trocars, 77, *78*
Diverticulitis, chronic, 92
Diverticulosis, 92
Drains, for cholecystectomy, 130
Droperidol, inguinal herniorrhaphy and, 261

Economic issues, 62, 62*t*
Electrocautery, 19
    cystic duct occlusion and, 213
    gastrointestinal injuries and, 80
Electrodes:
    contact area and current density and, 55, *55*
    needle, 55
Electrogenerators, 77
Electrosurgery, *48–50*, 48–56, *52–55*
    cautery differentiated from, *48*, 48–49
Embolism:
    carbon dioxide, anesthesia and, 70
    venous gas, anesthesia and, 70–71
Emphysema, subcutaneous, anesthesia and, 71
End colostomy, 320–321, *321–323*
Endobag, 26–27, *28*
Endocoagulation, 23
Endometriosis, 93, *93*
Endoscopic retrograde cholangiopancreatography (ERCP):
    bile duct transection and, 218, *220*
    bile leaks and bilomas and, 222, *229*
    common bile duct stones and, 146
Endotracheal intubation, 70
Energy concepts, 45–48, *46*, *47*
Epidural anesthesia, 69–70
Epigastric bleeding, as complication, 79
Equipment:
    compatibility of, 77–78
    disposable, cost of, 62
    failure of, 77–78, *78*
    for pediatric laparoscopic surgery, 327
    sterilization of, 81
    (*See also* Instruments)
Ergonomics, 83–88
    eye-hand coordination and paradoxical movement and, 83–85, *84*, *85*
    hand movements and their control during surgery and, 86
    skill acquisition and, 86–87
    systems approach and, *86*, 87, *87*

Ergonomics (Cont.)
    tactile feedback and, 86
    visual aspects of laparoscopic surgery and, 85–86
Esophageal hiatus, closure of, *250*, 252
Exploratory laparoscopy (*see* Diagnostic laparoscopy)
Extracorporeal knot tying, 25, *26*
Extracorporeal shock wave lithotripsy (ESWL), 206–211, *208*, *210*
Eye-hand coordination, 83–85, *84*, *85*

Falciform ligament, pediatric laparoscopic surgery and, 328, *329*
Fallopian tube disease, 92
Feedback, tactile, 86
Fetal monitoring, operating during pregnancy and, 163
Fibroids, uterine:
    observation of, 92
    subserosal, 92
Fistula, mucous, 321, *323*
Fluence, 47
Focus, troubleshooting and, 39
Focus adjustment, laparoscopes and, 34
Fogging, 15
    troubleshooting and, 39
Forms, preoperative patient education and, 66–67
Free beam lasers, 44–45

Gallbladder:
    difficult to remove, *164–167*, 167–168
    percutaneous ablation of, 213–214
    (*See also* Cholecystectomy)
Gallstone pancreatitis, cholecystectomy and, 132
Gallstones
    asymptomatic, 203–205
    contact dissolution of, *203*, 211–212
    cystic duct cholangiography and, 146
    difficult to extract, 176–179, *181*
    fragmented in duct, 179, 181
    impacted, 181
    lithotripsy and, 206–211, *208*, *210*
    oral dissolution of, 205, 205–206, *207*
    recurrence of, 212–213, *213*
    retained, as complication of cholecystectomy, 227–228
Gastroesophageal reflux, laparoscopic treatment of, 245–253, *246–252*
Gastrointestinal effects, of anesthesia, 72
Gastrointestinal injuries:
    as complication, 79–80
    as complication of cholecystectomy, 223, *230*

Gastrotomy, 237, *240*
General anesthesia, 70
    for inguinal herniorrhaphy, 261
Genitourinary complications, 80
Glare, troubleshooting and, 39
Glyceryl 1-monooctanoate (monooctanoin), stone dissolution and, 211
Grainy image, troubleshooting and, 39
Grasping instruments, 23, *24*
Groin herniation, postoperative, 81

Hand movements, control during surgery, 86
Heat, 41–42
Heat capacity, 42–43
Heat transfer, 42–43
Hematoma, cystic, 92–93
Hemipylorectomy, truncal vagotomy and, 235–237, *238–240*
Hemipylorectomy/pyloroplasty stapler, 243
Hemostasis, obtaining, 223
Hernia(s), diaphragmatic, congenital, 93–94
Herniation, as complication of cholecystectomy, 229, 232
Herniorrhaphy, inguinal(*see* Inguinal herniorrhaphy)
High definition television, 33
High energy surgery, 41
Highlighting, troubleshooting and, 39
Holmium:yttrium-aluminum-garnet (Ho:YAG) laser, 43
    for cholecystectomy, 129
Hot tip lasers, 44, 45, 46
Hue, video systems and, 36
Hydrosalpinx, 92
Hypercarbia, controlling, 71
Hypovolemic shock, as contraindication to laparoscopy, 76

Imaging, asymptomatic stones and, 204–205
Infants (*see* Pediatric surgery)
Infection, as complication of laparoscopy, 80–81
Informed consent, 67
    for pelvic lymphadenectomy, 272
    for upper urinary tract and retroperitoneal surgery, 295
    for varicocelectomy, 281, *283*
Inguinal herniorrhaphy, 255–269, *256*
    anatomy and, 258, *259*, *260*
    extraabdominal preperitoneal repair and, 255
    future of, 269
    historical review of, 256–258, *257*, *258*
    indications and contraindications for, 258, 260

Inguinal herniorrhaphy (*Cont.*)
   intraabdominal peritoneal onlay patch repair and, 255
   operative protocol for, 261, *262, 263*
   preoperative preparation for, 260
   procedure for, 261, 263, *264–267*, 266–267
   results and complications of, 267–268, 268t, *269*
   transabdominal preperitoneal repair and, 255, 257–258
Inguinal organs, survey of, 92–93, *93*
Instruments, 23, *24*, 61–62
   for varicocelectomy, 284t, 284–285, *285*, 285t
   (*See also* Equipment)
Insufflation pressure, monitoring, pediatric laparoscopic surgery and, 329
Insufflator, failure of, 77
Insurance coverage, 65, 339–340
Intestinal obstruction:
   as contraindication to laparoscopy, 76
   following inguinal herniorrhaphy, 268
   following laparoscopy, 80
Intraabdominal biopsies, technique for, 95, *96–98*
Intracorporeal knot tying, 25, *27*
Intraoperative bleeding, management of, 149–151, *150–157*, 154–155
Irradiance, of lasers, 45–47, *46, 47*
Irrigation, *22*, 23

Jaundice, cholecystectomy and, 131–132
Joules (J), 47

Keterolac tromethamine (Toradol), postoperative pain control and:
   cholecystectomy and, 124
   inguinal herniorrhaphy and, 261
Keterolac tromethamine (Toradol), postoperative pain control and, 72
Kidney:
   cystic disease of, surgery in, 301–303, *302*
   lacerations of, as complication of cholecystectomy, 223
   removal of, 299, *299–301*, 301
Knot tying, 23–25, *25–27*
   extracorporeal, 25, *26*
   intracorporeal, 25, *27*
KTP³ laser, 43, 45, 47

Laparoscope(s), 11, 14–16, *17, 18*
   flexible, video systems and, 35
   video systems and, 34

Laparoscope holders, mechanical, 17
Laparoscopy:
   contraindications to, 76t, 76–77, 77t
   physiology of, 76
Laser(s), 43–45, *44*
   biopsies using, 95, *98*
   color of, 36, 44, *45*
   free beam, 44–45
   holmium:yttrium-aluminum-garnet, 43
      for cholecystectomy, 129
   hot tip, 44, 45, 46
   neodymium:yttrium-aluminum-garnet, 43, 45, 47
      pulsed, 48
   parameters controlling delivery of energy to tissue and, 44
   power density of, 45–47, *46, 47*
   pulsing, 47–48
   safety of, 78
Laser injuries, gastrointestinal, 80
Laser laparolithic cholecystectomy, 134, *135*
Laser light, characteristics of, 43–44
Ligamentum teres, pediatric laparoscopic surgery and, 328, *329*
Ligatures, loop, 24–25, *25–27*
Light sources, 17, *19*
Lighting intensity, depth perception and, 85
Lines of resolution, 33
Lithotripsy, 206–211, *208, 210*
Lithotrite, 212
Liver:
   injuries to, intraoperative bleeding and, 150–151, *151*
   lesions of, 94–95
      cystic, 94, *94*
Loop ligature, 24–25, *25–27*
Lymphadenectomy:
   pelvic (*see* Pelvic lymphadenectomy)
   retroperitoneal, for testes cancer, *304*, 304–305
Lymphomas, hepatic, 95
Lysis of adhesions (*see* Adhesions)

Marketing, 62–63
Mechanical laparoscope holders, 17
Mesentery:
   bleeding from, as complication, 79
   transection and securing of, for bowel resection, 311, *311–313*, 313
Mesh "butterfly," in inguinal herniorrhaphy, 257
Mesoappendix, transection of, 107, *107*
Methyl tert-butyl ether (MTBE), stone dissolution and, 211–212, *212*

Metoclopramide hydrochloride (Reglan), postoperative pain control and:
 cholecystectomy and, 124, 132–133
 inguinal herniorrhaphy and, 261
Midazolam hydrochloride (Versed), postoperative pain control and, 124, 132–133
 cholecystectomy and, 124
 inguinal herniorrhaphy and, 261
Monitor, 35–36
Monochromaticity, of laser light, 43–44
Monopolar cautery, 19, 50, *50*
Morbidity (*see* Complications)
Mortality rates, 75
Mucous fistula, 321, *323*

Nasogastric intubation, 72
National Television Systems Committee (NTSC), 32
Nausea:
 following cholecystectomy, 132–133, 134*t*
 following inguinal herniorrhaphy, 267
Needle, Verres(*see* Verres needle)
Needle biopsies, technique for, 95, *96*, *97*
Needle electrode, 55
Neodymium:yttrium-aluminum-garnet (Nd:YAG) laser, 43, 45, 47
 pulsed, 48
Neurologic complications, 81
Nisson fundoplication (*see* Gastroesophageal reflux)
Nitrous oxide, 70
Nonsteroidal antiinflammatory drugs, postoperative pain control and, 72

Obesity:
 problems presented by, 159, *161*, 161–162
 procedure failure and, 78
Oophoropexy, 334–336, *335–337*
Operating room set-up, *60*, 60–61, *61*
 for cholecystectomy, 123, *123*
Opioids, postoperative pain control and, 72
Oral cholecystography (OCG), asymptomatic stones and, 204–205
Orogastric intubation, 72
Ovarian cysts, 93
Ovarian diseases, observation of, 92
Ovarian tumors, 93

Pain, postoperative, 81
 following cholecystectomy, 132
 control of, 72
 following inguinal herniorrhaphy, 267–268, 268*t*
Pancreatitis, gallstone, cholecystectomy and, 132
Paradoxical movement, 83–85, *84*, *85*
Parametritis, 92
Patient education, preoperative, 65–67, *66*
Patient positioning, for upper urinary tract and retroperitoneal surgery, 295–297, *296–298*
Patient preparation:
 for inguinal herniorrhaphy, 260
 for pelvic lymphadenectomy, 272
 for upper urinary tract and retroperitoneal surgery, 295
 for varicocelectomy, 281–282, *283*
Pediatric surgery, 327–338
 anatomic considerations and, *328*, 328–330, *329*
 cannula placement for, 330–331
 establishing pneumoperitoneum for, 330
 laparoscopic equipment for, 327
 for malignancies, 334
 oophoropexy and, 334–336, *335–337*
 pyloromyotomy and, 331–333, *331–333*
 for undescended testes, 333–334
Pelvic fluid, removal of, 106, *106*
Pelvic lymphadenectomy, 271–278
 informed consent and patient preparation for, 272
 results with, 275, 278
 technique for, *272*, 272–275, *273*, *275–277*
Pelvic organs, survey of, 92–93, *93*
Peptic ulcer surgery, 233–244
 anterior seromyotomy and, 238–239, *241–243*
 highly selective vagotomy and
  of anterior trunk, 237–238, *241*
  of posterior trunk, 242–244
 plication and, 233–235, *234*
  endoscopically assisted technique for, 235, *237*
  laparoscopic technique for, 234–235, *235*, *236*
 truncal vagotomy and hemipylorectomy/pyloroplasty and, 235–237, *238–240*
Percutaneous gallbladder ablation, 213–214
Periappendiceal abscess, ruptured appendicitis with, 113–115, *114*, *115*
Pericecal abscess, ruptured appendicitis with, 113–115, *114*, *115*
Peritoneal cavity, survey of, 91, 92–93, *93*
Peritonitis:
 as complication of laparoscopy, 81
 septic, as contraindication to laparoscopy, 76
Phase, video systems and, 36
Phase Alternation Line (PAL), 32

Phlogiston, 41
Photocautery units, 42
Pixels, 33
Plication, of perforated peptic ulcer, 233–235, *234*
    endoscopically assisted technique for, 235, *237*
    laparoscopic technique for, 234–235, *235*, *236*
Pneumoperitoneum, 7–11, *8–10*
    creation of, 104
    establishing, pediatric laparoscopic surgery and, 330
    failure of attain, 78
Pneumothorax, anesthesia and, 71
Portal vein:
    injuries to, as complication of cholecystectomy, 223
    intraoperative bleeding from, 154
Power density, of lasers, 45–47, *46*, *47*
Pregnancy, operating during, 163
Preoperative check, of video system, 37–39
Procedure, failure of, 78
Propofol, 70
Prostate cancer, pelvic lymphadenectomy and (*see* Pelvic lymphadenectomy)
Pulmonary artery wedge pressure, anesthesia and, 70
Pulmonary effects, of anesthesia, 71
Pulsing, of lasers, 47–48
Pyloromyotomy, pediatric, 331–333, *331–333*
Pyloroplasty, truncal vagotomy and, 235–237, *238–240*

Quality management, 62

Radiation heat transfer, 42
Ramstedt's operation, 331–333, *331–333*
Reanastomosis, for bowel resection (*see* Bowel resection, reanastomosis and)
Referred pain, postoperative, control of, 72
Reflux esophagitis (*see* Gastroesophageal reflux)
Reimbursement, 65, 339–340
Renal cystic disease, surgery in, 301–303, *302*
Renal lacerations, as complication of cholecystectomy, 223
Resection margins, for bowel resection, identification of, 308–309
Resistance, 51
Resolution, video system and, 33
Retrocecal abscess, ruptured appendicitis with, 113–115, *114*, *115*
Retrocecal appendicitis, *112*, 112–113, *113*
Retroperitoneal bleeding, as complication, 79, *79*

Retroperitoneal fibrosis, ureterolysis and, *303*, 303–304
Retroperitoneal surgery:
    informed consent and preoperative preparation for, 295
    midline retroperitoneal structures and, *304*, 304–305
    patient positioning for, 295–297, *296–298*
Room set-up, *60*, 60–61, *61*
    for cholecystectomy, 123, *123*
Ruptured appendicitis, with abscess, 113–115, *114*, *115*

Safety, laser, 78
Sapphire probes, 42
Scissors, 23
Sculptured fibers, 46–47
Septic peritonitis, as contraindication to laparoscopy, 76
Séquentiel Couleur à Mémoire (SECAM), 32
Seromyotomy, anterior, 238–239, *241–243*
Shock, hypovolemic, as contraindication to laparoscopy, 76
Shoulder strap pain:
    following inguinal herniorrhaphy, 267–268, 268t
    postoperative, 81
    cholecystectomy and, 132
Single-chip cameras, 34
Skill acquisition, 86–87
Small bowel obstruction, following inguinal herniorrhaphy, 268
Small bowel resection (*see* Bowel resection)
Smoke accumulation, 15–16
Society of Endoscopic Surgeons (SAGES), 58
Splenectomy, 95
Splenic injuries, as complication of cholecystectomy, 223
Spot brightness, of lasers, 45–47, *46*, *47*
Staplers:
    hemipylorectomy/pyloroplasty, 243
    inguinal herniorrhaphy and, 263, 266, *266*
    for pediatric laparoscopic surgery, 327
    for transection of appendix, *109*, 109–110
Still-image generator, 36
Stimulated emission, 43
Stones (*see* Gallstones)
Subcostal incision, *2*, 3
Subcutaneous emphysema, anesthesia and, 71
Subserosal fibroids, 92
Suction, *22*, 23
Suturing, 23–25, *25–27*
Systems approach, 86, *87*, 87

Team, training of, *59*, 59–60
Team approach, 58–59
Television, high definition, 33
Temperature, 41–42
Testes:
    cancer of, retroperitoneal lymphadenectomy for, *304*, 304–305
    undescended, laparoscopy for, 333–334
Thermal injuries, gastrointestinal, 80
Tint, video systems and, 36
Tissue and Organ Extractor, 27
Tissue removal, 26–27, *28*, *164–167*, 167–168
Toupe procedure, *252*, 252–253
Training:
    complications and, 75
    of team, *59*, 59–60
Transcystic choledochoscopy, 173, *175–177*, 185–186
Transcystic duct common bile duct access, 189–190, *190–198*, 192–193, 199–201, *200*
Transillumination, for bowel resection, 311, *311*
Tremor, control during surgery, 86
Trocar(s), 11
    disposable, 77, *78*
    for pediatric laparoscopic surgery, 327
    placement of, 77
        for antireflux surgery, 245–246
        for appendectomy, 104, *105*, 106, *106*
        for bowel resection, 307–308, *308*
        for varicocelectomy, 282, 284, *284*
    sharpening of, 77
Trocar site, intraoperative bleeding from, 154–155, *155–157*
Trolley, setting up, 36–37, *37*, *38*
Troubleshooting, video systems and, 39
Tumor(s):
    biopsy of, 94–95
    hepatic, biopsy of, 94–95
    ovarian, 93
    (*See also* Cancer)

Ulcers, peptic (*see* Peptic ulcer surgery)
Umbilical vein remnant, pediatric laparoscopic surgery and, 328, *329*
Umbilicus, pediatric laparoscopic surgery and, 328, *328*
Underpayment, 340
Unipolar cautery, intraoperative bleeding and, 150
Unipolar electrogenerators, 77
Upper abdominal survey, 93–94, *94*

Upper urinary tract surgery, 295–304
    informed consent and preoperative preparation for, 295
    kidney removal and, 299, *299–301*, 301
    patient positioning for, 295–297, *296–298*
    in renal cystic disease, 301–303, *302*
    ureterolysis and, *303*, 303–304
Ureter, reimplantation of, 304
Ureteric injuries, 80
Ureterolithotomy, open, 304
Ureterolysis, *303*, 303–304
Ureteroureterostomy, 304
Urinary tract surgery (*see* Upper urinary tract surgery)
Ursodeoxycholic acid (UDCA), 205–206
Uterine cancers, transmural, 92
Uterine fibroids, observation of, 92
Uterine sound, placement for appendectomy, 104, *104*

Vagotomy:
    highly selective
        of anterior trunk, 237–238, *241*
        of posterior trunk, 242–244
    truncal, hemipylorectomy/pyloplasty and, 235–237, *238–240*
Vapor accumulation, 15–16
Varicocelectomy, 279–293, *280*
    development of laparoscopic approach to, 281, *282*
    procedure for, 281–290
        instrumentation and, *284t*, 284–285, *285*, *285t*
        patient preparation and, 281–282, *283*
        patient selection and, 281
        surgical technique and, 285, *286–289*, 287–290, *291*, *292*
        trocar placement and, 282, 284, *284*
    results with, 290, 292
    standard approach to, 281
Vascular injuries, as complication of cholecystectomy, 223
Venographic occlusion, 281
Venous gas embolism, anesthesia and, 70–71
Verres needle, 7–10, *8*
    gastrointestinal injuries and, 79–80
    misplacement of, 9–10
    problems with, 77
    supraumbilical insertion of, *8*, 8–9
Video cassette recorders (VCR), 36
Video systems, 31–40, *32*
    anesthetic monitoring and, 71

Video systems (*Cont.*)
    basic principles of, 32
    camera and camera control unit and, 35
    color and, 33–34
    flexible scopes and, 35
    high definition television and, 33
    laparoscopes and, 34
    monitor and, 35–36
    preoperative check and, 37–39
    resolution and, 33
    setting up carts and trolleys for, 36–37, *37, 38*
    skill acquisition and, 86–87
    still image generator and, 36
    troubleshooting and, 39
    video recorder and, 36
    virtual reality and, 39–40
Videotapes, preoperative patient education and, 66, *66*
    for inguinal herniorrhaphy, 260
Virtual reality, video systems and, 39–40
Visual acuity, improving, 85–86
Visualization, prevention of complications with, 78
Voltage, 51
    "cut" and "coag" modes and, 52, *52, 54*

Wound hematomas, following inguinal herniorrhaphy, 268